D1465882

The History and Practice
of College Health

The

History and Practice

of

College Health

Edited by

H. Spencer Turner, MD, MS, FACPM

and

Janet L. Hurley, PhD

The University Press of Kentucky

Publication of this volume was made possible in part by a grant
from the National Endowment for the Humanities.

Editorial and Sales Offices: The University Press of Kentucky
663 South Limestone Street, Lexington, Kentucky 40508-4008

06 05 04 03 02   5 4 3 2 1

Library of Congress Cataloging-in-Publication Data

Turner, H. Spencer, 1938-
    The history and practice of college health / H. Spencer Turner and Janet L. Hurley.
        p. ; cm.
    Includes bibliographical references and index.
    ISBN 0-8131-2257-0 (cloth : alk. paper)
    1. College students, Health and hygiene, United States, History. 2.College students,
Medical care, United States, History.[DNLM: 1. Student Health Services, History, United
States. WA 11 AA1T947h 2002] I. Hurley, Janet L., 1948- II. Title.
LB3497.3 .T87 2002
378.1'971, dc21   2001007632

Manufactured in the United States of America.

Contents

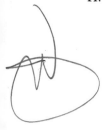

Acknowledgments

In early 1998 when we first conceived the idea of a textbook on the history and practice of college health, neither of us really understood the enormity of the task that lay before us. Nonetheless, with the cooperation of all the chapter authors, we have been able to finish very close to the original plan and have the text ready for publication in 2002.

Thanks are due to many individuals. First among these are the chapter authors. All the authors, who are busy persons in their own right, agreed to contribute their work without compensation. Further, they were willing to tolerate our phone calls, e-mails, letters, and demands to meet time schedules, receiving all requests with good humor. Further, they were willing to read, and reread, and finally reread again our editing efforts to produce a finished product.

A special thanks is also due to the Health Service staff at the University of Kentucky. Particularly important were our two administrative assistants, first, Ms. Angie Tomlin and then, upon her retirement (not because of the textbook), Ms. Libby Moss. Without the truly tireless efforts of these two talented women at typing and retyping and proof-reading manuscripts, this text would, in truth, never have become reality. Also, many of our staff members reviewed chapters and made suggestions—a special thanks to them.

Although this book represents the first textbook ever devoted solely to the history and practice of college health, we would be remiss not to recognize and say thanks to authors who preceded us. First, Dana Farnsworth's book from Harvard on college health administration (in the early 1960s) and Kevin Patrick's treatise on college health as part of a trilogy on school health (in the early 1990s) helped pave the way for this text. Just as important are all those individuals who, through the past 140 years of college health, assiduously recorded their observations, their findings, and their knowledge about our field. All these efforts have culminated in college and university health's first textbook devoted solely to the history and practice of the field, and designed for college and university practitioners and administrators involved with campus student health services.

A particular note about the format of this text is important. It was understood from the start that busy practitioners would not likely read this textbook from start to finish. Rather, we expected that those with a specific interest in a given topic at a given time might read or review the subject on which they had a specific interest or need to know and eventually cover the entire text. Thus, in many respects the book is designed as a series of monographs, any one of which could, under other circumstances, stand alone. The risk, of course, is repetition across chapters, but we believe that careful editing has minimized this concern. Further, this text is not written or designed to be a diagnostic or treatment guide for any specific condition. These issues are covered well in many other textbooks. Instead, each chapter examines its topic as it relates to college health—this focus is not available elsewhere. For similar reasons, in general, websites are not listed. It is expected that this text will be used far beyond the "life" of most named websites.

As a final note, it is important to reiterate that both editors and all authors contributed their time and efforts without compensation, so that profits realized from this book will be directed to the American College Health Foundation in support of the continued growth and support of programs of the American College Health Association.

Contributors

CO-EDITORS

H. Spencer Turner, MD, MS, FACPM, is Director of University Health Service, Administrative Head Team Physician, and a clinical professor of Preventive Medicine and Environmental Health at the University of Kentucky. He received a BA from Manchester College and earned his MD summa cum laude from The Ohio State University, where he was elected to Alpha Omega Alpha and where he earned a postdoctoral Master of Science. He completed a residency in preventive and aerospace medicine at Ohio State and was chief resident in 1968–69. Dr. Turner is board certified in preventive medicine and is a Fellow of the American College of Preventive Medicine. He was Director of University Health Service at Ohio State from 1970 to 1980 and in private practice from 1980 to 1990 in Dayton, Ohio. Dr. Turner is a Fellow and past president of the American College Health Association and holds that organization's two most prestigious awards—the Ruth E. Boynton Award and the Edward C. Hitchcock Award. He is a co-founder of the Kentucky College Health Association and of the Student Health Services at Academic Medical Centers group. He is Associate Editor for Clinical Medicine for the *Journal of American College Health.*

Janet L. Hurley, PhD, is Associate Director/Administrator at the University of Kentucky (UK) Health Service, a position she has held since 1993. Prior to that, she was Associate Dean for University Extension at UK. Before coming to UK in 1985, she worked in continuing education at Kansas State University. Dr. Hurley has a BS from Miami University (Ohio), an MS in student personnel and counseling from Kansas State University, and a PhD in higher education administration from UK. She is a recipient of the Adel Robertson National Professional Continuing Educator Award for Outstanding Leadership, Scholarship and Service for the University Continuing Education Association (UCEA), and is a Fellow of the American College Health Association. Dr. Hurley was a member of ACHA's Health Care Reform Advisory Council and co-chair of the ICD–9/CPT work group. She is a co-founder of the Kentucky College Health Association and conceived the idea for and co-founded the Student Health Services at Academic Medical Centers group.

CONTRIBUTING AUTHORS

Jean Benthien, CRNP, MSN, has been Director of Health Services at Point Loma Nazarene University since 1975. She did her undergraduate work at San Diego State and her graduate work at University of San Diego. She is certified as a college health nurse.

In 1991 Ms. Benthien published a Health Services Policy and Procedure Manual for small schools. She is an active member of ACHA and PCCHA and currently serves as president of California College Health Nurses Association.

Marthea J. Blewitt, Development Coordinator for the American College Health Foundation (ACHF), is a Certified Fundraising Specialist, having completed Goucher College's Fundraising Management Program in 1998. She has worked on a part-time basis for ACHF since 1994. Her seven years of development experience include managing planned giving programs, grant writing, and coordinating annual fund drives.

Karen M. Butler, RN, MSN, CNS, received a Bachelor of Science in Nursing from UNC-Chapel Hill and a Master of Science in Nursing from the University of Kentucky. She was Director of Nursing for University of Kentucky Health Service from 1992 to 2001. Prior to that time, most of her career in nursing was as a hematology/oncology nurse and nurse researcher. She has received multiple awards for academic achievement and is a member of Sigma Theta Tau International Honor Society. Currently, Ms. Butler is an instructor in the UK College of Nursing, where she is pursuing her doctorate with a research focus on the health of college students.

Stephen C. Caulfield is Chairman of the Chickering Group, a student health insurance company, where he has been employed since February 1997. Prior to this position, Mr. Caulfield was a partner of William M. Mercer, Inc., a management consulting firm, where he specialized in health care issues. He previously was employed as a faculty member and Assistant Dean of the Albert Einstein College of Medicine in New York, as the Director of Health Affairs and Regional Operations for the United Mine Workers Multi-Employer Trust, and as the President and Chief Executive Officer of the Government Research Corporation, a consulting firm previously located in Washington, D.C. He is currently a Director of the Tufts Managed Care Institute.

Pornthip Chalungsooth, EdD, LPC, a Licensed Professional Counselor, has worked at the University of Arkansas for eight years as a mental health clinician, with a specialty in cross-cultural counseling. He has been a liaison and a consultant for the University of Arkansas International Program Office since 1993.

William A. Christmas, MD, FACP, is a graduate of the Boston University School of Medicine. He is a board-certified internist with training in infectious diseases. Dr. Christmas has practiced college health for over 25 years at Bennington College, the University of Rochester (NY), the University of Vermont, and currently at Duke University, where he is an Associate Clinical Professor of Community and Family Medicine and Director of the Student Health Service. He is a past president of the American College Health Association, is currently chairman of the American College Health Foundation, and has served as a consultant to 14 institutions of higher education.

Thomas A. Dale II, MD, is a graduate of the University of Kentucky and the University of Kentucky College of Medicine. He interned in Savannah, GA and did his residency in family practice at Tallahassee Memorial Hospital. He is board certified in family practice. During the summers Dr. Dale performs volunteer work at Mashoko Hospital in Zimbabwe, Africa. Dr. Dale has been employed by University of Kentucky Health Service since 1976, where his primary responsibilities are in the Gynecology Clinic, where he supervises the clinical operation of that clinic.

John M. Dorman, MD, is an Associate Clinical Professor in Pediatrics and staff physician at Cowell Student Health Service at Stanford University. He was educated at Williams College and Harvard Medical School, with further training at Massachusetts General Hospital in Boston. He has been active in the Clinical Medicine Section of the American College Health Association, is a former executive editor of the *Journal of American College Health*, and continues as a consulting editor. He is a Fellow of the Association and received the Boynton Award in 1993 for service to the Association.

Wayne H. Ericson, PhD, obtained his doctorate in college student personnel administration from the University of Northern Colorado (UNC). From 1972 to 1980 he served as the Student Health Service Director at the UNC. He was employed by the Western Colorado Health Systems Agency as Associate Director from 1980 until 1982, when he became Director of Illinois State University (ISU) Student Health Service. Dr. Ericson, an ACHA Fellow, has been active in the American College Health Association (ACHA), having served as a faculty member in the Management Training Program and as treasurer of the Association.

Sarah M. Feiss is the former Communications Coordinator of the American College Health Association. Ms. Feiss holds bachelor's degrees in French and English from Franklin and Marshall College.

Sharon B. Fisher, MA, is the Communications Coordinator of the American College Health Association. A native of Baltimore, Ms. Fisher holds a bachelor's degree in advertising from Loyola College and a master's degree in publications design and writing from the University of Baltimore.

Mark R. Gardner, MD, holds a BS in Biology and an AB in Psychology from the University of Illinois. He earned his MD at Northwestern University Medical School in 1982 and completed a residency in Internal Medicine at Evanston Hospital in 1985. Dr. Gardner is an instructor of clinical medicine at Northwestern University Medical School and was formerly Director of the Northwestern University Health Service. He is a past president of the Mid-America College Health Association.

Ted W. Grace, MD, MPH, has been the Director of Student Health Services at Ohio State University since 1992. Previously he was the Director of Clinical Services at San Diego State University. He received his MD from Ohio State University and his MPH from San Diego State University, where he also completed a preventive medicine residency and a fellowship in student health administration. Dr. Grace is currently a clinical assistant professor in the Division of Health Services Management and Policy in the School of Public Health and in the Department of Family Practice, both at Ohio State. He is a Fellow of the American College of Physicians, American Academy of Family Practice, American College of Preventive Medicine, and the American College Health Association, which awarded him the E. Dean Lovett Award in 2000.

Wylie C. Hembree, MD, who received his MD from Washington University in St. Louis, is the Director of the Student Health Service on the Health Sciences Campus of Columbia University in New York City. He is an Associate Professor in the Departments of Medicine and of Obstetrics and Gynecology, and an Associate Attending Physician at the New York Presbyterian Hospital. During 30 years at Columbia, in addition to Student Health, Dr. Hembree has maintained a clinical practice and continued both basic and clinical research in medical andrology and reproductive endocrinology. He is a Fellow of the American College of Physicians.

Marlene Belew Huff, LCSW, PhD, received a BA in 1984, an MSW in 1987, and a PhD in 1999, all from the University of Kentucky. Dr. Huff is an Associate Professor and Director of the Social Work Program at Eastern Kentucky University in Richmond, Kentucky. In addition, she has a private practice where she provides individualized marital and family counseling state-wide. Prior to her employment at Eastern Kentucky University, Dr. Huff was an Assistant Professor at the University of Kentucky College of Social Work.

Mark A. Jenkins, MD, earned a BA from Rice University in 1983 and an MD from University of Texas Medical School in Houston in 1987. He performed a residency in internal medicine at University of Texas Affiliated Hospitals in Houston, and is board certified by the American Board of Internal Medicine. From 1992 to 1998 he was Associate Director of Student Health Service at Rice University and in 1998 was named Director at the same institution. He is currently co-chair of the Rice Institutional Review Board and since 1993 has been team physician for all NCAA sports.

Patricia R. Jennings, MHS, PA-C, is an Assistant Professor in the Department of Physician Assistant Studies with a joint appointment in the University of Kentucky College of Pharmacy. She is also a physician assistant with the UK Chandler Medical Center Infectious Disease Division. She received her Certificate in Physician Assistant Studies and master's in Health Sciences from Duke University and was awarded the Academy of Physician Assistant Program Faculty of the Year Award in 1998.

Betty Anne Johnson, MD, PhD, received her medical degree at Harvard Medical School, completed her internal medicine internship and residency at Brigham and Women's Hospital in Boston, Massachusetts, and received her PhD in microbiology from the University of Iowa. She is Professor of Medicine in the Division of General Medicine, Medical College of Virginia Campus of Virginia Commonwealth University (VCU), and directs the University Student Health Services at VCU.

Elaine C. Jong, MD, earned her doctorate from University of California, San Diego. She is trained in internal medicine and infectious diseases, and has a special interest in parasitic and exotic infections, refugee medicine, cross-cultural communication, vaccine-preventable diseases, and the health of international travelers. Dr. Jong is Director of the Student Health Service and Hall Health Primary Care Center at the University of Washington, Seattle, where she is Clinical Professor of Medicine. She also serves as Co-Director of the Travel and Tropical Medicine Service at the U.W. Medical Center.

Richard P. Keeling, MD, received his doctorate from Tufts University. He completed residency training in Internal Medicine/Hematology at the University of Virginia (UVA). He directed the UVA Health Service for 13 years. Subsequent to that he was director of the Health Service and professor of Medicine at University of Wisconsin-Madison until 1999, when he started his own private company. He is currently Chairman and Executive Consultant for his own health consulting and design firm in New York City, working to improve health and health-related services for young people. He is Editor of the Journal of American College Health and serves as Senior Scholar for the Program on Health in Higher Education and Senior Fellow for the Association of American Colleges and Universities. A past president of ACHA, Dr. Keeling has received the highest awards of both the American College Health Association and the National Association of Student Personnel administrators.

Gerald R. Ledlow, PhD, CHE, is a certified health care executive in the American College of Healthcare Executives, with over 12 years of practical experience as a health care administrator, having held several positions as the director of managed care operations for a health system and has served on numerous committees, including JCAHO accreditation committees. Dr. Ledlow has formed a preferred provider organization and has implemented resource utilization review systems, demand management systems, and referral management systems under a managed care model. He earned a PhD in organizational leadership with emphasis on health care system communication from the University of Oklahoma, a master's of health care administration from Baylor University, and a BA in economics from the Virginia Military Institute.

Joyce B. Meder, MPA, received an AS in Nursing in 1977, certification as an OB-GYN nurse practitioner from the University of Arizona in 1980, a BS in Health Service Administration in 1984 from the University of Phoenix, and a Master's of Public Administration from Golden Gate University in 1986. She was employed by the University of Arizona in 1977 and in 1999 was promoted to Assistant Vice President for Health and Wellness, a position she retained until her retirement in December 2001. She has been an active member of both the Pacific Coast College Health Association and the American College Health Association. She served as President of ACHA in 1996–1997, and received the Ruth E. Boynton Award in 1998. In addition to her work as a surveyor for the Accreditation Association for Ambulatory Health Care, she served as Chair of the ACHA Consultation Services Program.

Dana Mills, MPH, is the Director of the Student Health Service at Marquette University. He holds a master's degree in Public Health from the University of Michigan. Mr. Mills has been involved in college health for 27 years, with a combined 24 years in administration at University of Michigan, Northern Illinois University, and Marquette University, and three years working for a private consulting group specializing in higher education health care. He has consulted at numerous public and private colleges and universities across the nation and has given more than 25 presentations at ACHA and regional affiliate meetings. As a member of ACHA, he has participated on ACHA's Benchmarking Work Group, Bylaws Committee, and Administration Section Nominating Committee. He is a Fellow of ACHA.

Doyle E. Randol, MS, Col. USA (Ret.), is the Executive Director of ACHA. A native of the Washington, D.C., area, Mr. Randol is a 1972 graduate of Howard University. As an ROTC student at Howard, Mr. Randol was commissioned into the Army Medical Service Corps upon graduation and remained on active duty for 26 years, retiring in 1998. He held various command and staff positions within the Army Medical Department (AMEDD), reaching the rank of Colonel. Upon retirement from the United States Army, Mr. Randol assumed the position of Executive Director of the American College Health Association in May 1998.

Betty Reppert, PA-C, MPH, received her certification as a physician assistant from Bowman Gray School of Medicine/Wake Forest University, and her master's degree in Public Health from the Medical College of Virginia. She is the Director of the Office of Health Promotion for University Student Health Services at Virginia Commonwealth University. She serves as Chair of the University Substance Abuse Committee as well as the team leader for the JCAHO accreditation effort at the health services. She is a member of the Healthy Campus 2010 Task Force for the American College Health Association and has published and presented in the areas of quality improvement and accreditation in college health.

Christopher Sanford, MD, DTMH, is Co-Director of Hall Health Travel Clinic and Attending Physician, Department of Family Practice, University of Washington. He earned his BA at the University of California, Santa Barbara, and his MD at the University of California, San Diego, and completed a residency in Family Practice (in which he is board certified) at San Jose, California, Medical Center. In 2000 he earned his DTMH (Diploma in Tropical Medicine and Hygiene) at the Gorgas Course in Clinical Tropical Medicine, in Lima, Peru. He holds a Certificate of Knowledge in Tropical Medicine and Travelers' Health from the American Society of Tropical Medicine and Hygiene.

Mary Alice Serafini, MA, is Assistant Vice Chancellor for Student Affairs and Director of University Health Center at the University of Arkansas. She earned her MA in multicultural education at California State, Sacramento, and her BA at Knox College. Ms. Serafini is a member of the American College Health Association Task Force on Violence (Chair, 2001–2002), and the Administrative Section Program (Chair). She has 16 years of teaching and administrative experience in West Africa, including three years as a Peace Corps volunteer.

Alice C. Thornton, MD, earned her MD from Marshall University, and completed her internal medicine residency at Bowman-Gray School of Medicine. Additional training included a two-year fellowship in infectious disease at Indiana University. She is an Assistant Professor of Medicine in the Department of Medicine, Division of Infectious Diseases at the University of Kentucky College of Medicine. Her areas of interest are the treatment of HIV disease and STDs. She is currently researching trichomoniasis in women.

Peggy Ingram Veeser, EdD, APRN, BC, received her BSN from Vanderbilt University in 1971, her MS in Nursing from University of Tennessee-Memphis in 1978, and her EdD from University of Memphis in 1986. She has been certified since 1980 as a Family Nurse Practitioner. Since 1995 she has been a professor of nursing at University of Tennessee Health Science Center. From 1992 to 2000 she was Associate Dean for Academic Affairs, College of Nursing, and since 1986 has been Director of the University

Health Services, both at UT-Memphis. Dr. Veeser is the author of several publications in college health and in nursing, and is presently Chair of the Tennessee Health Center for Nursing. She is a 1998 recipient of the Lovett Award from the American College Health Association and was Vice President of ACHA, 2001–2002.

Robert Watson, EdD, FACHE, is Associate Director (Administrator), Student Health Care Center at the University of Florida, where he has been employed since 1989. After a 30-year career in the U.S. Army Medical Department, he retired as a Colonel, hospital administrator. His last assignment was as Assistant Dean, Army Medical Field Service School, San Antonio, Texas. Dr. Watson completed his MBA at the University of Hawaii and earned his MHA and Doctor of Education degrees from George Washington University, Washington, DC. His Fellowship in the American College of Healthcare Executives was conferred in 1982.

Leighton C. Whitaker, PhD, ABPP, earned his BA from Swarthmore College and PhD from Wayne State University. He is a Diplomate in Clinical Psychology of the American Board of Professional Psychology. He is currently an Adjunct Clinical Professor for the Institute for Graduate Clinical Psychology at Widener University, editor of the *Journal of College Student Psychotherapy,* consulting editor for mental health for the *Journal of American College Health,* and a Fellow of the American College Health Association. He teaches, writes, and presents on college mental health, schizophrenic disorders, and violence prevention. Previously he was Associate Professor and Director of Adult Psychology, University of Colorado Health Sciences Center; Professor and Director of the University of Massachusetts Mental Health Services; Director of Swarthmore College Psychological Services; and a consultant to the U.S. Department of Labor's Job Corps Program.

J. Robert Wirag, HSD, has served as the Director of the Student Health Service program at the University of North Carolina at Chapel Hill since January 1999. This is his third directorship, following The University of Texas at Austin, 1987–95, and the University of Arkansas, 1983–87. His professional career spans a period of over 30 years and includes faculty appointments at the University of Notre Dame, DePaul University, and The Pennsylvania State University. Dr. Wirag is past president of the American College Health Association, a board member of the American College Health Foundation, and an active participant in ACHA's Consultative Services Program.

Pamela Woodrum, RN, OGNP, is a graduate of St. Joseph Infirmary School of Nursing, Louisville, Kentucky, and the Gynecologic/Obstetric Nurse Practitioner Program at Emory University in Atlanta, Georgia. She began her clinical practice in gynecology in the University of Kentucky Health Service in 1973. Ms. Woodrum has precepted nurse practitioner students and midwifery students, and for a time was active in the teaching program for fourth-year medical students. She has lectured on contraception, sexually transmitted diseases, and other gynecological issues. Most recently, she has focused on issues of human sexuality, including patient education and counseling and program development and implementation in the campus community.

Christine G. Zimmer, MA, CHES, is Director, Office of Health Promotion and Education, at Sindecuse Health Center, Western Michigan University. She has served as Vice

President of the American College Health Association and as Co-Chair of the ACHA Task Force on Health Promotion in Higher Education, which developed "Standards of Practice for Health Promotion in Higher Education." She is a Fellow of the American College Health Association and is a member of the American College Health Foundation Board of Directors. Ms. Zimmer is a recipient of ACHA's Edward Hitchcock Award for outstanding contributions in the field of college health and the Ruth E. Boynton Award.

Chapter 1

The History and Development of College Health

H. Spencer Turner, MD, MS, FACPM, and Janet L. Hurley, PhD

The Early Years

"There shall be no scollar nor infaunt, of what country or shire so ev. he be of, beyng man child, be refused, except he have some horrible or contagious infirmyties wiche he, and shall alwaies be, remytted to the discretion of the Warden or deputie for the time beyng."[1, p. 1] This regulation was promulgated in the fifteenth century by regents of Manchester College, London, by which students with "horrible and contagious infirmities" were excluded from enrollment. Fortunately, by the beginning of the nineteenth century a more enlightened approach had developed for dealing with issues related to "infirmities" of one sort or the other. Thomas Jefferson, as Rector of the University of Virginia, reported in the minutes of the Board of Visitors, April 7, 1826:

> At a meeting of the Visitors of the University of Virginia held at the said University on Monday the 3rd and Tuesday the 4th of April 1826 at which were present Thomas Jefferson, Joseph C. Cabell, John H. Cocke, Chapman Johnson and James Madison the following proceedings were had.
>
> . . . There shall be established in the University a Dispensary which shall be attached to the Medical School, and shall be under the sole direction and government of the Professor of Medecine who shall attend personally at the Anatomical theatre, or such other place as he shall notify, from half after one to two oclock, on every Tuesday, Thursday and Saturday, for the purpose of dispensing medical advise, vaccination, and aid in Surgical cases of ordinary occurrence, to applicants needing them.
>
> All Poor, free, persons, disordered in body, topically or generally, and applying for advise, shall receive it gratis; all others, bond or free, shall receive it on the payment of half a Dollar at each attendance, for the use of the institution, and all persons shall be vaccinated

gratis, and the Students particularly shall be encouraged to be so, as a protection to the institution against the malady of the small pox."[2]

This plan, which obviously put particular emphasis on immunization, established a "public" and "private" clinic that medical students could attend, both as students and patients.

By 1825, Harvard had introduced methods of mass physical education in a manner adapted from practices in universities in Germany and Scandinavia. Following Harvard's example, Dartmouth, Williams, Yale, and Amherst introduced a gymnastics program, and, by mid-century gymnasiums filled with exercise equipment were common in most colleges and universities. The rationale for these programs apparently was alarm over the sedentary existence of the American college youth, whose diet was still the hearty one of the hard-working farmer but whose physical exertions were confined to walking, ball playing, and, in a few schools, rowing. Exercise, it was thought, was the best means of improving the students' health.[3] Thus, it was not unexpected that the development of college health during the latter part of the nineteenth century was an integral part of the growth of departments of physical education and hygiene in most colleges. Physicians were commonly employed as either chairs or senior staff members in these departments.

In 1840 William Alcott expressed doubt that schools would "ever become what they ought to be as places for the promotion of health . . . until they are brought under the care . . . of judicious medical men . . . .our schools ought to have their regular physicians as much as our houses of industry, our almshouses, or our penitentiaries."[1, p.1]

Such was the case at Amherst College, the institution which is generally acknowledged to have established the first college health service. In 1856, Amherst president William A. Stearns observed:

> Students of our colleges have bodies which need care and culture as well as the intellectual and moral powers and which need this care at the same time with higher education. The breaking down of the health of students, especially in the spring of the year, which is exceedingly common, involving the necessity of leaving college in many instances and crippling the energies and destroying the prospects of not a few who remain, is, in my opinion, wholly unnecessary if proper measures could be taken to prevent it."[4, p.37]

In August 1859, the Board of Trustees of Amherst College created a Department of Physical Education and Hygiene. Credit must be given to one particular member of the board, Nathan Allen, MD, for in describing the program to be initiated, Dr. Allen specified the following: a medical examination of every student on arrival at the college; a course of instruction in hygiene; treatment for the sick; and a regularly conducted program in physical exercise for all students during their four-year curriculum. Further, Dr. Allen requested "an annual report including particularly the kind and number of sicknesses from which the college students were suffering."[5, p.278]

Subsequently, Stearns appointed Dr. John W. Hooker as Professor of Hygiene at Amherst. Hooker thereby became, so far as has been recorded, the first physician directly employed by any college in the United States.[6] Subsequent to Hooker's resignation within the year because of illness, the board appointed Dr. Edward C. Hitchcock Jr., son of a previous president of the college and an 1853 graduate of Harvard Medical School, to the position. Under his guidance, the program at Amherst seems to have been successful from the beginning. It is that successful beginning and Hitchcock's long years of service that have given Edward Hitchcock the deserved title "Father of American College Health."

Hitchcock, as did others of his time, placed a great emphasis on anthropometric measurements and the belief that physical measurements were the best indices of the health status of an individual. His detailed measurements and records became a model for others.

Of particular interest is Hitchcock's responsibility as a co-founder, in 1885, of the American Association for the Advancement of Physical Education and his presidency of that organization for its first three years. This association included health and physical education staff from several colleges and universities and was a precursor to the American School Health Association (later the American College Health Association). Hitchcock served Amherst as Professor of Hygiene and Physical Education until 1898. From 1898 to 1910, he was dean of the faculty. He died in February of 1911.

At nearby sister schools there were similar programs being created. A resident physician, Dr. Mary A. B. Homer, was added to the staff of Mount Holyoke in 1860, and in 1862 she was made a teacher of physiology.[7] At Vassar, Dr. Alida C. Avery was in residence from its beginning in 1865; she also served as Professor of Physiology and Hygiene.[8]

> When students are ill they are placed under her (Avery's)' professional care, unless previous arrangements, approved by the President, have been made to secure the attendance of other physicians. When other physicians are engaged, their visits must be made knowledge and they must be in communication with the resident physician in regard to the treatment of the patient in order that she may discharge her duty as health officer of the institution. In the infirmary, complete arrangements are made for the comfort of the sick and a competent nurse is in constant attendance. The infirmary, a consultation office and full-time medical staff may qualify Vassar as the "first" true health service for women. Wellesley was not far behind and in 1876, in its first circular noted that "a lady physician will reside in the college and will have the general care of the health of students."[1, p.4]

In 1885, Dr. J. W. Seaver was appointed Medical Director of the Yale gymnasium, where a "thorough physical examination and measurement of each student is made yearly by the medical director and a record of these results is kept as a basis of advice as to exercise and regimen."[1, p.4] Similar procedures were developed about the same time at Harvard under Dr. D. A. Sargent and at Johns Hopkins under Dr. E. M. Hartwell. Hartwell reported that by 1886, of the principal colleges and universities in the United States, physicians in charge of student health were employed by Amherst, Harvard, Yale, Johns Hopkins, Haverford, Vassar, and Wellesley.[9] He did not include Mount Holyoke, and it is likely there were other institutions employing physicians, as well. Nonetheless, by the late 1800s only approximately a dozen colleges employed full-time physicians, chiefly in connection with their departments of physical training.

Dr. R. S. Canuteson summed up the early association between college health and physical education noting oldest perhaps of the cornerstones of a health program was physical education, and later its offsprings, intercollegiate and then intramural sports. Apparently this one activity did not satisfy the growing interest in physical welfare of college students, and so the next step was, almost simultaneously, the introduction of classes in personal hygiene, the forerunner of what we today prefer to call health education, with emphasis on the factors making for healthful living or environmental hygiene. [10, p. 7]

It was to be expected, then, that college health programs before the turn of the century placed a major emphasis on intercollegiate athletics. College health and intercollegiate athletics were to remain very closely associated for the next 50 years. (The relationship between health service, physical education, and athletics was perhaps no better exemplified than at The Ohio State University, where Dr. John W. Wilce [after whom the current health services building is named] coached football for 15 years, completing his medical studies on the side, then spent the next 30 years as director of Student Health Services.)

In 1909, G. L. Mylan, as chairman of a committee of the American Physical Education Association on the Status of Hygiene in Colleges and Universities, sent a questionnaire to 138 institutions, receiving replies from 124.[11] The data indicated that 75% of students were given a medical examination before participating in gymnastics or athletics, with 14% having the exam by the college physician, 30% by the medical director or advisor, and the remainder by the director of physical education, who was, most usually, a physician. In some cases the exam was repeated annually. In others it was "when expedient." In addition, medical or surgical treatment was provided in about half of the institutions; 15% provided care for emergencies only; 12% provided infirmary care; and 4% provided care for athletes only. Anthropometry, which had been so important in the latter half of the nineteenth century, was declining, while the medical examination was increasing in importance and in detail.

In the latter half of the nineteenth century, some colleges began to establish infirmaries to care for ill students, particularly as isolation wards for students with communicable diseases. As has been noted, Vassar and Wellesley colleges were the first to furnish infirmaries for the care and isolation of women students, followed by infirmary care for men at Princeton in 1893 and at the College of William and Mary in 1894. The combination of the development of infirmaries and the move away from anthropometric measurements and gymnastics to detailed medical examinations, was a reflection not only of need as defined by the internal events of the colleges and universities themselves, but also of the external influence of the changes occurring in medicine during this same period of time.

The University of California was one of the first schools to develop a comprehensive student health program (as it might be defined today), providing both medical care and infirmary care beginning in 1901. Dr. G. F. Reinhardt wrote in 1913,

It may be a surprising statement that the University of California Infirmary with its large daily clinic and its hospital facilities owes its existence less to a direct effort to improve student health than an effort to improve class attendance. In 1900, the faculty of the University of California became dissatisfied with the average attendance of students upon [*sic*] classes and investigated the cause of absence with a view to meting out proper discipline to delinquents. The discovery was an unexpected one: that sickness and not idleness or lack of interest was at the bottom of the trouble.[12, p. 295]

In addition to the usual illnesses affecting the young adult population, epidemics of typhoid were common in the early 1900s. Cornell University's Health Service experienced major growth as a result of a typhoid epidemic in 1903, in which 291 students became ill. Following a typhoid epidemic at the University of Wisconsin, a comprehensive program was established in 1907. As Boynton has noted:

> Perhaps these colleges and universities which had epidemics in those early days were fortunate, for in the majority of schools the general pattern continued to be that of a physician attached to the department of physical education with the health program consisting almost exclusively of physical examination on admission, the results of which were used largely to assign students to physical activity classes and the teaching of classes in hygiene.[12, p. 296]

A word regarding funding of these early college health services is important. At the outset, health services were funded almost entirely from tuition and/or general fees. This pattern continued until the mid–twentieth century. It was not until after World War II and the rapid expansion of health services that alternative funding sources began to be seriously explored. (More discussion on funding will follow later in this chapter.)

In the early part of the twentieth century, many institutions believed that physical education, health service, health teaching, and environmental health should be under one administrative head. This was often the director of physical education or athletics and usually a non-medical person. As the medical aspects of the total health program began to develop, this organizational pattern shifted and health services became their own entities responsible for the total health program, with the exception of physical education and athletics.[12] This was an important development because it represents a clear change in the responsibilities of the "campus physician" from physical education and athletic activities on campus to a more comprehensive health program.

Perhaps the most radical event influencing the direction and development of college health services on the national scene was World War I. Boynton notes:

> Historically, wars have always created concern on the part of nations for the health of their young people. In England, for example, the Boer War resulted in the first national legislation to protect the health of children. Likewise, in this country, the first World War caused national concern for the health of our young people because of the large numbers of young men found to be physically unfit for military service . . . we find that World War I had a very direct effect on focusing attention on the need for college health programs. Inspired by pre–induction physicals which identified physical defects in young men, colleges and universities began to set up (or expand) programs to prevent and correct physical defects which might interfere with academic programs.[12, p. 296]

THE STOREY YEARS

While Dr. Edward Hitchcock Jr. has generally been acclaimed as the first person employed full-time as a college health physician in the United States, the unsung hero of the continuing growth and development of college health is Dr. Thomas Andrew Storey. Storey, who was born in Kansas in 1875, entered Stanford in 1892 as a pre-law student. In this second class of the university were two other men who had a major influence upon the direction of Storey's career and with whom Storey would interact over the next 50 years. Further, each of them would be important to the evolution of college health programs in the United States during the first half of the twentieth century.

One of these two was Dr. Ray L. Wilbur, who became the first dean of the Stanford Medical School, president of Stanford from 1916 to 1943 and chancellor from 1943 until his death in 1949. Wilbur was also a president of the American Medical Association and served as Secretary of the Interior under Herbert Hoover.

The second classmate was Dr. William F. Snow, who was director of the Student Health Service at Stanford for a short period. Then, in 1914, he became a founding member of the American Social Hygiene Association (ASHA). In 1915, he left Stanford to become the first Director of the ASHA. Snow received the assignment of combating venereal diseases in the military by "1) provision of modern diagnosis, treatment, and chemical prophylaxis, 2) vigorous repression of prostitution in the vicinity of training camps, 3) instruction of the soldiers in the prevention and avoidance of infection, and 4) provision of wholesome entertainment in and near training camps."[13, p. 29] In 1918, at the urging of the ASHA and Snow, Congress was persuaded to appropriate funds to carry out these four charges.

The funds were distributed to state health departments and to the U.S. Public Health Service to establish the first Division of Venereal Disease Control and, most importantly to college health, to distribute $537,900 to colleges and universities to assist in developing educational measures for venereal disease prevention. The vehicle for distribution was the development of a new board, the United States Interdepartmental Social Hygiene Board. Dr. Thomas Storey, with a PhD in physiology from Stanford and an MD from Harvard, who had left California in 1907 to accept a position at the College of the City of New York, where he organized the Department of Hygiene, was named the executive secretary of this group. In later summarizing the work of the board, Storey believed the board's most important effort was distributing money to colleges and universities, because educating future leaders of society would have the most lasting effect on the control of venereal diseases. He further pointed out that "departments of hygiene" had been established or enlarged at 39 schools, colleges, and universities as a result of this program.[14]

Despite the discontinuation in 1921 of congressional funding for the interdepartmental board, Snow and ASHA recognized the need to continue programs for venereal-disease control on college campuses. As a direct result, one year later, ASHA financed the formation and operation of the "President's Committee of Fifty on College Hygiene." This committee was formed to "stimulate the development and extension of instruction and training in hygiene in normal schools, colleges, and universities."[15, p. 3] Storey was named executive secretary of the committee, thereby continuing his work from the "old" U.S. Interdepartmental Board. Also on the committee were Snow and Wilbur, Storey's old classmates from Stanford.

Significantly, also on this committee was Dr. John Sundwall, who convened the group which became the American College Health Association. The American Student Health Association (later to change its name to the American College Health Association [ACHA]) was established and held its first meeting on March 4, 1920, in Chicago.

Although Storey was unable to attend this meeting, he was elected in absentia to a one-year term on the executive committee and had a paper read at the first meeting. He attended the next year and again the third year, where he presented a paper entitled "Objectives in the Organization of College Departments of Hygiene." Although he missed the fourth meeting, he was still installed for a two-year term at the fifth meeting (in 1925) as the fourth president of ASHA (ACHA). Of note is that Snow was also in attendance at this meeting; in fact, ASHA was a prominent program participant.

The President's Committee continued to be active for many years and, as noted by Christmas and Dorman:

> The committee was an important instrument for the advancement of health centers on college campuses because it brought together university presidents and ACHA leaders. In 1927, Storey published *The Status of Hygiene Programs in Institutions of Higher Education in the United States; a Report for the President's Committee of Fifty on College Health.* The survey found many deficiencies and defects in these programs, concluding that "under these conditions our institutions of higher education will be a long time in producing a scientific public opinion in favor of periodic examination and the selection of scientific health service."[13, p. 32]

Storey returned to Stanford in 1926, where he not only became director of the Department of Hygiene, but also filled the position of executive officer of the Board of Athletic Control, which included Stanford's athletic affairs, health service, infirmary, and public health programs for the campus.[11] In 1931, Storey was named chairman of the First National Conference on College Hygiene, which was sponsored by the President's Committee of Fifty, the American Student Health Association, the National Health Council, and the National Tuberculosis Association. Its purpose was "to focus the attention of our most competent authorities upon the identification of the basic problems of college hygiene; secure their expert analysis of those problems; and then have them formulate a consequent statement of their conclusions."[16, p. 5] The published proceedings of the conference were deemed as a useful "measuring rod" of the growing responsibilities of every college for the protection, maintenance, and promotion of the health of the students. The conference, for the first time, "pointed out the need for an agreement upon desirable minimum standards for colleges and universities in the areas of health service, health teaching, physical education and environmental health."[12, p. 301]

The Second National Conference on College Hygiene, sponsored by the same organizations, was held the following year. The second national conference emphasized the legal, social, and educational responsibilities of presidents and governing boards of colleges and universities to provide for the establishment and maintenance of hygiene instruction in health services.[17] Also at the second conference, the importance of the contribution that "mental hygiene" can make to the well-being of college students was emphasized. Further, the conference emphasized the importance of teaching social hygiene, nutrition, and the whole area of physical education. In this latter context, it was noted that "in many colleges, athletics is a real problem . . . emphasis upon any single phase of physical education, including intercollegiate athletics is deplored."[16, p. 11]

Thomas Storey was on the organizing committee for the second conference when he retired from Stanford at age 65. He then accepted a job with ASHA (of which Wilbur was then president of the board). Storey's friend Snow, although retired, remained active in ASHA. As mobilization began for World War II, Storey, with his prior experience, was placed in charge of the Atlanta office of ASHA and focused his efforts on issues related to prevention and treatment of venereal diseases. He died of heart disease at age 68 in Atlanta in 1943.

THE WAR YEARS

In the summer of 1936, an international conference on the issue of college and university student health services was held in Athens, Greece. Seventeen countries, including the United States, were represented at the meeting, and the following statement of views represented one of its outcomes.[1]

- Very careful attention should be given to the health of students by the State and the universities.
- Students should participate not only financially but also actively in services designed to care for those who are ill. Such participation is indispensable for obtaining positive results.
- In addition to medical care for sick students, special care should be given to prophylactic means for bettering the health of students and for increasing their endurance in case of illness. Also, very special care should be taken to provide measures against tuberculosis which endangers our university young people.
- Administrative supervision should be imposed obligatorily in anything that concerns the physical activities of young people and their state of health should be regularly checked.
- In all European nations it is considered a national right to take measures necessary for developing and supervising the physical activities of youth.
- Every measure having for its purpose the conservation of the health of students should, in order that it may be efficacious, depend not only on administrative or legislative organization but also and especially on the physicians who should apply these measures. These physicians ought to have a training of such a kind that they will be in condition to take adequate measures in any circumstances not only for each separate case but for all students.
- It is indispensable to organize the services of hygiene in such a way that it may be possible to derive exact statistics as to the health of the students. These statistics are necessary for determining the policies required and indispensable in each country, a policy which ought to be based upon positive and comparative data.

- The basis for such statistics may be obtained by keeping a special record of the health of each student taken from careful and periodic medical examinations.
- That college physicians may be better prepared for their work, we consider that each country possessing a well-organized health department should take the initiative in developing adequate facilities for the training of an especially chosen personnel.
- The work of the conference has demonstrated the absolute necessity for similar conferences of specialists occupied with questions of the health of students; therefore, the members of the Congress propose the convocation of an international congress for the health of students every 4 years at the time of the Olympiads. In order to promote such a project we are establishing a central bureau in the University of Athens with the collaboration of the German secretariat. This bureau invites the cooperation of appropriate departments or organizations in carrying on this work, and will serve as a clearing house of information. [1, p. 7, 8]

Unfortunately, it appears that despite plans for further meetings, no such further collaborations were held, which one must assume would be related to the beginning of World War II.

In 1937, the federal government's Office of Education (then part of the United States Department of the Interior) conducted a survey of student health services to "furnish a general picture of provisions and practices in the important field of medical supervision and care" in college and university health services.[1, p. 2] Of 656 institutions surveyed, 352 responded. While the results were reported primarily based upon school size (with some breakout for women's, men's, co-educational, junior colleges, and professional and technical schools), several summary conclusions were reported.

> From one college, the establishment of such a service has extended in some degree to practically all institutions of higher education, especially those which have the responsibility of parental care for youth far removed from home. These services, however, represent all degrees of development. They vary all the way from an examination of the heart of those who expect to participate in strenuous athletics . . . to the most detailed investigation of bodily and mental conditions now possible.
>
> From the crude picture painted by statistics, we find as follows:
>
> a) of coeducational colleges and universities . . . having an enrollment of fewer than 500, 10% employ full-time and 55% part-time physicians. . . . In half these institutions, efforts are made of furnishing ample care of ailing students.
>
> b) in coeducational institutions with 500 or a 1000 students, there is a rise in the number having full-time physicians to 40% . . . 35% or more have part-time doctors . . . in 20% special efforts are made in the field of mental hygiene.
>
> c) 1000 to 2000 students . . . 90% employ one or more physicians . . . treatment of ambulatory cases is offered in 60%.
>
> d) in larger institutions of this group an increase in proportion of full-time workers and in the total number of physicians and nurses . . . more than 50% have developed special activities in mental hygiene.[1, p. 57]

Information concerning his physical condition is furnished the student as an outcome of his medical examination and in many schools he is free to consult the school physician at any time regarding the "accidents in his own body" and with regard to more general matters of hygiene. This is not quite enough, however, for the student should be informed concerning the structure and functions of his body and with regard to the general principles underlying personal and community health.[1, p. 61]

No doubt the great depression and World War II caused the interruption of the Third National Conference on College Health, which was not held until 1947. The meeting had the following objectives:

A. To review the progress and status of college health programs
B. To identify and define the major health problems of college students and the responsibilities of the college administration for the health of students and others on the campus.
C. To suggest adaptable programs that will provide health education, physical education in health service and healthy environment for students during college years and in preparation for later individual and community resources
D. To publish these recommendations in a suitable form to serve as a guide to administrators and others interested in college health. [18, p. 3]

This third conference was particularly important in that, for the first time (and perhaps because of the openness following the war years), there were discussions of special health problems including "social hygiene," a euphemism for issues related to sexuality. It was noted that sexual hygiene had too often been regarded as aiming at freedom from venereal diseases and freedom from non-venereal disorders of the sexual organs. The committee charged with this area noted that "the larger review of social health should be stressed in social hygiene in college. This view includes all physical, environmental and social aspects of sex in human life."[18, p. 100]

The report of the conference also included a summary of the findings of health practices of various colleges and universities, reporting a survey of over 300 institutions, 132 publically controlled and 168 privately controlled. Of these, 270 institutions offered medical care for ambulatory illnesses, 152 gave counseling in mental hygiene, 274 offered physical education activity courses, 281 defined themselves as having a student health service office or dispensary, and 163 had a student infirmary.

THE POST-WAR ERA AND THE MOORE-SUMMERSKILL REPORT

In 1953, the most accurate and comprehensive survey of college health services ever undertaken was carried out by Norman Moore, MD, and John Summerskill, PhD, of Cornell University.[19] The data give a clear, concise overview of college health in the United States nearly 100 years into its development. While previous surveys had used a mailed questionnaire, this survey employed a personal interview technique, assuring complete and uniform reports. Letters were sent from the president of ACHA to 1,157 colleges. Each letter requested the name of the person in charge of the health service, i.e., the one being interviewed. Field representatives of the Continental Casualty Company interviewed health service directors (or their equivalents) on behalf of ACHA. Data for each college were reported in two ways; first, by means of a questionnaire filled out by the insurance company representative during the interview, and, second, by means of another questionnaire that the health service director filled out as a confidential report after the interview.

The findings reported were based on responses from 61% of the recognized colleges in the country. The incidence of colleges without health programs was *highest* among two-year colleges, colleges offering a specialized academic program, and colleges with enrollments under 500. The incidence of colleges without health programs was *lowest* among western colleges, women's colleges, four-year colleges with graduate training, and colleges with enrollments of over 2000. (Of the 1,157 respondents, 200 claimed no responsibility for health of students in any way; thus findings are based on 957 colleges).

Findings included the following:

- Detection of Disease—90% of colleges required entrance physical exams with half of these carried out by college health service physicians and the other half by students' own physicians. Sixty percent required entering students to have an entrance chest X-ray. Entrance medical histories were required at 60% of the institutions.
- Prevention of Disease—less than half of the colleges required some kind of vaccination or immunization for new students.
- Health Records—three-quarters of the health services kept cumulative health records for individual students.
- Clinical Care—80% reported a clinical program for care of accidents or illness.
- Health Education—Courses were offered at 80% of the colleges with a student health service. Most included instruction on both physical and mental health.
- Physical Education—90% of colleges with a health service offered a PE program (supervised by health service personnel at 20%).
- Athletic Medical Care—three quarters of colleges with a health service provided medical care for athletes, supervised by the health service at two-thirds of these.
- Sanitation and Nutrition—50% of health service had responsibility for sanitation in dorms, lodgings, pools, washrooms, and eating places (actual inspection often carried out by the local governmental agency).
- Health Service Research—less than 20% engaged in research of any kind.
- Health Service Personnel—director was a physician at 40% of colleges, nurse director at 25%, directors from general or physical education at 25%; two-thirds of directors worked full-time at the college; 40% worked full-time at the health service; 20% had no physician on health service staff.
- Finances—30% paid specified health fees; 60% financed through general or tuition income; remaining financed through insurance or fee-for-service.

This survey also found that 85% of four-year colleges and 90% of universities with graduate training programs furnished clinical care, with the average number of annual visits being 3,170 per 1,000 students. Ancillary services were provided by more than

50% of the survey respondents and typically included laboratory, pharmacy, radiology, and, less often, physical therapy, and vision and hearing testing services. Responsibility for medical care beyond outpatient care was assumed by three-quarters of the institutions, with one-third having infirmaries and the remainder assuming the responsibility for students hospitalized in community hospitals. Of note is that nearly all campuses provided student health care for less than $10 per student per year.

The results of the Moore-Summerskill survey were used as a basis for a fourth national conference on health and colleges, which was held in 1954, again under the sponsorship of the National Tuberculosis Association. The focus of the meeting was "team work and meeting the health needs of college students."[20, p. 303]

In addition to discussion of teamwork, one particularly important concept endorsed by the conference was that the "cost of medical care and hospitalization whether provided by the student health service or by community physicians and hospital facilities, should be borne by the student through payment of a health fee designated as such."[21, p. 5] This represented a significant change in the issue of financing student health services, because, as previously noted, from the mid-1800s until recent times, college health services had been funded almost without exception from general funds and/or tuition. However, with the expansion of services, particularly following World War II, other funding sources were necessary. In fact, Ralph Canuteson, MD, in his ASHA (ACHA) presidential address in 1946 had stated that "provision for any type of prepaid medical care was a radical departure in the field of medicine and it was not immediately accepted as an ethical procedure" by the medical profession and that "health services for many years had been providing prepaid medical care with considerable success and many difficulties."[7, p. 7] In response to the concerns about financing student health care, which were emerging during the late 1940s, the first student health insurance program was inaugurated during the fall quarter of 1948 at the University of Denver, which thereby became the first institution of higher education to afford an opportunity for health insurance for students.[22]

Two other important developments occurred in college health during the 1950s. In October 1952, Dr. Norman Moore (two years later to be co-author of the report just described) began publication twice yearly of a small journal entitled *Student Medicine*. In 1958, Dr. Moore recommended that *Student Medicine* become the official journal of the American College Health Association. In 1962, the name *Student Medicine* was changed to *Journal of the American College Health Association*.

A second major development during the 1950s was the appointment, in 1955, of a special committee to study the possibility of a permanent association office for ACHA. Ten years later, in 1965, Dr. Ben Reiter became the first paid executive director but died after serving only one year. Subsequently, in July 1966, Lee Stauffer was named the executive director of the American College Health Association and served in the position for one and a half years.[23] He was followed by James Dilley, who served for 18 years, by Stephen Blom for 6 years, and Charles Hartman for 8 years. As of the time of this treatise, Randal Doyle has been executive director since 1998.

In 1960, Dr. Samuel Fuenning, president of ACHA, appointed a committee to develop a document specifying recommended standards and practices for a college health program following the groundwork laid by the four national conferences on college hygiene. (This first such document was published by ACHA in 1961.[1] It has had many revisions—1969, 1977, 1984, and 1991—with the most recent revision published in the summer of 1999.)[24]

THE SIXTIES AND SEVENTIES

Farnsworth summarized the progress of the American College Health Association in 1962:

> The factor mainly responsible for increasing the standards of performance of college health services. . .has been the revitalization of the American College Health Association. This organization, now more than 40 years old, had become somewhat routine and perfunctory in the pursuit of its goals of improving college health services, and it was seriously handicapped by lack of funds. During the latter part of the last decade it changed its format from that of an institutional membership alone to a combination of institutional and individual membership. It developed its own quarterly journal, the *Journal of the American College Health Association*. . .stimulated activity in its regional affiliated health associations, broadened the scope of subjects discussed at its annual meetings and presented a series of guidelines designed to aid institutions seeking to improve or establish their health services. In 1962 it had 397 institutional and 800 individual members. . .The association adopted in 1961 a statement of recommended standards and practices for a college health program. This formulation, reasonably detailed in its recommendation, propounds a philosophy that a good college health program should provide much more than first aid for accidents and medical care for acute illness. . .the idea that colleges have a responsibility for the health needs of their students is apparently gaining acceptance, in part because of internal developments and part because students and their parents are taking it for granted."[25, p. 1290-1291]

By the mid-1960s Farnsworth could report that college health services were becoming large business organizations, noting that the time had passed when a lone physician aided by a nurse could adequately provide health care. He emphasized the use of preventive medicine and heath education as a means to decrease the need for treatment and noted that health education programs have preceded and were often more effective and are better organized than the health services."[26, p. 1]

The year 1960 began the second century of college health in the United States, as the arrival of the "baby boomers" on campuses marked a period of unparalleled growth. As Christmas noted:

> When the baby boom generation entered college in the mid 1960's they caused an unprecedented expansion of higher education, including the need for student services. At this time, the health fee gained wide acceptance as a means of financing campus health centers, which in turn came to be administratively designated cost centers or auxiliary enterprises. At the larger institutions, health centers were significantly expanding their roles on campus by more comprehensively addressing the emotional needs of students and by establishing environ-

mental health and safety programs that offered services to faculty and staff, as well as to students . . . As health care has become more complex and more expensive, infirmaries have been phased out at many institutions. The emphasis on athletic medicine that had once characterized college health centers has also diminished as intercollegiate athletics has become big business and athletic departments have become much more involved in providing care for the athletes.[27, p. 243]

In 1976, the Josiah Macy Jr. Foundation sponsored a conference on college health programs. Dr. Willard Dalrymple, chair of the program, noted the problem of the impact of limited national resources and decreasing financial support for institutions of higher education causing scrutiny of health service budgets.[28, viii] In this context, this conference recognized the continuing conflict (which nearly 25 years later has again raised its head) between two major schools of thought, one which sees education primarily as concerned with cognitive processes as opposed to a more encompassing, integrated view of the college period, with its intellectual development being intimately associated with personal, psychological, and sociological growth. [28, p. viii] Points of concern discussed at the Macy Conference included the relationship of health programs with the university, the campus, and the general community; staffing; extending opportunities and responsibilities; special needs of women, special needs of minority groups; and organization and support of health service programs. Also of particular interest in this conference was the discussion of the context of practice for university health services in relationship to the developing HMO movement.

James Dilley, then executive director of ACHA, noted that in actuality, college and university health services had been working with the model that was, in essence, an HMO. He explained that, "because Section 1310 of the law [the Health Maintenance Organization Act of 1973] requires that all employers subject to the Fair Labor Standards Act and employing more than 25 persons must make available a health maintenance option in addition to their insurance plan it has now become a matter of national policy that such a system for the provision of health services be universally available."[28, p. 152,153] He was concerned that a national health insurance plan might be enacted that would ignore the special concerns/issues of college students. He continued: "We in the college health services are concerned that the program enacted will make it possible for the present health care system in colleges and universities, which is currently serving the approximately 9.3 million students in that segment of post-secondary education known as higher education, to be nurtured and permitted to grow . . . we must become more adroit in our justification of a health service delivery system that serves a unique segment of that society."[28, p. 154] Those early warnings in 1976 were foreshadowing for the future.

THE EIGHTIES

By the 1980s, college health services had continued to expand programs and reach larger numbers of people. But the winds of change were beginning to blow. In his presidential address to the ACHA annual meeting in 1981, Dr. H.S. Turner stated, "The past and our progress notwithstanding, I genuinely believe that if we are to make the point of the need for our continued existence at institutions of higher education, we must again indicate to administrators, to organized medicine . . . . that we do have a role to play and that we are viable."[29, p. 7] Turner continued by pointing out at least four major areas which he believed needed attention. These included (1) a changing student body with an increasing number of older students, particularly women and part-time students; (2) concern about changes in fiscal support for higher education, pointing out that "it is quite clear that the days of free-flowing money to institutions of higher education, be they public or private, are a thing of the past . . . . We must not only be creative and innovative in the utilization of limited budgets, but we must become masters at communicating the value of our activities to those who control budgetary allocations"[29, p. 8];(3) environmental health and safety activities, particularly when viewed in the face of new and changing regulations and the impact of multiple regulatory agencies; and (4) health insurance issues, including national health insurance, portability and financing. He pointed out that none of the proposed methods for financing national health insurance, whether they were "catastrophic insurance" or "cradle to grave insurance," recognize the special contributions of college health services.

Dr. Harold Enarson, then president of The Ohio State University, keynote speaker at ACHA's 59th convention in 1981, made the following observations about college health from a university president's perspective.

> Given today's fiscal realities, maintaining quality will require that health services include in their efforts the promotion of health as well as the treatment of injury and disease. Communicable diseases . . . have largely been brought under control, while the chronic ones . . . .can best be avoided given our current state of knowledge by changes in life style . . . .The promotion of wellness is one [aim] we must pursue more vigorously in the '80s . . . .better diet, more exercise, learning to cope with stress in one's academic and personal life, awareness of the effects of tobacco, alcohol and other drugs on the body, and understanding of human sexuality . . . better control of toxic agents . . . .protective immunization for (health science) students . . . more attention to conditioning to prevent athletic injuries in both men and women—these too can make a positive contribution to good health. Such a broad commitment to wellness demands closer links between the university health service and other campus units—physical education, recreation, athletics, perhaps home economics, health education, nutrition. The mission of the student health service—to keep the most students at the most books the most time—can no longer be carried out in isolation. We need health care pioneers who can forge new alliances and new partnerships, who can accept the challenge of doing more with less, and doing it exceedingly well."[3, p. 13]

In the mid-1980s, a worldwide event occurred which had (and will continue to have) a lasting impact on medicine and, particularly, on college health. "AIDS, it has been said, put ACHA on the map."[30, p. 271] With the emergence of HIV during the 1980s, ACHA found itself at the center of increased visibility and, indeed, some "fame." ACHA responded by establishing an ACHA Task Force on HIV Disease in September 1985, chaired by Dr. Richard Keeling, who became president of ACHA in 1989. This task force (which was still active at the end of the 1990s) produced a series of prevention materials, at least two editions of a special report, many years of grant support for regional workshops, grants to institutions, a number of important publications, and, particularly important, a definitive seroprevalence survey describing the patterns of HIV infection among students.[30]

An excellent picture of college and university health in the late 1980s was painted in Kevin Patrick's report in the Journal of the American Medical Association[31] and his textbook, *Principles and Practices of Student Health,* the third part of a trilogy on school health."[32] This textbook represented the first (and only, so far as the authors can determine) comprehensive textbook ever published on college health practice.

Patrick reported student health services were available to approximately 10 million of the 12.5 million university and college students throughout the United States in the late 1980s. Some 27,000 persons were employed in college health, including approximately 3,000 physicians. In larger institutions, each student health center employed an average of 3.7 physicians per 10,000 students, and about 70% of these were full-time. The average age of students was 26 years; over 50% were financially independent; 40% were uninsured or underinsured; and 20 to 30 million student visits were made yearly to student health centers.[31] In regard to financing, Patrick noted that by the late 1980s sources of financing for health services had changed little since 1950—with a continued mix of prepaid health fees, general or university funds, fee–for–service revenue, and insurance reimbursement. He noted one study which suggested the majority of small campuses (3,000 or fewer students) fund their health centers mainly through general fund resources but noted that "many large institutions have developed sophisticated health maintenance organization models."[32, p. 3304] Of particular note was the reported variation in the level of investment in student health among different campuses. Among the private institutions annual support ranged from $28 to $415 per year per student, compared with $34 to $206 per year per student for public schools.[32]

Patrick felt that student health services were still suffering from an image problem in the late 1980s:

> . . . student health has . . . lacked a real identity and a positive image. Commonly held beliefs about student health practice are that it is retirement or part-time practice for many physicians and the professionals of lesser quality are drawn to the field, perhaps after failing in practice or in efforts to obtain employment elsewhere . . . the description of student health as the "backwater of medicine" has become a difficult image to dispel."[29, p. 3304]

However, it was Patrick's observation (and it is the observation of the authors) that by the late 1980s this "backwater image" (which may in the very early years have had validity in some institutions which were unwilling to commit the resources to hire active, bright, and well-trained physicians) is no longer correct and, in fact, has not been true for many years.

On the positive side, Patrick noted many areas of strength in student health services: the quality of physician staffs improving, having to do with an increasing supply of physicians and their willingness to accept salaried positions for flexibility in working hours; the contribution of student health centers to teaching and research in their parent institutions, particularly at the larger schools; the accreditation of student health centers by the two national ambulatory care accreditation agencies; the very strong national network of student health personnel, noting that the American College Health Association, as of May 1988, consisted of nearly 1,000 individual and 650 institutional members; and the strength of the *Journal of American College Health* with peer-reviewed articles. Most importantly, he pointed out the continued opportunity for student health services to alter risk factors for many of the causes of premature morbidity by health education/prevention programs that assist in altering behavorial lifestyles.

Patrick very concisely summarized medical developments of the third quarter of the twentieth century in terms of their impact on college health:[30]

- The growth in the number of college students had not only created the demand for space in higher education, but the need for student services of all types including development of full-service comprehensive student health facilities.
- The development of medical science and, therefore, the solidification of the "medical model" approach to disease within student health centers (similar to other sectors of medical practice) and moving away from an emphasis on health education and prevention.
- ". . . athletic medical services, especially on campuses with substantial intercollegiate athletic programs, experienced a marked drift away from this sphere of influence of mainstream student health concern. The need for a balance between medical care for the athletic student and services for the student athlete, a common desire throughout the entire history of college health and higher education, was overwhelmed by the impact of television and the revenues it produced upon college athletic endeavors. Although certainly not universal, this phenomenon was common enough to further alienate most remaining individuals whose sentiment might have wedded college health, physical education and physical fitness."[30, p. 508]
- The social changes occurring in society related to sexual activity, alcohol and drug use, unplanned pregnancy, and abortion, and the impact of these factors on health and health care needs of college students. Campus administrators who had disavowed the precepts of in loco parentis could not escape the needs of addressing health issues created by these phenomena.[30, p. 508]

Patrick summarized by noting:

It is becoming increasing clear . . . that we cannot afford to have our every medical technologic wish come true . . . most of the benefits of high technology medicine are realized by the very sick and the very old. This is also where most of the resources go . . . a directly related problem is the current crisis in health insurance and access to medical care. College students are among the most poorly insured group in America with from 20-30 % without any medical coverage. The escalating cost of medical care is not making this problem better. This creates an unconscionable circumstance in which many of our nation's youth are effectively denied access to even simple health care. Also, student health services, while not traditionally heavily dependent upon insurance reimbursement for support, may be more so in the future as college administrators attempt to hold the line on cost. Lack of health insurance will then create even more disenfranchisement. [32, p. 508]

This issue is one that still plagues health services in the new century.

THE NINETIES TO THE YEAR TWO THOUSAND

College health finds itself at one of its inimitable crossroads. During the 1990s, with increasing costs of medical care, related in a large way to increasing technology, and with decreasing resources in higher education, health services have been forced to examine ways in which they can become more cost efficient, as well as to assume more responsibility for the uninsured or underinsured student. Simultaneously, health services recognize that health promotion and disease prevention might be the most important thing that we need to do. In that context, we see increasing efforts in health education and health promotion activities among college health services.

Because of the concern about financing, college health services began, in the early 1990s, to be introduced to a new word—"outsourcing." Outsourcing happens when an institution allows a private vendor onto campus to offer a needed service to its students, rather than the university, per se, offering the services. Examples include food service, bookstores, computing services, and, since 1995, health services. With the increasing demand for dollars, college and university administrators have begun a serious effort to make decisions about what was considered "core" to the educational mission and to redirect institutional financial support towards those core functions. In many institutions, the health service has made a successful case for being part of the core function. Other institutions have been less successful, and some student health services are, indeed, outsourced to local health maintenance organizations or other physician groups, and to at least one commercial enterprise endeavor (although this company ceased operation rather abruptly in March 2000 and relinquished the operation of 10 health services to their respective institutions).

At the same time, however, changes in financing of health services were also affected by the medical community at large. In 1994, in response to developments in Washington, when it appeared that the enactment of national health insurance was a distinct possibility, ACHA formed a Health Care Reform Task Force. A Health Care Reform Advisory Kit was developed, with the admonishment that college health professionals had not been well connected to "the decision makers" and that these professionals would have to become proactive to ensure that health interests of college students were considered in any debates about health care reform. An additional task of this health care reform committee was to develop ways to inform the "decision makers" in Washington that "we do what others say the nation's health care system should do."[33, p. 2] College health professionals were encouraged to inform legislators to view the college health model as an example—one that effectively and intricately links primary health care, psychological services, and community health, and one which functions as a managed care capitated plan.

Unfortunately, this effort met with little initial success, since (in the opinion of the authors) it did not seem that the voice of college health was heard. What could have been a major crisis for college health services was averted by the failure during the first Clinton administration of national insurance planning to ever really become effective. Since that time, efforts at national health care reform have been much more piecemeal and have focused most recently on development of health maintenance organizations and managed care models. These developments do not, however, absolve college health services of responsibility and concern for their future.

Beyond 2000

A snapshot of college health at year 2000 reveals a very different student body than was seen even 50 years before.[33, 34]

- Of 14.5 million college students in the country, only 58% are between the ages of 18 and 24; the average age of students in a college university in the United States is 26.
- Minorities comprise 28% of the 14.5 million college students; i.e., 19.9% of all students attending public and private four-year institutions; 25–29% at community colleges. These students are characteristically more likely to be without health care coverage than their white counterparts.
- Fifty-six percent of all college students receive some financial aid; 29.5% come from families that earn less than $30,000; 11% of their parents work at semiskilled or unskilled jobs or are unemployed.
- Forty-five percent of all those between 18 and 24 experience extended periods with no health insurance coverage; estimates are that 25% of all college students are without any health insurance.

William Christmas, considering issues for the future of college health, has made several recommendations and predictions. He noted that "college health centers will need to adopt the managed care model quickly, particularly if they are located near a large medical center."[34] He emphasized the need for college health centers to align themselves with outside providers who offer specialist care beyond that available at the health service. There will need to be significant restructuring of college health centers in order to meet the challenge of competition with other medical communities that see college students as a healthy population who will subsidize the less healthy older population. Christmas also suggested that physician directors will very likely become medical directors and be replaced in their "business" role by medical administrators. Increasing numbers of nurse practitioners and physician assistants will be employed as clinicians in response to the shortage and high cost of primary care physicians.[24, p.245] In addition, there will be colleges and universities, faced with uncertainty of the future of financing of the health care system on a national level, which will continue to be interested in privatizing campus health centers.

Although the American College Health Association continues to grow and remains a strong, viable organization with its national offices and its seven regional affiliates, the increasing demands and extended responsibilities placed on college health services have created the need for "non-official" college health organizations to bring together like institutions to discuss common problems and to develop solutions.

Two examples of such informal organizations are the "Sunbelt Group," which began as a one-day summer meeting in the 1980s but has now evolved into a three-day meeting devoted to discussing common problems among schools in the southeastern United States, and a second group, Student Health Services at Academic Medical Centers (SHSAAMc), which was organized in February 1997 by the editors of this text. While only about 20 institutions were represented by 35 professionals attending the first SHSAAMc meeting, by the third meeting, these numbers had doubled and the programming had progressed from informal discussions about need for such a group to discussions of such importance that they attracted representatives from the Centers for Disease Control and Prevention (e.g., on bloodborne pathogen exposures). Whether these fledgling groups will continue to be independent of ACHA and whether similar "unique need" groups will evolve remains to be seen.

Another development that began in the 1990s reflects not only evolving technology but the response of college health to the utilization of new technological resources. Dr. Jo Sweet at the University of Tennessee–Knoxville established the first electronic listserve for college health professionals. It became, in a very short period of time, and continues to be, a major source of information, discussion, and debate on college health issues throughout the United States and, indeed, the world. This listserv currently has over 1,600 individual members, representing over 400 institutional members.

All the problems notwithstanding, the authors believe strongly that college health services will survive. The very problems which created the need for college health services still exist, perhaps even more so than 140 years ago. Although many college health service personnel might have thought they were invincible, they now realize the need to change how we do business—particularly how we relate to the rest of the higher education community and to the "outside" medical community.

We must have an impact on the social setting in which education occurs. This is related to arresting the risky health behaviors of students by returning to our roots of primary and secondary prevention for the individual student, albeit with a great deal more sophistication than anthropometric measurements. In addition, we must continue the excellent clinical care, which has now become the expected norm for college health services.

We submit that the overall responsibilities of a health service cannot effectively be outsourced and that if we do them well, while continuing our easily accessible, relatively inexpensive, and high-quality care for injuries and illnesses along with strong and effective programs in health promotion, college health services' future is indeed bright. In 1860, good health was considered essential to academic achievement. It still is.

REFERENCES

1. Rogers JF. Student Health Services in Institutions of Higher Education. Washington, DC: US Department of Interior, Office of Education. Bulletin. 1937; No. 7.

2. Minutes of the Rector and Visitors of the University of Virginia, Vol. 1, April 7, 1826, Thomas Jefferson, Rector.

3. Enarson HL. Perspective on College Health in the 80's: A President's View. J Am Coll Health. 1981; 30:11–13.

4. Raycroft JE. History and Development of Student Health Programs in College and Universities. In: Proceedings of the 21st Annual Meeting of the American School Health Association. Ann Arbor; 1940; 37–43.

5. Bruyn HB. Edward Hitchcock, Jr., MD. Student Medicine. 1962; 10(3), 277–285.

6. Bruyn HB. Staff (Hitchcock Museum, Amherst College). Student Medicine. 1962; 10(3), 186–293.

7. Electronic Mail. RG 7.17, Mount Holyoke College Archives and Special Collections. Health Service Records, Annual Reports, Report of the Sanitary Committee. July 1861.

8. Electronic Mail. Gita Nadas, Special Collections, Vassar College Libraries.

9. Hartwell EM. Physical Training in American Colleges and Universities. Bureau of Education. 1886; Washington DC.

10. Canuteson RI. Looking Ahead in College Health. In: Proceedings of the 24th Annual Meeting of the American School Health Association. Minneapolis; 1946; 7–8.

11. Mylan GL. Report of the Committee on the Status of Hygiene in American Colleges and Universities. American Physical Education Review. 1916; 15, 446–452.

12. Boynton RE. Historical Development of College Health Services. Student Medicine. 1962; 10(3), 294–305.

13. Christmas WA, Dorman, JM. The Storey of College Health Hygiene: Thomas A. Storey, MD, and the Promotion of Hygiene. J Am Coll Health. 1996; 45:27–34.

14. Storey TA. A Summary of the Work of the United States Interdepartmental Social Hygiene Board. 1919-1920. Social Hygiene. 1921; 7:59–76.

15. Storey TA. The Status of Hygiene Programs in Institutions of Higher Education in the United States: A Report of the President's Committee of Fifty on College Hygiene. Stanford University Press; 1927.

16. Proceedings of the First National Conference on College Hygiene, National Tuberculosis Association. New York; 1931.

17. Health in Colleges: Proceedings of the Second National Conference on College Hygiene, National Tuberculosis Association. New York; 1937.

18. A Health Program for Colleges: Report of the Third National Conference on Health in Colleges, National Tuberculosis Association. New York; 1948.

19. Moore NS, Summerskill, J. Health Services in American Colleges and Universities, Cornell University, Ithaca, New York; 1954.

20. Team Work in Meeting the Health Needs of College Students: Report of the Fourth National Conference on Health in Colleges, National Tuberculosis Association. New York; 1954.

21. Ginsburg EL. The College and Student Health, National Tuberculosis Society. New York; 1955.

22. Barbato L. Some Flashbacks to the Early Years of ACHA. J Am Coll Health. 1995;43:283-284.

23. Cooper DL. Personal Recollections of College Health and the ACHA. J Am Coll Health. 1995;43:285–286.

24. Guidelines for a College Health Program, The American College Health Association. Baltimore; 1999.

25. Farnsworth DL, Prout C, Munter PK. Health in Colleges and Universities. N Engl J Med. 1962;267(25):1290–1295.

26. Farnsworth DL, Editor. College Health Administration. New York; Appleton–Century-Crofts; 1964.

27. Christmas WA. The Evolution of Medical Service for Students at Colleges and Universities in the United States. J Am Coll Health. 1995; 43:241–246.

28. Dalrymple W, Purcell EF. Campus Health Programs. New York; Joseph Macy Foundation; 1976.

29. Turner HS. The Challenge to Change. J Am Coll Health. 1981;30:7-9.

30. Keeling, RP. College Health Regards to HIV: Hard Lessons and a Rich Heritage. J Am Coll Health. 1995;43 (May):272.

31. Patrick K. Student Health: Medical Care Within Institutions of Higher Education. J Am Med Assoc. 1988;26(22):3301-3305.

32. Patrick K. The History and Current Status of College Health: Principles and Practices of Student Health. Volume 3, 1992; Oakland, CA; Third Party Publishing Company; 501-514.

33. Health Care Reform and College Health: A Call to Action, American College Health Association. 1994.

34. Christmas WA. The Evolution of Medical Services for Students at Colleges and Universities in the United States. J Am Coll Health. 1995;43 (May):241–246.

CHAPTER 2

COLLEGE HEALTH AT THE NATIONAL LEVEL

The American College Health Association
Doyle Randol, MS, Col. USA (Ret.), Sarah Feiss, BA,
and Sharon Fisher, MA

The Journal of American College Health
Richard P. Keeling, MD

The American College Health Foundation
Marthea Blewitt

THE AMERICAN COLLEGE HEALTH ASSOCIATION

The American College Health Association (ACHA), founded in 1920, is dedicated to serving the health needs of students at colleges and universities. It is the principal leadership organization for the field of college health and provides services, communications, and advocacy that help its members to advance the health of their campus communities.

Today, ACHA's membership has grown from the original 20 institutions of higher education to more than 900. These member institutions represent the diversity of the higher education community: two-and four-year, public and private, large and small. ACHA also serves more than 2,000 individual college health care professionals: administrators, support staff, physicians, nurses, nurse directors, health educators, mental health providers, and pharmacists, as well as students dedicated to health promotion on their campuses. To better address individual needs, the membership is divided into regional affiliates and discipline-specific sections.

Although the issues in college health and the structure of the association have changed dramatically in the last 80 years, ACHA's purpose has always remained the same—to advance the health of students and to serve as the principal advocate for college health.

Establishing an Association

By 1920, some 60 years after the first college health program was established, college health programs had developed on numerous campuses throughout the country but were without a national professional association to provide leadership and direction. Their medical directors, including physicians and nurses at some smaller institutions, often attended the annual meetings of other associations (notably the National Collegiate Athletic Association), but met among themselves at these meetings to discuss issues relevant to college health. Eventually, interest developed in forming a national organization to focus specifically on issues related to college health programs, such as environmental health, health education, medical exams, and mental health.

At an organizational meeting held in 1920, an agreement was reached to form an association dedicated to the field of college health—the American Student Health Association (ASHA). The newly elected president, Dr. John Sundwall, and other officers were charged with drafting bylaws.[1]

The first ASHA Annual Meeting took place in Chicago on December 31, 1920. The meeting was held in conjunction with other associations' meetings to allow members to attend sessions coordinated by these other organizations. Representatives from 53 institutions in attendance signed and adopted the first ASHA constitution and bylaws.[1] Topics addressed at this first meeting included interaction with other departments on campus, the need for a permanent records system, mental hygiene, and sanitation in living quarters. The pattern of meeting during the time of other associations' meetings was to continue for the next several years, with a single day allotted for ASHA concerns.

Until the sixth annual meeting, members of the executive committee had been the only individuals involved in managing the affairs of the association. That year (1926), the executive committee recommended a change in the bylaws to establish five other committees to assist with ASHA's activities.[1] Also in the same year, the Ohio Section of ASHA was formed, joined by the New England Section in 1927; these became the first regional sections (now called affiliates).[2]

1930s & 1940s: An Independent Annual Meeting and a New Name

One of the main goals of the association during the 1930s was to further develop the regional sections. Thus 15 geographic sections were established throughout the United States, each intended to include relatively equal numbers of colleges and universities. A portion of each ASHA member's dues ($2.50) was given to the section to which the member belonged for programming within that region.[2]

The First National Conference on College Hygiene, held in 1931 (see Chapter 1), served as an impetus for the growth of ASHA. The conference report provided the first written guidelines and minimum requirements for a college health program.[1] Shortly thereafter, a council of the association was created to act for ASHA between annual meetings. It was composed of all past presidents, the officers, and six members-at-large. The executive committee included the officers and two other members elected by the council. At the 15th Annual Meeting in 1935, the journal *Lancet*, a monthly medical journal, became the official news organ of ASHA. The arrangement stipulated that the journal *Lancet* would publish the business proceedings from the annual meeting and in each issue would publish one scientific paper which had been presented at the annual meeting.[1]

The format of the ASHA annual meetings began to change during the late 1930s and the early 1940s. In 1937, the decision was made to no longer schedule ASHA meetings in conjunction with other associations; the first independent annual meeting took place in 1938. Additionally, beginning the same year, the scientific sessions were no longer entirely presentations of papers. Instead, one half of the sessions were designated as paper presentations and the other half as roundtable discussions, in an effort to involve as many members as possible in the meeting activities.

The Second World War had a significant effect on ASHA and health centers on college campuses. Only one annual meeting was held between 1941 and 1945. Health centers on campus lost many health professionals to the military services. At the same time, the military requested many college health care facilities to provide medical care for military personnel in training on campus. After the war, health services had to deal, as indeed did all of society, with a large influx of returning veterans, and their facilities had to be made accessible to disabled veterans.

For ASHA, the years after the war were a period of transition. In 1948, the name of the association was changed to the American College Health Association (ACHA) to avoid confusion with the American School Health Association (ASHA), which had just changed its named from the Association of School Physicians. The office of president-elect was established, and it was at this time that the annual meeting changed its meeting time from December to May.[1]

1950s: A Journal Is Begun and a National Office Is Organized

The *Journal of American College Health* began its life in October 1952 as a modest, semi-annual publication called *Student Medicine,* the creation of Dr. Norman Moore, with Dr. Ralph Alexander, who headed the Department of Clinical and Preventive Medicine at Cornell University, as its editor. In late 1962 the American College Health Association, upon transfer of the copyrights from Cornell University, assumed responsibility for managing and publishing the journal.

The 1950s were years of remarkable expansion and change in higher education: the G.I. Bill brought thousands of new students to campus; the democratization of colleges accelerated (providing access to higher education for more women, students of color, and students from a wider spectrum of socioeconomic status); and the Cold War's stimulus to engineering, aeronautics, and space exploration, coupled with general optimism about the possibilities of science and technology, led to extraordinary increases in federal funding and public support. The same trends that contributed to the growth of college health as a field stimulated interest in research about college students and gave

ACHA a stronger foundation. Accordingly, ACHA changed the name of *Student Medicine* to the *Journal of the American College Health Association* (JACHA) and increased its publication frequency to quarterly.

The early 1950s were also a time when the need for a national office became evident. All board members had full-time positions at their respective institutions and were unable to devote sufficient time to the advancement of the association. Further, the need to increase services, research, publications, and other activities was clear. ACHA began to garner funds for this purpose. In 1957, Dr. Carl R. Wise, the incumbent president of ACHA, received an anonymous gift of $5,000 that was intended to be used to establish a national office. The secretary-treasurer was John Summerskill, PhD, of Cornell University. Cornell donated office space in its health center for the ACHA national office, and the gift that Dr. Wise had received was used to purchase office supplies and hire a part-time secretary.

ACHA, working with several other associations to plan and fund the event, sponsored the Fourth National Conference on Health in Colleges in 1954. The relationship of different disciplines within and outside college health was discussed, as was student health insurance. The results of a national survey on current practices in college health (the Moore-Summerskill Report) were presented at this meeting and proved extremely valuable to the field.[2] (See Chapter 1.)

In 1957, eight sections representing different disciplines in college health were created within the association. Many of these sections, which varied from the Section on Administration to the Section on Tuberculosis Control, still exist. It was also agreed that a new section could be formed whenever interest was expressed by at least 15 members of ACHA who were not already members of another section. At the same time, membership was expanded to include individual members and associates or junior colleges. Dues for institutional membership were based on the number of students enrolled at the institution and ranged from $20 to $50 per year. Annual meeting registration was set at $3 but was assessed only to individuals who did not pay dues or did not represent a member institution.[1]

1960s: Structure and Finances Are Determined

Throughout the 1950s it had become increasingly apparent to many members and officers that there was a need to evaluate health centers for accreditation or certification. In 1961 President S. I. Fuenning charged a committee with developing standards for a college health program. After being reviewed and edited by the council, the final version of *Recommended Standards and Practices for a College Health Program* was approved. During this time, liaisons with other national organizations such as the American Personnel and Guidance Association and the American Medical Association were established.[1]

Also in 1961, the 100th anniversary of Dr. Edward Hitchcock's appointment at Amherst College was commemorated by creating the Hitchcock Award to honor an individual who had made an outstanding contribution to the field of college health. The executive committee selected Dr. Harold S. Diehl to be the first recipient of this award.[1]

Another significant change for ACHA occurred in 1961 when the national office moved to the University of Miami (Florida). The university donated office space, furniture, and supplies. Dr. Ruth Boynton, who had been elected secretary-treasurer and had moved to Miami after retiring from the University of Minnesota, became the first person working only (part-time) for the association. In 1962, the first formal budget for ACHA was drafted. Dues for institutional members were increased in 1963 and ranged from $15 for junior colleges to $75 for institutions with an enrollment of over 5,000. The association included 397 institutional members and 800 individual members.[1]

The theme of the 41st annual meeting, "Ethical and Professional Relationships," was important, as ACHA had now come to be recognized as *the* national organization devoted entirely to the advancement of college health. Other organizations sought assistance from ACHA as the association began to earn recognition for its work in programs such as athletic medicine and health promotion.

Two years later, in 1965, the goal of hiring a full-time executive director was realized. ACHA had accumulated a cash balance that permitted the appointment of Dr. Benjamin R. Reiter as the first executive director. Other achievements reported at the annual meeting that year included an increase in membership, the establishment of a program for accrediting college health services, and the creation of a fellowship category in ACHA membership. Dr. Reiter died shortly after his appointment, and interim arrangements were made until the next annual meeting, when Lee Stauffer, MPH, was chosen as his replacement.[1]

The United States Public Health Service awarded ACHA a grant to examine the smoking patterns of college students during the 1966–67 school year. With the $49,000 from this project, the association was able to hire a full-time project coordinator and secretary as well as increase office space.[1] Dr. Ruth Boynton announced her retirement from the position of secretary-treasurer in 1965. In her honor, the Ruth E. Boynton Award was created in 1968 to recognize her distinguished service to the association.

A year after assuming the position of executive secretary, Mr. Stauffer submitted his resignation and Mr. James Dilley, who had been the project coordinator of the smoking survey, was appointed the new executive secretary in 1968. The national office moved to Evanston, Illinois, where for the first time it existed independent of a member institution.[2]

1970s: A Complete Reorganization

In 1969, with Dr. Lewis Barbato as chair, the Long-Range Planning Committee created a plan to completely reorganize the association in order to meet the upcoming challenges of the 1970s, and in 1970 a new constitution and bylaws were adopted. The Council of Delegates was to be composed of the officers (the president, president-elect, six vice-presidents, and the treasurer), delegates from the member institutions, delegates from the affiliates, delegates from the sections, past-presidents of the association, and the executive director. The six vice-presidents would chair various commissions addressing issues within the association. For the first time in the history of ACHA, all three major constituencies of the association—member institutions, sections, and affiliates—were represented in the governing body.[2]

At the 1971 annual meeting, the business meeting of the institutional representatives was renamed the Representative Assembly. This group retained the authority to amend the constitution and bylaws and to elect officers and delegates. The ACHA Executive Board was also established at this time, and included the president, president-elect, vice-presidents, immediate past-president, treasurer, two members of the Council of Delegates appointed by the president, and the executive director (voice but without vote).[2]

Organizational changes continued to accommodate the changing needs of the membership. The Section on Students and the Section on Junior/Community Colleges were established in 1974. In 1975, the Executive Committee, which consisted of the presidential officers, the treasurer, and the executive director, was established under the authority of the Executive Board. At the same time, the Program Planning Group was formed to coordinate the annual meeting.[2] In 1976, the Representative Assembly transferred the responsibility of electing officers and making changes to the constitution and bylaws from itself to the Council of Delegates.

In 1977, membership was expanded to include health care organizations that contracted with colleges to provide health care to the campus community. At the annual meeting that year, the number of vice-presidents was reduced to three. One year later, the ability to change the constitution or bylaws was divided between the Council of Delegates and the Representative Assembly, so that both bodies would have to concur before changes were made to either document.[2]

From 1976 to 1980, the executive board reviewed the committee structure annually, and by the end of the decade there were 12 committees. In 1979, since many members felt that there would be a growing relationship between ACHA and the federal government, the national office moved its headquarters from Evanston, Illinois, to Rockville, Maryland, near Washington, D.C.[2]

During these years of change and growth in the association, the *Journal* had continued to grow and improve as well. Dr. Ralph Alexander, who had been editor since the first issue in 1952, served in that position until 1973, when Willard Dalrymple, MD, director of the health service at Princeton University, succeeded him. Dalrymple's inauguration as editor—at the end of another decade of growth and confidence in higher education—was marked by a further increase in the *Journal*'s frequency, to bimonthly. In 1977, Robert Gage, MD, of the University of Massachusetts, Amherst, replaced Dalrymple as editor. During Dr. Gage's three-year tenure, *JACHA* formalized and made regular two previously occasional types of articles, "Clinical and Program Notes" and "Viewpoints." Dr. Gage also first encouraged letters to the editor. The development of routine Clinical and Program Notes reflected the *Journal*'s need to continue to serve practitioners—in a broadening variety of disciplines—with practical, applied knowledge, while publishing, as major articles, research studies that increasingly focused on health behavior and its determinants. Clinical and Program Notes also provided a more realistic publishing opportunity for busy clinicians and health educators, who usually did not have the necessary resources and requisite institutional support to conduct the kind of rigorous research that would survive critical editorial review. By the late 1970s , the *Journal* had developed the forms and structures for almost all its current major categories of articles.

1980s: Increased Visibility and a Growing Membership

The year 1982 was an especially critical one financially for ACHA. The move to Rockville had proved to be costly, and the association's financial resources had gradually eroded. Consideration was given to the dissolution of ACHA, but at the annual meeting in Seattle, Washington, the board voted not to disband. ACHA managed to survive a $100,000 deficit through the efforts of a core group of committed members and colleges.[3] In the same year, in part because of the financial situation but also coupled with the recognition of the need for experienced, professional management, the Helen Dwight Reed Educational Foundation, through its educational publishing division, Heldref Publications, acquired the *Journal of the American College Health Association* from ACHA and changed its name to the *Journal of American College Health (JACH)*. This last change of name reflected not only the transfer of the publication's ownership but also the broadening and diversification of its audience. By the early 1980s, most of the major articles were being submitted by researchers and scholars in academic departments, rather than by practitioners in health centers—the clinical, counseling, and prevention professionals whose continued participation was the goal of the Clinical and Program Notes.

Meanwhile, in addition to the changes in the *Journal,* the association was experiencing a resurgence in other ways, under the direction of a new executive director, Stephen Blom. In 1983, the first Prematriculation Immunization Requirement (PIR) was adopted. Five years later, the association would become a partner with the new National Coalition on Adult Immunization. In 1984, the Mental Health Section established the Dorosin Memorial Lecture fund in honor of Dr. David Dorosin, a Stanford University psychiatrist.

The AIDS Task Force was also established in 1984. Dr. Richard Keeling, whose work in AIDS-related issues was earning national recognition, chaired the task force. Two years later, ACHA received its first HIV-related Centers for Disease Control (CDC) cooperative agreement.

At the 1987 annual meeting in Chicago, ACHA's new governance and structure model was approved and implemented. The new model created a streamlined structure by placing day-to-day operational authority with the board of directors. Also, six regional representatives elected by the affiliate ACHA organizations were added to the board to more efficiently bring issues from the affiliates to the national level for discussion and action.

Also that year, two other important changes occurred. The Section on Junior/Community Colleges became the Nurse-Directed Health Services Section, and the Pharmacy Section was formed to improve programming efforts for college health pharmacists. By the end of 1987, ACHA had total revenue in excess of $300,000 and had reestablished itself as an organization "in the black."[4] And, by 1988, the association had nearly 1,000 institutional members and 650 individual members.[5]

In 1988, the board of directors of the ACHA voted to establish a foundation to serve as the development branch of the association. This new organization, which would be separate from the association, was named the Foundation for Health in Higher Education (FHHE).[3] A group of ACHA leaders, including the executive director met in September 1989 to discuss plans for the foundation. Subsequently, ACHA loaned FHHE funds to help launch fundraising operations.

During the fall of 1989, the national office moved to a bigger office space in Rockville, Maryland, to accommodate the growing number of ACHA employees. In October of that same year, Miguel Garcia-Tunon, coordinator of the ACHA/CDC-HIV Seroprevalence Project, died after a year-long battle with AIDS. An annual award was established in his honor.[6]

THE COMING OF AGE OF THE *JOURNAL OF AMERICAN COLLEGE HEALTH*

With the move of the *Journal* to the publishing firm Heldref, a managing editor was installed. Mary Anna Bloch held the position from 1982 to 1988; subsequently, Martha H. Wedeman was appointed and has managed the *Journal* through periods of significant change, growth, and redirection. ACHA retained some influence on *JACH* after its acquisition by Heldref through a formally appointed *JACH* Affairs Committee, chaired by one of the senior editors, which relates to the association's board of directors through a designated liaison. The board of directors advises and consents to the nomination of senior editors and, through its JACH Affairs committee, interacts with the *Journal*, its editors, and Heldref in matters of policy. Neither ACHA's board of directors nor the Committee have, or have sought, any influence on, or control over, editorial matters.

After Dr. Gage's tenure as editor from 1977 to 1980, there was only one more single editor, James B. McClanahan, MD, of Stanford University (who served from 1980 to 1983), until Dr. Richard Keeling's appointment in 1997. Dr. McClanahan had not one successor but three: the position of editor was temporarily discontinued in 1983 in favor of a group of three executive editors. This important change was primarily in response to the increasingly multidisciplinary nature of college health scholarship and practice. During the 1970s, "college health" came to encompass not just clinical medicine, but also mental health, health education (more recently called health promotion), and administration. Having three executive editors recognized the differing epistemologies and languages of these disciplines and divided the editorial workload—an increasingly important issue for an all-volunteer editorial staff, each member of which also had full-time responsibilities in college health—as the quantity (and, eventually, the quality) of manuscripts submitted to *JACH* improved.

Clifford B. Reifler, MD, MPH, director of the University Health Service at the University of Rochester and a longtime advocate, supporter, reviewer, and associate editor for the *Journal*, became "first among equals," representing the *Journal's* interests and coordinating the work of the other executive editors (initially, Jane Zapka, MEd, from the University of Massachusetts, Amherst, and John Dorman, MD, from Stanford University). Each of the three executive editors presided over manuscripts and articles in an appropriate area of research and practice, matching their experience and training: Initially, Reifler covered mental health and administration, Dorman was responsible for clinical medicine, and Zapka was senior reviewer for health education.

Over the years, Beverlie Conant Sloane, PhD, of Dartmouth University, replaced Zapka (1985), Paula L. Swinford, MS, of the University of Southern California, replaced Conant Sloane (1989), and Richard P. Keeling, MD (then of the University of Virginia), succeeded Dorman (1992). In 1992, a fourth executive editor, for nursing, was appointed;

Mary-Kate Heffern, MSN, RN-C, of Princeton University, was the first nurse to serve in that role, and Jean Garling, EdD, RN-CS, ANC, of the University of Rochester, succeeded her (with the revised title of associate editor) in 1998. Among the most essential, enduring, and consistent of the *Journal*'s senior editors was Allan J. Schwartz, PhD, who began reviewing quantitative methods and statistical analyses in submissions long before he was officially named statistical editor in 1989. Dr. Schwartz, who started his work with the *Journal* in the early 1980s as a colleague of Dr. Reifler's at Rochester, set high standards that materially improved the scientific value of major articles.

In 1997, after the death of Dr. Reifler (who, as the capstone to a distinguished career with *JACH,* had served 14 years as an executive editor), the *Journal* once again modified its editorial structure, returning to a single-editor model; the executive editors became associate editors, each with responsibility, as before, for a major content area. This new strategy supported the *Journal*'s intention to improve the overall quality of articles published and to bring greater consistency to its editorial processes, standards of review, and voice. By retaining the discipline-specific associate editors, it could do so without sacrificing the value of an interdisciplinary perspective. Dr. Keeling, by then director of University Health Services at the University of Wisconsin-Madison, began his first four-year term as editor that year. Paula Swinford continued as associate editor for health promotion until 1998, when Joanne B. Auth, MHEd, CHES, assumed that role in 1999. After the 1997 restructuring of the editorial team, there was no specific associate editor for mental health until 2000, when Eric L. Heiligenstein, MD, of the University of Wisconsin-Madison was appointed; similarly, there was no associate editor for clinical medicine until the same year, when H. Spencer Turner, MD, Director of the University Health Service at the University of Kentucky in Lexington, assumed those responsibilities. By mid-2000, the *Journal* once again had a full complement of senior editors. In addition, 18 consulting editors and at least as many ad hoc reviewers shared responsibility for reading and evaluating the manuscripts submitted to the *Journal.*

By the late 1990s, *JACH,* having without question become recognized and accepted as a significant peer-reviewed journal, was routinely receiving important submissions from distinguished researchers who could easily have published their work in other, more mainstream journals. The *Journal* published the results of the National College Health Risk Behavior Survey (NCHRBS) of the Centers for Disease Control and Prevention (CDC) in 1997. From 1997 through 2000, it brought to print eight excellent reports on drinking, drug use, and smoking on campus from the Harvard School of Public Health. Authoritative studies of suicide, nutrition, tobacco abuse, sexual behavior, and occupational health and safety (especially, protection against bloodborne pathogens) in higher education now regularly appear in its pages. It has now become common for *JACH* articles to be the subject of press releases, media interviews, and public debate as an important voice for health issues in higher education. A detailed description of the philosophy and layout of *JACH* is presented in Appendix 2.

1990s: The Foundation Grows

Subsequent to its establishment by the ACHA Board of Directors in 1988, the first official meeting of the Foundation for Health in Higher Education (FHHE) board was held in May of 1991. Original members of the FHHE Board of Directors were: C. Barbara Driscoll, RN-C, ANP; Richard P. Keeling, MD; W. David Burns; John Longest, MD; William Christmas, MD; Charles Hartman, EdD, ACHA executive director; and Catherine Tassan (1992). At that time, FHHE began soliciting and accepting donations from members, affiliates, and others for specific projects and for establishment of the Miguel Garcia-Tunon Fund.

In 1993, following the implementation of ACHA's Resource Development Plan, the foundation began focusing more intensely on seeking funding from both individuals and organizations. In order to provide new direction and focus for the foundation, the FHHE board voted to change the organization's name to the American College Health Foundation (ACHF), and shortly thereafter Marthea Blewitt was hired to support both ACHA resource development and ACHF activities. The ACHF board began regular meetings during the ACHA annual meetings and, when possible, in January of each year at the national office of ACHA. The newly named organization and its board of directors faced the challenge of redefining and renewing the mission and intent of ACHF and spent considerable effort educating both ACHA members and its leaders about the purpose and the goals of the foundation.

Since its inception, the goal of the foundation had been to focus on obtaining funding for specific projects to benefit ACHA and the field of college health. In an effort to further clarify this intent to potential donors, in June 1999, the ACHF board revised the foundation's mission statement. The revised statement reads: "The mission of the American College Health Foundation is to provide long-term financial support for the American College Health Association by building endowments through charitable gifts and contributions."

To accomplish this mission, members of the ACHF board identify and contact individuals and organizations interested in supporting the foundation and invite them to become contributors. In the early days of the foundation, all cash contributions were commingled in an account with ACHA funds. In July 1998, all ACHF funds were transferred to a separate account, facilitating foundation record-keeping while assuring donors that ACHF funds would be used only for the purpose specified by the donor or, if unrestricted, by action of the ACHF board. In January 1999, ACHF funds were transferred to an account with an investment firm, and the ACHF board established an investment policy, specifying the types of funds in which to invest, and specified clear guidelines for the disbursement of foundation funds. If requested by the ACHA board, funds to support specified purposes or programs may be transferred to ACHA with the approval by a majority of the ACHF board. The maximum amount available for annual disbursement is 5 percent of the portfolio's average market value over the past three years, ensuring that spending amounts will not interfere with the stability or growth of the fund.

Within the investment portfolio, ACHF has established six separate named funds, providing various giving opportunities for donors while helping to meet the needs of the association. The funds provide various giving options while funding important areas of college health. The funds are:

- Foundation Endowment Fund—This is an unrestricted fund supporting specific needs of the association and the field of college health.
- Health Promotion in Higher Education Fund—This restricted fund, established in 2001, supports and enhances health promotion and prevention services in higher education.
- Josh Kaplan Fund for Clinical Medicine—This restricted fund, established in 2001, supports presentations and professional development activities focusing on the practice of clinical medicine.
- Student Resources Fund—This fund was established through a major corporate gift given by Student Resources and supports ACHA annual meeting programming and professional decelopment activities benefiting ACHA members.
- Clifford B. Reifler Fund—This fund was established from a bequest made by the late Dr. Reifler. Earnings from this fund are used to enhance the *Journal of American College Health.*
- Murray DeArmond Student Activity Fund—This fund was established through a gift from Joyce B. Meder, RNP, MPA. Earnings from this fund are used specifically for student activities at ACHA annual meetings.

Named funds can be established by individuals or organizations with a minimum investment. All new donor-restricted funds must first be approved by the ACHF board to ensure their purpose agrees with the mission of the foundation.

With various giving opportunities in place for prospective donors, ACHF leadership is now faced with the challenge of convincing ACHA members to consider making voluntary contributions in addition to paying membership dues. From the time the foundation was renamed, the ACHF board focused on the goal of educating members of ACHA regarding the value of making gifts to the foundation, to ensure that the mission of ACHA continues, and began a concentrated effort to make members aware of the foundation's goals and activities. Through articles in various ACHA publications, mailings, and by exhibiting a more visible presence at the ACHA annual meetings, those in the college health field have now become more aware of the purpose and goals of the foundation. As a result, by June 2000, total foundation cash assets totaled $67,865, with an additional $5,500 in cash pledges and another $65,000 in pledged bequests. The foundation board set a goal to surpass $100,000 in cash assets by the end of the year 2001. (All royalties from this textbook are donated to ACHF.)

The 1990s Continued: Setting New Standards

Perhaps the vision of those beginning ACHF influenced the selection of ACHA's 1990–91 theme: "Vision 2000: Setting New Standards." To guide the association through the changes sure to come in the next decade, two important documents which had been prepared by ACHA committees were made available at the 1991 annual meeting in Boston: *College Health 2000: A Perspective Statement in Higher Education* and *Recommended Standards for a College Health Program* (a revised version). Also during 1991, Charles Hartman assumed the position of executive director.[7]

A year later, at the 1992 annual meeting in San Francisco, several important changes in the bylaws were made in direct response to member comments. Voting delegates agreed to open up the process of election of officers to all regular and student members and, for the first time in ACHA's history, to hold the election by mail. Three new task forces were established, and board members were no longer permitted to hold task force or committee chair positions. The year 1992 also marked another move for the national office, to its present-day (2001) location in Linthicum, Maryland.[8]

ACHA has always recognized the need to improve its communication with members by making full use of changing technology. In the fall of 1993, the association began communicating on-line via the Student Health Services listserv, an e-mail discussion group launched by Dr. Jo Sweet at the University of Tennessee-Knoxville. And in March of the same year, Fax on Demand, a way for members to quickly receive requested information 24 hours a day, was begun.

The ACHA staff and board spent a significant portion of 1993–94 responding to the developments occurring nationally related to health care reform. The Health Care Reform Advisory Council was appointed, workshops were held, and at the 1994 annual meeting the board reallocated budget monies to focus on health care reform initiatives. In 1994, the Vaccine-Preventable Diseases Task Force paved the way for institutional members to receive discounts on the hepatitis B vaccine in a new Vaccine Discount Program. Additionally, the year 1994–95 marked the initial adoption and use of ACHA's Strategic Plan, which looked toward new revenue streams as more traditional income sources were gradually decreasing. ACHA celebrated its 75th anniversary in 1995 with the annual meeting theme, "Celebrate College Health: Past, Present, and Future." During the mid-1990s the association began to develop more diverse programming and formed subcommittees to focus on ethnic minority and gay, lesbian, bisexual, and transgender issues.

During this time not only were efforts directed toward internal reorganization, but ACHA increased its collaboration with other national associations, becoming a member of the Council for the Advancement of Standards in Higher Education as well as the newly formed National Benchmarking Council for Higher Education and solidifying its liaisons with the National Association of Student Personnel Administrators (NASPA), the BACCHUS/GAMMA Peer Education Network, the Joint Commission on Accreditation of Healthcare Organizations (JCAHO), and the Accreditation Association for Ambulatory Health Care (AAAHC).

In 1996, in order to keep pace with the costs of doing business, ACHA increased its institutional dues, the first full-scale increase in more than 10 years.[9] Much of the early part of 1997 was focused on the Health Insurance Portability and Accountability Act (HIPAA) of 1996. Because of the participation of college health professionals and students, the Student Health Insurance Portability and Protection Act (SHIPPA) was introduced in the House of Representatives in 1997 to ensure that college-sponsored insurance plans would be covered under the HIPAA law.[10] Also beginning in 1997, ACHA launched a major student awareness campaign on meningococcal disease, with support from an unrestricted educational grant. Since the association intended to cultivate more corporate and government support in the coming years, guidelines for corporate and federal relationships were devised and later adopted in 1999.

As part of its goal to promote research, ACHA conducted surveys to collect data regarding activities of college health centers and student health. The Benchmarking Data Share Survey, the annual Pap Smear and STD Survey, and the National College Health Assessment (NCHA) were all instituted during the 1990s to advance college health and help campus communities.

Doyle Randol, MS, Col. USA (Ret.), was appointed the new executive director in May 1998, following Charles Hartman's resignation. A new, more forward-looking Strategic Plan was adopted in 1999, with a revised set of goals.[11]

As the 1990s drew to a close, the Fax on Demand system was phased out as the Internet's use exploded. The ACHA Internet home page debuted at the 1996 annual meeting in Orlando, and the web site has continued to expand and be improved upon as a communications tool for the membership.

Year 2000: A Current Snapshot

Today, ACHA's Board of Directors is comprised of the executive committee (president, president-elect, vice-president, treasurer, pastpresident, and executive director), four members-at-large, six regional representatives, and two student representatives. Section officers represent the individual members participating in one of the nine ACHA professional interest sections: administration, athletic medicine, clinical medicine, health education, mental health, nursing, nurse-directed, pharmacy, and students/consumers. The association has nine standing committees and 22 ad hoc committees, covering issues such as alcohol, drugs, tobacco, campus violence, ethics, HIV/STDs, and immunization.

ACHA recognizes six regions comprised of a total of 11 affiliate organizations, which are governed by their own elected officers. These affiliates play an important role in helping college health care providers forge strong links with colleagues in their state or region. The affiliates are Central, Mid-America, Mid-Atlantic, New England, New York, North Central, Ohio, Southern, Southwest, Pacific Coast, and Rocky Mountain.

While the association is still chartered in the state of Illinois, the ACHA national office is located, as previously noted, in Linthicum, Maryland. The headquarters has a modest staff of 21 employees, led by Executive Director Doyle Randol, who reports to the board. The executive director is supported by an executive assistant/board liaison. The national office has four departments: Member Programs and Services, Finance and Business Operations, Research, and Federal Cooperative Agreements. Member Programs and Services includes a director, a program development coordinator, a web/production manager, a communications coordinator, a membership coordinator, a continuing education coordinator, and a production coordinator. The Finance and Business Operations Department includes a director, an administrative services coordinator, an administrative services assistant, a staff accountant, and a network systems administrator. Under Research, there is a director and a health education research coordinator. Additionally, a development coordinator is employed to assist with fundraising management for the American College Health Foundation.

ACHA is currently involved in two cooperative agreements with the Centers for Disease Control and Prevention (CDC) that address HIV and AIDS education and prevention on the college campus. The first agreement is a five-year HIV Prevention Project in collaboration with the National Association of Student Personnel Administrators. The goal of the project is to institutionalize integrated HIV prevention education efforts. ACHA's second CDC cooperative agreement, "College Students in High-Risk Situations," is another five-year project, which primarily targets men who have sex with men. This project disseminates information in a train-the-trainer format to five innovative campuses that serve as "models" to other local schools over the project period. Each cooperative agreement has a project director and an assistant project director.

Membership in ACHA, based on the calendar year, includes three categories:

- Individual, for college health care providers and students
- Institutional, for any institution of higher education
- Sustaining, for other health and business organizations who wish to support college health and cooperate with ACHA

For the 1999–2000 year, individual membership dues at a member institution are $125; at a non-member institution, $155. Student membership is $35. Institutional membership dues begin with a base fee of $260. Beyond this base, each institution pays an additional amount equal to .058 percent of its total health service budget. Sustaining membership dues are $250 for non-profit organizations and $1,500 for for-profit organizations. Total revenues and expenses for the 1999 fiscal year (January 1–December 31, 1999) were over $2.3 million, with gross revenues from both membership dues and the 1999 annual meeting each totaling over $595,000.[12]

During the 2000 membership year, ACHA had over 2,200 individual members, approximately 900 institutional members, and 16 sustaining members. Seventeen new institutions, 225 new individuals, and six new sustaining members joined in the 2000 membership year. Members who have earned Fellowship in the association now total 141.

Education and training is an important component of the association's services. ACHA-sponsored events provide continuing education (CE) credits and contact hours for physicians, physician assistants, nurses, certified health education specialists, pharmacists, and psychologists. This professional development ensures that health centers maintain the highest standard of quality for their staff and services. ACHA helps its institutional members provide continuing education credits and contact hours to health services staff at no cost. Continuing education details are found in ACHA's *Approver Handbook for Affiliate, Regional, and Institutional Program Planners* and in the *Provider Handbook*.

The national annual meeting continues to take place after Memorial Day. The meeting is the primary source of continuing education credits, professional development, peer-recognition activities, and networking opportunities for most ACHA members. The educational programming is coordinated by the Program Planning Committee, which is chaired by the president-elect and made up of the section chairs, advisors on research, diversity, and student issues, CE reviewers, the vice-president, and two representatives of the national office. The several continuing education reviewers on the committee review the program submissions for their disciplines and assign appropriate credit. At the meeting, task forces, sections, and affiliates hold their business meetings and discuss their agendas for the upcoming year. At the Open Forum, members have a chance to make presentations and voice their opinions to the board of directors.

ACHA's web site has become a primary means of communication with its members. The site provides information about membership, networking opportunities, the annual meeting and affiliate meetings, research projects, continuing education, publications and guidelines, professional and volunteer opportunities, and a variety of programs and services for today's college health professional. Web-design services are offered to affiliates, and the association hosts three affiliate sites (New England, Southern, and Mid-America). It also provides links to the Mid-Atlantic, Southwest, Pacific Coast, and New York web sites. In 2001, ACHA will have a redesigned site with "members-only" features, so members have special online access to resources, products, and services, as well as increased networking opportunities.

In 2000 the annual meeting was for the first time held outside of the United States, in Toronto, Ontario, Canada. This successful meeting drew over 1,700 attendees and featured over 130 programs. The Program Planning Committee was praised for the variety of programs, which included a "Social Justice and Health" track, "Hot Topic" sessions targeted to specific disciplines, and an increased number of marketing and technology-focused programs. The five-day meeting had many opportunities for networking and meeting with colleagues. Corporate sponsors provided funding for sessions, special events, and promotional materials. Almost 70 exhibitors gave attendees the opportunity to view the latest products and services in the Exhibit Hall.

ACHA: A Vision for the Future

Entering the new millennium, ACHA has a renewed sense of unity and purpose within the association. To promote healthy communities and healthy individuals as critical components of student learning, the association will always value:

- Social justice, human dignity, and respect for all persons
- Provision of student-centered services
- Professional excellence, responsiveness, and ethical practice
- Multidisciplinary and collaborative approaches to health care delivery
- The commitment and participation of those who advance health care
- The active involvement of students

Through the ongoing efforts of its members and staff, ACHA will continue to serve as the primary advocate for the health of college students by striving to integrate the critical role of college health into the mission of higher education.

APPENDIX 1

American College Health Association Awards and Honors 1920–2000

During its 80 years of existence, the American College Health Association has developed a number of awards to honor those who have served the association and college health in a specific exemplary manner. This recognition falls into two categories: named awards and fellowship. ACHA has eight named awards, and the following descriptions come from that organization.

- **Edward Hitchcock Award**—This award commemorates the work of Edward Hitchcock Jr., MD, who founded the first college health service at Amherst College in 1861 and was established in the 1961 centennial year of college health. The award honors ACHA members who have made outstanding contributions to advancing the health of all college students.
- **Ruth E. Boynton Award**—This award is named for Ruth E. Boynton, MD, who was an inspiration and guiding force as ACHA president (1940-41) and treasurer (1961-65), and who directed the University of Minnesota Student Health Service, which bears her name. The award honors ACHA members who have provided distinguished service to the association.
- **Ollie B. Moten Award**—This award commemorates the work of Ollie B. Moten, RN, past chairwoman of the Nursing Section of ACHA and former director of the Student Health Center at Texas Southern University in Houston. This award, established in 1992, honors ACHA members who have made a significant impact on the institution of higher education in which they work, regardless of whether the individuals have been active beyond their institutions.
- **Lewis Barbato Award**—This award is named in honor of ACHA past president, emeritus member and Fellow, Lewis Barbato, MD, former director of the University of Denver Health Service. The award honors students (ACHA members or non-members) who have made major contributions to college health as reflected in the association's mission and vision statements.
- **Miguel Garcia-Tunon Memorial Award in Human Dignity**—This award was established in 1989 to memorialize Miguel Garcia-Tunon, coordinator of the ACHA/CDC Seroprevalence Project from April 1988 to October 1989, and whose life and work exemplified dignity and integrity. This award honors ACHA members whose work, life, writing, research, or way of living have promoted the cause of human dignity and nurtured the appreciation of human differences.
- **E. Dean Lovett Award**—The E. Dean Lovett Award was created in 1990 to honor Dr. Lovett, past president of the Pacific Coast College Health Association and former director of the University of Hawaii Health Service. Dr. Lovett was an advocate of nurses in community colleges, small colleges, and university health services. This award, created by the ACHA Nurse-Directed Section, honors ACHA members who have directed a college health service or contributed significantly to the development of a college health service program in an exemplary manner.

- **The Clifford B. Reifler Award**—This award was created to honor Clifford B. Reifler, MD, MPH, who was former executive editor emeritus of the *Journal of American College Health,* former Director of the University of Rochester Health Service, and past president of ACHA. This award honors ACHA members and non-members who have made outstanding contributions to the *Journal of American College Health.*
- **The Hannibal E. Howell Award**—This award was created in 1998 to honor Hannibal E. Howell, MD, who has been involved with leading the association to increase its efforts toward inclusiveness and addressing ethnic minority concerns since he became director of Hampton University Health Center in 1960. This award honors ACHA members who have made outstanding proactive contributions to their campus communities and ACHA by promoting health care and preventive health relevant to ethnic minorities.
- **Outstanding Research Publication**—This award was created in 2000 to recognize and support the research publication endeavors of individual ACHA members or an individual at an ACHA member institution. This award recognizes and encourages the efforts of ACHA members and individuals at ACHA member institutions who have published their research activities and therefore have advanced the field of college health.

The second honored category includes Association Fellows. Fellowship in ACHA requires two major areas of qualification. The first is professional achievements in the field of college health. These include such areas as:

- original contributions to the advancement of knowledge in the field
- distinguished educational, professional, or administrative ability
- publication in professional journals other than the *Journal of American College Health*
- service to employing institution(s)
- academic (teaching) responsibilities
- research activities
- recognition by other related organizations

The second area of qualifications requires service to ACHA. This includes such areas as:

- annual meeting participation, including presentations, panels, program planning
- service to the association; acting as an officer of the association, section, or an affiliate
- publication in the *Journal of American College Health*
- attendance at ACHA and/or affiliate annual meetings
- full-time commitment to the field of college health for most of the requisite period of ACHA membership (membership for at least five years)
- other outstanding service to ACHA

APPENDIX 2

The *Journal of American College Health (JACH)* is the only scholarly journal that focuses exclusively on health in higher education. Like other professional journals, *JACH* provides a system of reviewing, assessing, and reporting important research, a medium for evaluating and describing current trends in practice, and a forum for the expression of opinion on current issues and controversies. Unlike many otherwise similar publications, however, *JACH* is fundamentally both multidisciplinary (responding to scholarship and practice in several disciplines) and interdisciplinary (integrating knowledge across those disciplines). Whereas many professional journals serve the members and interests of a particular discipline (for example, the *American Journal of Nursing*) or a specific professional group, *JACH* is published to serve a broadly defined field that includes researchers, scholars, and practitioners whose major shared interest is health as it is experienced, lived, determined, and served in higher education.

The authors and readers of the *Journal*'s articles include not only the whole range of practitioners, educators, and administrators who respond directly to students' health needs (including physicians, nurses, physician assistants, pharmacists, dentists, health educators, counselors, and allied health professionals), but also the researchers and scholars in education, psychology, public health, environmental health, community health, nursing, and medicine (among others) who discover new knowledge about health concerns and opportunities among students; senior academic officers and administrators; the student affairs professionals who develop and provide programs and services on campus; and students themselves (especially peer educators, student health advocates, and members of student health advisory boards). The paid circulation of the *Journal* has, in recent years, hovered around 3,000 subscribers, half or more of whom receive the publication as a benefit of their membership in ACHA.

JACH publishes six kinds of articles:

1. **Major articles.** The heart of the *Journal*'s scholarship, the Major Articles are original research studies, theory-based manuscripts, and state-of-the-art reviews that make significant new contributions to knowledge in college health. Major Articles always include detailed reviews of the relevant literature, careful descriptions of the chosen research method, a completely explained analysis of the results, and a concluding Comment that explicates the study's limitations and puts its findings in context. Before their acceptance for publication, these articles must have passed a rigorous, multi-layer review process, often including a statistical review. The *Journal*'s most frequently quoted and cited studies have been Major Articles.

2. **Clinical and Program Notes.** The Clinical and Program Notes are briefer and less formal than Major Articles; although they also undergo rigorous editorial review before acceptance, they are more practical and experiential. They provide practitioners, educators, administrators, and researchers the opportunity to report on interesting programs and services, new applications of technology, clinical cases with educational value, or management techniques (as examples).

3. **Viewpoints.** The Viewpoints provide authors (students, college health professionals, faculty, and others) a forum for expressing ideas, opinions, and perspectives. The purpose of editorial review of Viewpoints is not to stifle any author's point of view, but to guarantee that the submission is relevant to the field, cogently argued, logical and sound in its reasoning, and clear in its writing.

4. **Editorials.** The editor—or, occasionally, a guest editor—writes an editorial for each

issue. Its purpose is to focus the reader's attention on the most important points in each of the articles in that issue. The editorials usually draw out themes that are common to the pieces and relate those themes to other research, programs, and perspectives.

5. **Emerging Issues in College Health Practice.** Through special articles that bring readers up to date about important, evolving concerns that affect many of the disciplines in college health, the Emerging Issues series allows the *Journal* to focus intensively on issues that have broad relevance. Although a single article may qualify for publication in the Emerging Issues category, more likely the *Journal* will publish a series of related pieces in series in successive issues.

6. **Letters to the Editor.** The *Journal* encourages the submission of letters to the editor, either in response to articles published in earlier issues or as a way to make a very brief report of an interesting finding, program, or service. Given the relative infrequency of publication, though, it has been difficult for *JACH* to sustain continuing dialogue or debate through these letters.

Editorial Philosophy and Process

Like other major professional journals of academic significance, *JACH* employs a stratified, sequential, highly structured, systematic review process to guarantee the quality and value of the articles it publishes. All manuscripts that are candidates for publication as Major Articles, Clinical and Program Notes, and Emerging Issues in College Health Practice are submitted for detailed editorial review. A more limited process is used to evaluate submissions for Viewpoints and Letters to the Editor. In recent years, about 125 new manuscripts have required review and decision annually; of those, only 15-20 percent will (eventually) be accepted for publication.

The *Journal* uses its review process not only to assess the value of submissions, but also to improve them before publication and, regardless of the eventual outcome (publication or not), to develop the skills of the authors. A significant percentage of the manuscripts *JACH* receives come from relatively inexperienced researchers and scholars. Many of the practitioners, educators, and administrators who submit Clinical and Program Notes, especially, have had little training in preparing and editing manuscripts. *JACH*'s reviewers take very seriously their obligation to assist authors in improving their work; even rejected manuscripts arrive in their authors' hands with detailed comments that may improve the prospects of publication of other work later. In most circumstances, the process of review, revision, and reassessment becomes truly collaborative.

For almost 50 years, *JACH* and its predecessors have provided a platform for research, intellectual growth, and improvements in practice in college health. In 1989, the *Journal* won its first award-a distinguished achievement award from the Educational Press Association of America for an article by Robert J. Berson, PhD, on bereavement groups for college students. A second, similar award came in 1992, for an editorial by Jay Friedman on male roles and the quality of campus life. The Washington EdPress has given *JACH* three awards: an honorable mention for the theme issue on campus violence (1992; Brett Steenbarger, PhD, and Christine Zimmer, MS, guest editors), another honorable mention for the theme issue on peer education (1993; Jeffrey M. Gould, MEd,

MA, guest editor), and the silver award for the theme issue on substance use and abuse (1994; Richard P. Keeling, MD, guest editor).

REFERENCES

1. Boynton R. The First Fifty Years: A History of the American College Health Association. *J Am Coll Health.* 1971;19:269-281.

2. Dilley J. Development of the Structure of the American College Health Association. *J Am Coll Health.* 1980;28:354-358.

3. *Action Newsletter.* May-June 1990; 29.

4. *Action Newsletter.* May-June 1988; 26.

5. Patrick K. Student Health: Medical Care Within Institutions of Higher Education. *J Am Med Assoc.* 260;3305.

6. *Action Newsletter,* November-December 1989; 29.

7. *The Annual Report of the American College Health Association.* 1991-92.

8. *The Annual Report of the American College Health Association.* 1992-93.

9. *The Annual Report of the American College Health Association.* 1995-96.

10. *The Annual Report of the American College Health Association.* 1996-97.

11. *The Annual Report of the American College Health Association.* 1997-98.

12. *The Annual Report of the American College Health Association.* 1999-2000.

CHAPTER 3

ADMINISTRATION AND FINANCING
OF COLLEGE HEALTH

Wayne H. Ericson, PhD, Dana M. Mills, MPH,
and Gerald R. Ledlow, PhD, CHE

INTRODUCTION AND OVERVIEW

The practice of college health is essentially an unrecognized specialty in the broader health care system. The population being served is traditional college-aged students and a growing number of non-traditional students who, collectively, present significant challenges from both clinical care and marketing standpoints. Because of the ongoing developmental nature of this population, there are also challenges to effective preventive health care.

Health care services are among the most complicated organizational structures in society. The college health service on most campuses is not only a microcosm of the health care and prevention activities existing in society and thus subject to the influence of external health care market and regulatory forces, but also must function within a complex institution of higher education. Leading and managing such an organization requires competence in several multidisciplinary areas; an administrator must master both the science and art of leadership and management.

Within this framework, important guiding principles for college health professionals include service quality and economy, patient sensitivity, enabling student personal growth and development, continuous evaluation and improvement, ethical decision-making, and the removal of barriers to access by students relating to cost, hours of service, facilities, location, scope of care, and referrals.

College health services are diverse; "If you've seen one health service, you've seen them all" is clearly not correct. The reality is that "if you've seen one health service . . . you've seen ONE health service." Campus sizes range from less than 100 to over 50,000 students. Many health services employ only a single nurse and have limited hours of service and (perhaps) a relationship with a local private physician or hospital. Though the systems are small and uncomplicated in structure, these nurses offer an incredible amount of care, sensitivity, and guidance for those seeking service. Resources are stretched to the maximum, yet there is consumer demand for more.

At the other end of the spectrum are college health services that function as large multi-specialty clinics with a full array of ancillary services, caring for populations including students, faculty, staff, spouses, dependents, and in some cases, the general public. The budgets of these "mega" services can reach tens of millions of dollars with staffing of over two hundred individuals. This great diversity in college health is one of the profession's greatest strengths. It enables those in college health to find multiple ways to serve their populations.

In order to further understand the practice of college health, and thus the administrative skills necessary to manage such organizations, it is important to list certain assumptions about the campus environment. These assumptions demonstrate certain "universal truths" about college health and what administrators, regardless of health service size, will invariably experience. These assumptions are:

- Students will become ill or injured whether or not the college has a health program, and students/parents should be prepared to pay for care.
- Students and parents expect that some form of health care (i.e., non-emergency, ambulatory care) will be provided or otherwise arranged for.
- Institutions want (or need) to make health services available.
- There is no such thing as free health care.
- There are three major ways to pay for health care: prepay (tuition or health fee), fee-for-service, insurance
- Medical costs will continue to increase.
- Students will need information on how to improve/maintain health status.

Whether the reader is from a "nurse-only" campus clinic or a "mega" service, there are commonalities in purpose and thus in administrative skills needed. This chapter is designed to identify and briefly explain key administrative and financial skills necessary for successful management of a college health service. The material covered includes the "five Ps" (personnel, problems, politics, policies, and procedures) and more. However, it is not intended to be exhaustive on any of these subjects, as new or improved methods and strategies are regularly being developed.

ADMINISTRATION

Most dictionaries define "administration" as "management." In the thesaurus included in common word-processing software, the term is also synonymous with "direction," "running," "supervision," "government," "organization," and (perhaps the all-too-familiar term) "paperwork."[1] In essence the job of "administration" is one of providing resources for the work to be accomplished within an environment of fiscal accountability and responsibility. It has been predetermined that the work to be done is important, and that through some organized manner, the proper resources are applied in order to achieve a desirable product or outcome. In the case of college health clinical work, for example, "administration" is the bringing together of provider and patient in a proper environment to achieve a desirable endstate: proper diagnosis, effective treatment, and, ultimately, improved health. This implies that administrators must serve both providers of care and patients by removing barriers to access, performance of work, and problem-solving.

The fact that administrators must play that vital barrier-removal role is their principal way to add value to the healthcare operation; administrators do not diagnose, treat, or perform procedures on patients (that activity feeds the revenue engine of the operation). That simple reality makes all the difference. Administrators have critical roles that are grounded in leadership and management competence; those competencies are required to ensure the healthcare operation's survival. Leaders and managers perform their work in four areas: 1) building relationships; 2) exchanging information; 3) decision making; and 4) influencing.[2,p.43] The resulting outcomes of quality administration are improved patient health outcomes due to barrier-free (or barrier-reduced) provider—patient relationships (increased efficacy and effectiveness); increased productivity of the operation (efficiency); improved patient, provider, and staff satisfaction; responsible financial performance and resource acquisition; and effective image building and marketing. The corollary for a college health promotion program in the image-building and marketing arena might be the design of media pieces with consumer input resulting in widely distributed knowledge of preventive health behaviors. Thus, administration is not only a multifaceted supportive activity but also one that intends to create positive outcomes. In an ever-changing environment, leadership becomes critical to organizational success.

The term "leadership" is often described as "management" as well. Leadership and management, however, are two distinctly different, albeit related, sets of activities and behaviors. Management is more intent on maintaining the status quo and following the procedures and policies of the organization. Again, from the same common word-processing software, the terms "control," "guidance," and "direction" are also listed with this term.[1] Leadership is much more. It means not only taking responsibility, as in being charged with charting a direction, but is also associated with "style" and adaptation of this style to help the organization reach its full potential by creating an organizational culture that is effective, efficient and efficacious as it responds to the external environment. Management is briefly discussed, then followed by a set of leadership imperatives.

THE NATURE OF MANAGERIAL WORK[2]

Research by Mintzberg (1973), McCall, Morrison, & Hannan (1978), and Hales (1986) shows that popular conceptions of manager activities of careful planning, sitting in their office waiting for the exception to normal operations, and careful orchestration of events are a myth. Actually, the nature of a manager's work is very different from the perception:

- Content of work is varied and fragmented. Work is varied and very brief in duration (most activities last less than two minutes); average number of activities increases at lower levels of management; interruptions are frequent, conversations disjointed, and important activities are interspersed with the trivial; mood swings are radical.

- Many activities are reactive. Manager behavior is reactive rather than proactive in nature; more problems are identified than can be solved (chaotic rather than rational decision-making); problems that have immediacy, deadlines attached, or superior attention get worked/solved quicker. Managers spend little time in reflective planning; "fire fighting" takes over for team-building, planning, and training.
- Interactions often involve peers and outsiders. Managers spend more time with persons other than direct reports or superiors. Kanter (1983) found that managers with innovative changes/programs require lateral relationships to implement programs.
- Interactions typically involve oral communications. Managers have five prominent ways to obtain/transfer information: 1) written messages, 2) telephone messages, 3) scheduled meetings, 4) unscheduled meetings, and 5) observational tours. Managers show a strong preference for oral communication, with the most involved being face-to-face interaction (scheduled/unscheduled meetings).
- Decision processes are disorderly and political. Much of managerial literature describes decision-making as discrete events made by a single manager or group in an orderly and rational manner. This is sharply contradicted by descriptive research on managerial decision-making (Cohen & March, 1974; McCall & Kaplan, 1985; Schweiger, Anderson, & Locke, 1985; and Simon, 1987). Some major decisions are the result of many small actions (incremental processes) taken without regard to larger strategic issues. Decision processes are really characterized by confusion, disorder, and emotionality rather than rational orderly decision-making. For decisions involving major change or having strategic implications, Kanter (1982) and Kotter (1982 and 1985) found that outcomes depend on influence skills and persistence of individual managers and the relative power of coalitions involved.
- Most planning is informal and adaptive. Kotter (1982) found that general managers developed agendas consisting of loosely connected goals and plans related to their job responsibilities and involving a variety of short- and long-term issues; also, Kotter found that the implementation of agenda items is a gradual and continuous process. Quinn's (1980) study found that top executives made most important strategic decisions outside the formal planning process and that strategies were formulated in an incremental, flexible, and intuitive manner. In short, managers spend most of their effort in maintaining the organization and "running" the operation properly.

Leaders, on the other hand, are more future-oriented and prepare the organization to meet future challenges. Managers can be leaders and vice versa, although mindset and focus are different. Both efforts are for the good of the organization.

Leadership is a multidisciplinary journey in study, creation, synthesis of ideas, situational consideration, refinement, team-building and decision-making. Leadership can be borne by a single individual or by a cohesive team. The study of leadership has its roots in trait theory (leaders are born not made) and behavioral theory (leaders can be made), and currently embraces contingency theory (leaders must understand the situation and select the appropriate style at the right time to be effective). "Since the effectiveness of the leader has frequently determined the survival or demise of a group, organization, or an entire nation, it has been of concern to some of the foremost thinkers in history, like Plato, Machiavelli, or von Clausewitz. If leadership were easy to understand, we would have had all the answers long before now."[3,p.242] Contemporary leadership theory supports situational leadership (also called contingency leadership). That means a leader must adapt his or her style to the situation presented while maintaining the focused direction for the healthcare operation. A good leader works with staff to identify and pursue common goals. Leaders determine what must be done but let the team determine how to do it within a framework of coaching and mentoring.

Many leadership models, guides, books, and websites are available. No matter what leadership model is revered in the pop or scholarly cultures, the science and artistry of leadership is implied. Most leadership models, in some form or fashion, include the six agencies of leadership: 1) communication; 2) participation; 3) preparation; 4) identification of options; 5) closure (moving beyond past conflicts, negativity, and inequity); and 6) celebration.[4] A good leader is a teacher, cheerleader, critical evaluator, visionary, and perpetual source of energy for the organization. Leaders who do their jobs well can develop their organizations from within or create an effective organization starting with the first person hired. They objectively analyze organizational status and, if necessary, act as the driving force to challenge staff to achieve higher levels of performance and, especially in college health, consumer and provider satisfaction; in essence a leader positively transforms an organization. The transformational leader is an individual who embraces the following tenets:

- a strong emotional state (e.g., charisma, passion, selling organizational vision to stakeholders);
- intellectual stimulation (e.g., creation of challenges, relating importance of work to competence and skill, awareness of problems or limitations);
- individualized consideration (e.g., knowing one's staff, external constituents, and other stakeholders well, coaching, support and encouragement to those one leads);
- inspirational goals (e.g., set challenging yet attainable goals, set standards of excellence, create a learning environment, and again, achieve vision ownership from those being led and from external stakeholders); and
- transactional behavior (e.g., merit pay or bonuses or time off for excellent performance).[5]

The challenge is to lead effectively within a constantly changing environment (simply consider changes in health care over the past decade). The challenge is to know what styles and behaviors to utilize within a changing environment while maintaining organizational focus and values.

Dynamic environments require leadership. Leaders are required amid constant change; if organizations and environments were static, only managers would be needed to maintain the status quo. Leaders change the status quo to improve the organization, with the catalyst being constant change. At the personal, team, and organizational levels, leadership is a critical element in the recipe for organizational success. At whatever level one occupies in an organization, leadership makes a difference. The challenge is to focus one's knowledge and skills to empower the total organization to complete its mission, reach its vision, and compete successfully in an environment that constantly changes. Conceptually, leadership tends to be a self-contained domain; this traditional thinking does not contribute to the organizational feeding required to succeed in dynamic industries like health care. In essence a leader develops the appropriate organizational culture that fosters organizational success within a dynamic environment. The unique and important function of leadership, contrasted with management or administration, is the conceptualization, creation, and management of organizational culture.[6] Leaders develop and reinforce organizational culture through consistent communication, actions, and behaviors. Leaders communicate both explicitly and implicitly the assumptions they really hold. If they are conflicted, the conflicts and inconsistencies also get communicated and become part of the culture.

An absolutely essential factor in creating organizational culture and successful management of a college health service is the establishment of and adherence to ethical standards and principles. Many health care organizations, including the American College Health Association (ACHA), in its "Guidelines for a College Health Program," have already developed such standards.[7] As organizations grow and develop, especially with the use of new technology and management information systems, there is the need to regularly review and update policies, procedures, and decision-making with regard to equity and fairness.

Administrative skills and leadership qualities come quite naturally to some individuals. Other persons have the capacity and inclination to develop these skills and abilities. But, universally, all individuals can sharpen their talents in managing resources and being a leader of an organization through formal training or self-study and progressively more responsible and demanding experiences.

In the remainder of this chapter, the authors present what they believe are the essential skills and abilities for strong administration and leadership functions in the college health environment. Arguably, these skills and abilities prepare one for the broader health care environment, but the emphasis is on those traits that should serve well in a campus community. Sources of information include a survey of "management competencies,"[8] accreditation standards,[9,10] and the authors' individual experiences in managing and consulting for college health services over two decades.

COMMUNICATION

All leadership and management start with effective communication. In fact, everything a leader or manager says or does, or does not say or do, communicates a message. The planning, work, and evaluation process depends on communication. Personal and organizational communication effectiveness is salient.

Personal communication must be clear, consistent, and focused on building teamwork, reducing ambiguity, and alleviating uncertainty. Ambiguity in simple terms relates to knowing what questions to ask; if one is at a loss as to where to start or what to ask, ambiguity is present. Uncertainty deals with the level of information one has available to answer questions. A short list of personal communication improvement strategies is foundational, yet powerful.

- Use descriptive language rather than evaluative language. Descriptive language tends to be "we-oriented" and describes the situation. Evaluative language relates to finger-pointing. If evaluative language is required, always hold a private conversation rather than a public discussion.
- Use confirming language rather than disconfirming language. Confirming language makes people value themselves more, whereas disconfirming language devalues people. Successful healthcare administrators need team-oriented performance; that is best accomplished within a confirming environment.
- Reduce ambiguity and uncertainty in your words and actions. Be clear in your communication. If your level of ambiguity and uncertainty is high, let others know that learning, research, and collaboration are required to improve decision-making information. Related heavily to reduction in ambiguity and uncertainty is the concept of media richness. Rich media (such as face-to face conversation) allow quick feedback (to include nonverbal feedback) between parties, while media low in richness (flyer or memorandum) tend to be one-way, feedback-poor, or slow. Email is only slightly rich, and the telephone is moderately rich. Use richer media when ambiguity and/or uncertainty are moderate to high.[11,12,13]
- Spend time, face-to-face, with key stakeholders such as providers, staff, patients, institutional administration, and other constituents to build trust and relationships to learn what issues and barriers to care or performance exist. Communicate frequently and with a purpose for short durations.

Organizational communication can be improved by similar approaches, such as fostering confirming communication environments and facilitating effective conflict management approaches. Again, reducing ambiguity and uncertainty and improving team-oriented communication are keys to success.

Effective, relational, and honest communication at the interpersonal and organizational levels builds trust. Trust is a key element in building relationships and is especially important to administrators.

LEADERSHIP AND STRATEGIC MANAGEMENT

A major task of a college health service leader is to chart a course of action. One of the most important functions of a leader is to critically and objectively analyze the organization's environment and performance and decide if the organization's *activities* are congruent with the organization's own *goals and objectives,* and the *mission* of the institution. An objective, credible evaluation of the environment and of organizational performance is absolutely critical to developing and keeping current a strategic plan, especially if a significant change in direction is anticipated.

Most often this analysis occurs when there is a change in leadership, but periodic evaluation and assessment is vital to the long-term success of any organization, even if only to validate the status quo. Formal analysis is generally participative and should involve organizational staff, consumers, stakeholders from other campus constituencies, and representatives from the broader health care marketplace. A comprehensive review of the organization (e.g., every 3 to 5 years) involves a variety of people with multiple skills functioning at different levels and with different responsibilities, in order to have a satisfactory evaluation.

Occasionally, in order to ensure objectivity, it may be more appropriate to have the review done by sources external to the health service. This will be further considered when assessment, evaluation, and comparison are discussed later in the chapter. For now, it is presumed that a comprehensive evaluation for "strategic planning" purposes is appropriately performed by college health administration.

Strategic planning has certain essential elements. A basic understanding of the process minimizes the time and effort spent on the planning process and provides objective analysis of the final product. This is particularly important if individuals other than college health personnel assist in, or perform, the review.

Strategic planning is a continuous process. The process involves moving an organization along a predetermined path based upon the organization's values and the realities of the external environment. Similar to deciding what road to take, what stops to make, and who will drive, the process involves deciding upon what goals are important to the organization and what objectives must be met to reach those goals. Also, strategic planning has an outcome—to pave the way for a better future state based on organizational values and the external environment. Improving effectiveness and efficiency; customer, provider, and staff satisfaction; and financial performance, as well as many other similar improvements, are a part of moving the organization to reach a better future state. The future state is the vision of the organization. The vision is what the combined staff of the organization strives to become. If the destination is clear and defined, planning the trip and getting commitment from staff become much easier. Also, organizational resources, including energy and time, can be devoted to reaching set goals and having a positive outcome, i.e., making the vision of the organization a reality. Thus, while strategic planning is a continuous process that uses living documents (such as the strategic plan), it is also a mindset of the entire team. The team must be focused on the important goals and objectives of the organization and must feel ownership in the process. Team-building is as much a part of strategic planning as the plan and process itself; successful administrators concentrate on improving communication and building teams before and during the strategic planning process.

THE ESSENTIAL ELEMENTS OF STRATEGIC PLANNING[14]

Successful strategic planning requires careful consideration of nine essential elements.

Outline of Elements

- Identify the target market: Describe the group of customers to be served.
- Identify mandates: Consider statutory regulations and institutional requirements.
- Develop a mission statement: Create a framework for the organization and articulate organizational philosophy.

- Assess the environment: Describe external constituents (e.g., students) and internal constituents (e.g., key employees).
- Use SWOT analysis: Measure internal *s*trengths and *w*eaknesses and external *o*pportunities and *t*hreats.
- Formulate goals and objectives: Define desirable outcomes (goals) and steps necessary to achieve those goals (objectives).
- Identify strategies: Promote the accomplishment of objectives.
- Implement programs: Apply the strategies.
- Evaluate programs: Analyze the accomplishment of objectives.

Identify the target market

At first glance the target market may seem obvious for a student health service. However, rather than assuming a market base, a college health administrator needs to critically evaluate the philosophical basis for the service. For example: For whom do we exist? What is our "overall" market? How can/should we segment this market (e.g., undergraduates, graduates, part-time and full-time students, international students, student spouses and dependents, employees, and visitors) and which segments do we wish to serve?

Identify mandates

It is essential to establish any mandatory requirements of the service so that, at the least, the minimal expectations of the organization are clear. For example, who is the college health service required to serve? What is the college health service required to do according to institutional policy or statutory regulation?

Develop a mission statement

Once a basis for service has been established, a clear, concise mission statement must be developed to create a framework for the organization and a foundation for the strategic plan, and to articulate organizational philosophy and clinical, educational, and promotional values with stakeholders. (An excellent source for the development of an organizational mission statement is the paper "College Health: A Model for Our Nation's Health" from the American College Health Association. The document describes the value of college health for each institution and the collective value college health has for our nation's college population.)

Criteria for the evaluation of the mission statement are:

- Does it answer the question "What business are we in?"
- Is it results-oriented rather than activity-oriented?
- Does it state the reason for what an organization *does;* not what it *can do?*
- Is it outward- or client (service)-oriented as opposed to inward-or organization-oriented?
- Does it reflect a collective value judgment?

Assess the environment

In order for an organization to adapt to its surroundings, an assessment of the environment is essential. The purpose of the environmental assessment is to:

- Be aware of influences (positive and negative) and the "political tendencies" of the environment.
- Prepare the college health service to respond to the health care marketplace (i.e., the "outside world").
- Help the college health service find the best "fit" between itself and the surrounding environment (similar to an organism in nature).
- Take advantage of strengths and opportunities while minimizing weaknesses and threats.

External Environment

An assessment of the external environment provides an opportunity to increase sensitivity to the environment in which the college health service functions, to turn organizational energy outward to meet needs, and to generate support for future directions.

Constituencies included in the external environment include students, faculty, administration, the media, the local health care system, local governments, and the community at large. The local health care system may include hospitals, clinics, and medical schools as competitors and/or collaborators.

In order to gather information regarding consumer satisfaction, market penetration, and reasons for non-use, a "market audit" is commonly performed. Marketing, in simple terms, is an exchange of information between the provider and the consumer. The emphasis is on gathering information that an organization (e.g., a college health service) can use to better meet the needs of the consumers (e.g., student patients). Marketing can be differentiated from selling (or unabashed advertising) in that selling tries to persuade the consumer to want what the organization offers, while marketing tries to persuade the organization to offer what the consumer wants (or needs, as in the case of college health services or health promotion). It is not uncommon for college health administrators to perform this phase of strategic planning first, to clarify needs and expectations, before deciding on goals and objectives.

This phase of the process can be as simple or complex as the college health administrator finds useful. However, to be done objectively and credibly, research skills are required (i.e., random sampling, survey development skills, and data analysis), which may necessitate assistance from the institution's survey research division or other trained researchers. Sophisticated techniques for designing surveys, collecting information, and analyzing results may make the process more complicated than the average college health administrator might find desirable, but the increased credibility and objectivity of results generally outweighs the extra efforts and expense.

Internal Environment

The internal assessment is designed to obtain a realistic understanding of existing strengths and weaknesses. Examples of constituencies comprising the internal environment include general and key administrative staff, health care providers, and student advisory groups. Fundamental resources in this phase of organizational assessment include number of employees, physical facilities, and supplies and equipment. Important output (or performance) data include quality measurements (as compared to accreditation standards), patient-satisfaction survey results, clinical outcomes, market penetration, and utilization trends.

Use SWOT analysis

This is the classic exercise to measure internal "*s*trengths and *w*eaknesses" and external "*o*pportunities and *t*hreats." It is sometimes difficult and time-consuming to do a SWOT self-analysis, but when done objectively, the process can provide compelling arguments for strategic plans and, ultimately, constructive change. The process utilizes the information obtained from the external and internal assessments, including a market audit. In the college health environment, strengths are likely to be the ability to satisfy students' needs, sensitivity toward patients, economy of operation, and accessibility. Weaknesses may include financing (i.e., amount and source), staff compensation, physical facilities, information systems, and lack of institutional administrative support.

Opportunities for a college health service are likely to be collaborations with the local health care community (e.g., hospitals, clinics, jurisdictional public health departments), and other colleges and universities. Threats may be outsourcing proposals from some members of the same group mentioned under "opportunities" or from legislation (e.g., eliminating funding sources, restricting services or eligibility, or applying unfunded mandates).

Formulate goals and objectives

A *goal* represents a desirable outcome which may or may not be achievable. For example, a goal might be the elimination of meningitis as a disease threat at one's institution, or ensuring that all enrolled students have adequate health insurance coverage. An *objective,* on the other hand, describes an activity or state of affairs that is achievable within a specified time frame and which is done in pursuit of a goal. For example, objectives relative to the two goals stated above might be the vaccination of at least 60 percent of residential students by the end of the academic year, or the development and presentation of a proposal to require all students to provide evidence of adequate health insurance coverage or be required to buy the college-sponsored plan. The establishment of "SMART" objectives is recommended (i.e., *s*pecific, *m*easurable, *a*ttainable, *r*ealistic, and *t*ime-framed components) in order to clarify intent and provide proper focus to organizational efforts.

Identify strategies

This step is to identify those strategies (activities) which, if performed correctly, should result in the achievement of objectives. It is a classic "brainstorming" session to evaluate all possibilities to solve problems and issues of concern while preserving those programs which are working well. Choosing a strategy can be described as the "reality testing" phase of the strategic planning. Normally there is at least one strategy for each objective. For clarification, strategies are activities which promote the accomplishment of an objective. During this stage, a review of objectives and goals is in order to make sure that the identified strategy (or strategies) can arguably succeed in satisfying the objectives while being consistent with existing organizational (and institutional) aims. Given the difference in sizes and resources of college health services and the differences in institutional direction and philosophies (e.g., public vs. private, sectarian vs. nonsectarian), strategies to reach similar goals may be markedly different among institutions. In some cases goals or objectives may need to be changed to adapt to the new information. Careful review of the results of the previous exercises may help determine which ideas or strategies are feasible from operational, financial, and philosophical perspectives. The final activity of this exercise is to prioritize the workable strategies.

Implement programs

The application of strategies is called "program implementation." This may be as complicated as establishing a new computer system or as simple as changing a form. But in either case, the strategy should be adequately described before implementation, and a starting date needs to be established.

Evaluate programs

In the final phase of strategic planning, an evaluation of outcome is performed to determine if the strategy was applied correctly and whether or not it actually accomplished the objective.

Organizational success and individual leader success are greatly related to strategic planning. Developing an organizational mission statement, a plan based on goals and objectives, a vision, and implementing the plan to attain the vision are the steps essential in the prescription for success.

EMPLOYEE ENHANCEMENT AND RELATIONSHIP MANAGEMENT

Health care is a people-intensive environment. Thus it is no surprise that effective health care administration recognizes and actively supports the contribution that staff make toward the attainment of clinical and operating goals and objectives, and overall consumer satisfaction. By and large, a competent, well-adjusted, customer-oriented staff makes for contented patients. However, a customer-oriented staff does not happen by accident. Staff relationships must be managed as any other valued resource in the organization.

College health administrators generally have four primary goals in the management of staff relationships in their organizations:

- Team-building, i.e., development of shared goals, is an ongoing process that changes with the introduction of new staff and the departure of incumbent staff. The team recreates itself after staff changes by imparting organizational culture to new arrivals and adapting to new personalities and professional skills to enhance the value and performance of the group. Team-building can also be formalized through orientation and training.

- Customer relations or, specifically, performance that is student-and service-oriented. And the "golden rule" of relations (i.e., treat others the way one wants to be treated) applies whether dealing with students or other staff.
- Workforce diversity (multicultural, multiracial) strengthens a college health staff. The nature of the work, i.e., serving an educationally, racially, and culturally diverse campus population, is enhanced by a commitment to diversity in the college health service workforce. Employing staff who are diverse in training, race, orientation, and culture mandates in-services on communications, group interactions, problem-solving, and conflict management.
- Empowerment gives staff and others the responsibility that is appropriate for their education and experience; empowering leaders tend to be more transformational.
- Effective multi-disciplinary communication is the key to positive staff interactions and therein, good routine information flow, problem-solving, and conflict management. And health services, whether campus based or not, require the work of a variety of staff trained in a variety of disciplines.

College health administrators set the tone for staff interactions through role modeling in meetings and individual discussions, and by what is written and communicated. It is generally expected that individuals trained in different disciplines will think and act differently than those of similar backgrounds. In fact, that variance in thinking and behavior may be a major factor in the success of an organization's strategic planning efforts. It is also a given that individuals trained in the same discipline often disagree; (e.g., physicians on medical treatments). The goal should not be to always avoid staff conflicts, but to use them creatively and fairly when they do occur, to reach positive outcomes for all concerned.[15]

Group Decision-Making Techniques

A helpful technique for college health administrators to use in group decision-making is to apply Tannenbaum and Schmidt's "Continuum of Leader Decision-making Authority."[16] This technique informs the group how an important decision will be made and who will ultimately make it. The process is based on the assumption that there are levels of decision-making authority (or a continuum) from 1 to 7. "Level 1" decisions are made by the director. "Level 7" decisions are delegated to the group for a decision. The closeness of the decision-making authority to either 1 or 7 determines the degree of administrative autonomy or group participation in the final decision. For example, if a director needs to make a decision on an associate director position, he or she may form a search committee and ask the group to screen, interview, and rank the top three candidates. This represents a "level 5" decision in that the director asked the group to make a tentative choice (i.e., top-ranked candidate) for his or her final approval. Another example might be the presentation of the final budget by the director to the executive team. The final budget would represent the collective wisdom of the group with some changes by the director. The director's intent would be to solicit input to see if there are any compelling reasons to change the proposal (i.e., the director has essentially made the decisions but doesn't want to leave any stone unturned). This would represent a "level 3" decision. Sometimes it is useful for the director to negotiate with the executive team at which level the decision will be made. This discussion helps to establish organizational significance of decisions to all concerned and apply the proper process to ensure the best possible outcome and staff involvement.

Another decision-making technique which is particularly helpful for clinical staff with administrative responsibilities is an adaptation of the clinical charting process designed by Lawrence Weed.[17] Clinicians are often trained to handle patients using the "SOAP" process; i.e., to evaluate patients according to "*s*ubjective" and "*o*bjective" findings, make an independent "*a*ssessment" of the problem, and then formulate a treatment "*p*lan." This "SOAP" process can also be used to help clinical staff regard administrative problems and issues in the same context as clinical decision-making. The "subjective and objective" analysis process can be used to relate to problems with patient flow as well as patient care; the "assessment" could equate to a potential solution or solutions; and, the "plan" could be the action to implement the solution. This technique is particularly helpful for busy clinicians and/or those who are new to the administrative decision-making process.

Chaotic Decision-Making [18,19,20,21]

Not all decision-making processes are rational and orderly. Chaotic decision-making is common in most organizations. The basic premise is that time, attention, decision-making load (number of decisions within a time interval), ambiguity, uncertainty, and technology issues all constrain and stress the organization's ability to make rational and controlled decisions. This "garbage can model of decision-making" can be stressful to administrators, but there are ways to create some semblance of order amid chaos and anarchy. Organizations with a high propensity for "garbage can" processes can proactively foster better decision-making by empowering employees, by planning, and by recognizing and training for the inevitable chaotic decision making environment. There are certain basic rules for influencing the course of decisions in a chaotic environment:[18]

- Spend time. Since time is a scarce commodity, someone who is prepared to spend time is offering a valuable resource.
- Persist. Losses and victories are partly fortuitous, due to the particular pattern of attention generated on a particular occasion.
- Exchange status for substance. Symbolic issues are likely to be more important to some participants than substantive issues. Thus, someone willing to trade "in the opposite direction" is in a favorable trading position.
- Facilitate opposition participation. The frustrations of chaotic decision processes tend to reduce aspirations.

- Overload the system. Any individual proposal may easily be defeated in a chaotic environment, but someone with a large number of projects will find some fraction of them being successful. Deadlines can also be used to manage the flow of problems.
- Segment decisions. If a problem is routine and results in the same or similar decisions each time, develop a policy or standing procedure for that problem. If a problem is not a critical organizational issue, decentralize the decision to trained staff members (empower subordinates), and spend time and effort on critical and important problems at the senior levels of the organization.
- Manage unobtrusively. "Sail" the organization, rather than "powerboat" it, through the use of high-leverage minor interventions.
- Interpret history. Control definitions of what is happening and what has happened to take advantage of the changing patterns of participation.

RESOURCE MANAGEMENT

Resource management encompasses all of the resources necessary to produce our product (broadly defined as good health care for the campus community), including financing and budget building, budget management, the "numbers side" of human resource management, organizational structure and interactions, information systems, and managing liability.

There are innumerable ways to manage the budget-building process, but a process that is consistent, participative, and objective generally produces the best product. A sample budget-building process which has been effective in many college health programs in requesting and acquiring adequate financial resources is presented below.

Typical Budget Building Process

As the first step of the typical budget-building process, a "fee (review) committee" should be appointed. This committee typically consists of representatives from student government, the student health advisory committee (SHAC), the campus budget office, the office of the vice president for student affairs (or a parallel administrator at this level), faculty, and the college health service. Ideally, the group should be chaired by a health service representative or the representative from the office of the vice president. This configuration builds credibility in the process, with all three political factions in a college or university represented, i.e., students, administration, and faculty.

The "fee committee" should meet regularly during the fall academic term with the following agenda:

- First Meeting: review workload objectives; outline the process and timetable; review health service demographics.
- Second Meeting: present financial history and current year's budget and utilization experience; project year-end figures.
- Third Meeting: present next year's budget (absent any changes in programs or services but including inflationary increases for supplies); review institutional projections for

merit increase funding and capital equipment replacement requests; present enrollment projections for next year; discuss operational problems needing attention (with cost scenarios); ask committee members to contribute any problems or issues.

- Fourth Meeting: provide the budget implications of any issue presented by the committee members; generate listing of budget options and financial (i.e., health fee) implications for next year and discuss priority; vote on those items to be included in next year's budget request; finish discussions on any new requests.
- Fifth Meeting: finalize a clear, concise financial strategy, with supporting documentation to recommend to the institution's administration.

This type of budget-building process generates "critical advocacy" from the major stakeholders on campus, which is essential for budget approval at higher levels. It allows students to become well informed about college health service issues without losing credibility with their peers. Sometimes members of the "fee committee" (e.g., student, faculty, or administration representatives) are also members of higher-level committees that review campus-wide budget requests. If so, they are in key positions to explain and advocate for health service budget approval.

FINANCIAL MANAGEMENT

For most college health services, the process for handling cash, accounting, and budget transactions is carefully prescribed in an institutional business procedures manual.

Financial management relates to the proper allocation and use of funds so that the organization can meet its financial goals and objectives and maintain or become (in the language of the corporate world) "a going concern." However, this does not mean that financial management for college health necessarily applies the same philosophies and strategies as the broader corporate health care environment. Rather, the analogy is made to encourage the application of sound financial management principles so that any college health service not only simply continues to exist but also is afforded the opportunity to grow and develop. Resources included in this category relate to personnel, operating expenses, capital funding, and for some college health services, investment funds.

Financial management also means enabling those programs that are within the planned budget and discouraging (or saying "no" to) those programs not budgeted (which emerge but are not rationally considered a priority). Managing the finances of a health care organization is often very difficult, because the efficient expenditure of funds is largely based on utilization of services, something over which the "manager," whether independent practitioner or a medical administrator for a large group practice, does not have complete control. Good fiscal managers will make carefully considered assumptions about the use of and need for resources in the budget-building process; nonetheless, they are assumptions. As the budget is administered, the assumptions may or may not be correct and may necessitate the need for adjustment.

Further, most college health services have a "global budget"; that is, there is a finite limit to funds available for the operating year. This is in contrast to the flexible budgets common in external health care organizations which rely on fee-for-service as the primary financing mechanism. Most college health services establish a budget based on tuition or health fees and have to "live with it" for the year, while fee-for-service entities typically have the option to raise charges.

Budget Accountability

In some college health services, budget accountability typically falls to the director or business manager. In this environment, there is an aggregate budget which serves as the only budget entity to manage. In other health services, there is often a process to disperse accountability so that persons most able to control expenditures are given the authority to do so. For example, cost centers (or revenue centers if income is generated) are established for the main services or functions of the college health service. Common cost centers are specific clinics (e.g., medical clinic, acute care clinic, women's clinic, allergy and immunizations, and sports medicine), ancillary services (e.g., laboratory, pharmacy, physical therapy, and x-ray), and health promotion. The responsibility for managing resources falls on those persons in charge of the specific cost center area. These individuals commonly have the authority to spend the dollars in their budgets according to previously approved plans and to make reallocation adjustments (within existing budget parameters) as necessary according to unanticipated changes in operating conditions.

Accounting and Internal Control

The actual responsibility for handling and recording purchasing transactions, paying bills, collecting receivables, making payroll, and timekeeping usually falls to a business/accounting office. On a manual or electronic basis, transactions are recorded in a general ledger, separate line-item accounts are debited or credited, and periodic reports of financial condition are generated (e.g., monthly aggregate and cost center reports). In smaller college health services, this entity is in one office and all activities may be performed by one or two people. In larger organizations, there may be separate offices and staffs for each function. The separation of duties and record-keeping for quality control and auditing purposes ("internal control") is much easier in larger organizations. The question of internal control may become an issue in smaller organizations because separation of functions is not possible. In this instance, an administrator should oversee the activities and/or randomly spot-check transactions, and request periodic audits from campus internal auditors.

Managing Funds in Institutions of Higher Education

There is a good deal of support for the notion that managing funds in a college health service in higher education is more difficult than in some other health care entities because of the narrow "tolerance for error" and the disincentives for prudent management of funds. For example, at many colleges or universities the college health administrator must finish the year-end budget within a certain range. Of course, the budget cannot be overspent, but neither may it be permissible to generate "surpluses" beyond a certain level. A fortunate few college health services can carry over funds from year to year with impunity.

Further, disincentives come with the budget-building process at some institutions. Prudent college health administrators who leave some funds unspent by year-end are "punished" in the following year's budget in two ways: first, the unspent funds fall to the institution's bottom line and can't be carried over, and, second, the next year's request for funds in that account line or lines might be cut due to seemingly "reduced" need. College health administrators may not be in a position to change the rules for fund balances, but effective oversight of funds over the long term will establish credibility with budget requests and gather institutional support for operational effectiveness. It will also establish and maintain credibility with student leaders who need to feel comfortable with their support of fees assessed to the student community.

Grant Funding

Many health-related activities are not reimbursed or are not reimbursed adequately. Some of these activities include health promotion and preventive services. One approach to fund such activities is by public and private grant opportunities. Partnering with university departments and faculty, community organizations, and other healthcare facilities can lead to grant funding, which can help cover the financial gap in providing unfunded or underfunded activities. This is an avenue worth pursuing on a university or college campus, since the infrastructure, databases, and knowledge exist in reasonable quality and quantity.

HUMAN RESOURCE MANAGEMENT

Human resource management is differentiated from relationship management in that it is concerned with "what" and "how" personnel record-keeping is performed. Managing staff resources is essential to good overall management (of labor-intensive organizations such as college health services), since the average college health service spends about 65–75 percent of its financial resources on the cost of staff.

Most college health services can rely in some measure on their campus human resources department for assistance with staffing processes and record keeping. However, the college health administrator needs to keep the following in mind:

- All staff, whether regular or part-time, should have a current position description.
- Written performance evaluations should be done on at least an annual basis, in an objective manner, by immediate supervisors.
- Account records for work and vacation/sick-leave time accruals must be kept accurately and current.
- Periodic compensation benchmarks are important to ensure that productive staff are paid fairly. (This most likely is controlled by central human resources.)
- Staff personnel files should include (at least) the original job application, notice of ser-

vice awards, professional recognition, all appointment papers and changes in appointment or rate of pay, performance evaluations, licensure or certification where required, and continuing education activities sponsored or otherwise subsidized by the college health service.

- Record-keeping of positions by a unique and individual code for each position is important to ensuring that all positions are accounted for. (Staff turnover, fractionation, recombination, and/or dormancy of positions can create misunderstandings between health service administration and institutional entities exercising control regarding approved positions.)

Continuing Education

For clinical staff and certain other professional staff there are legal requirements for continuing education. There is also arguably a "requirement" for other staff to stay current with changes in the field or to periodically upgrade their education and expertise. From an administrative standpoint, the responsibility for legally mandated continuing (e.g., medical) education is best defined as a joint responsibility. The staff member needs the continuing education credits to stay licensed, registered, or certified, and the organization can employ only staff who are in compliance with applicable practice laws.

For purposes of equity, the case can be argued that all other staff should have access to some form of periodic continuing education to be more effective in their jobs. For many college health services, provision of adequate funding and opportunity for continuing education credits is also a strategy to remain competitive for staff recruiting and retention. Therefore, continuing education resources should be included in the organizational budget. They may be allocated uniformly across clinical professions or distributed by category of staffing and potential cost of educational opportunities. Continuing education contributions by the organization may or may not include all resources to cover program registration, travel, and accommodations as well as time away from work. Monetary incentives supporting travel may also be used to encourage staff to develop proposals and presentations for professional association meetings.

ORGANIZATIONAL MANAGEMENT

A college health service's organizational chart generally displays reporting relationships and the flow of information in the organization. Depending upon the level of complexity of a function and the supervision necessary, an organizational chart may be "hierarchical" (i.e., more responsibility conveyed down through the organization to establish a deeper, more extensive chain of command with more layers of accountability, and decentralized decision-making). The opposite organizational chart would be less "hierarchical" (i.e., a shallower organizational structure with fewer layers of delegated responsibility and more centralized decision-making). The size, complexity, and developmental cycle of the college health service, and the leadership style of the college health director will influence whether a more or less hierarchical strategy is used.

Which organizational strategy used depends upon how the organization is best able to perform. If more extensive authority is delegated from the director, a more hierarchical chart will be necessary to reflect more defined channels of accountability. More complex or larger college health services may require additional layers of hierarchy (e.g., staff who report to frontline supervisors who in turn report to middle managers). Sometimes it is important to demonstrate both administrative and clinical reporting relationships. This may be particularly helpful if there are non-clinical managers with responsibilities for clinical entities which ultimately require some form of clinical oversight (e.g., lab as a functional area reporting to a non-clinical administrator while reporting to a clinician for "clinical" concerns). Ultimately, however, the best organizational chart depends on the people involved; the college health director's responsibility is to find a configuration which meets the needs for structure and achieves maximum organizational performance.

Organizational Development Cycles

College health services, like all other organizations, have a "life cycle" and a need for periodic renewal. The attentive college health administrator will recognize the life cycle stage that her/his organization is in and be prepared to make changes as appropriate. The life cycle continuum of a college health service includes:

- The "emerging service"—This organizational phase is characterized by a new mandate from the institution to develop a new program or accomplish a major overhaul of an established program. This change includes developing core staffing, services, hours of operation, marketing plans, facility space, and, sometimes, financing.
- The "growing service"—This organizational phase is characterized by development beyond the basic service in response to need. The needs may include, for example, additional staffing, space, new financing strategies, computer systems, and new eligible populations.
- The "mature service"—This organizational phase is initially characterized by relative stability in staffing, financing, service performance and satisfaction, information system development, space adequacy, established and written policy and procedures, and market penetration.
- The "regenerated service"—This organizational phase is characterized by a renewal of service performance, based on objective and critical review of organizational functions and consumer satisfaction. This phase will likely be repeated numerous times over the life of an energetic college health service.
- The "declining service"—This organizational phase is a service that has lost touch with its mission. Consumers are served below their expectations, morale is low, and staff turnover may be high. The organizational culture is that problems cannot be resolved and that self-fulfilling prophecies of doom become true.

These organizational stages either evolve over time or can be changed abruptly by new leadership or new institutional mandates. The challenge to a college health administrator is to provide opportunities for assessment and evaluation of services and then be able to act on the results. As noted, even the mature college health service requires regular re-newal and recommitment. Group participation in organizational performance evaluation is helpful if objectivity can be maintained. Comparison with other benchmark schools and accreditation standards, and thorough consumer population surveys, are valuable tools for objective, credible evaluation.

INFORMATION SYSTEMS MANAGEMENT

Information management, whether manual or automated (with computerized internal management systems, email, Internet connections, and more) is one of the most impor-tant technical responsibilities of college health administrators. For health services with clinical computer systems which handle administrative and clinical programs, the fed-eral regulations such as the Health Insurance Portability and Accountability Act (HIPAA)[22] have the potential to force significant changes in access and overall security of health record systems.

Often, one of the most complex undertakings of college health administration is the development, installation, or replacement of a computerized information system. The complexity of the task arises from several factors:

- Computer technology is in a constant state of change, in terms of both capabilities and cost.
- Effective computer systems must be used by a diverse staff population including clinical and non-clinical staff.
- The need for information is driven by clinical, administrative, and regulatory concerns.

General objectives of the information system include:

- To uniformly and efficiently gather and archive information relevant to the delivery of health care and health education services (e.g., patient registration, appointments, diag-noses, chart summaries, preventive health programs).
- To uniformly and efficiently gather information relevant to organizational performance (e.g., visits, diagnoses, productivity, outcomes, and quality assurance).

The requirements for a software system are dependent on how a specific college health service functions. For example, one health service's requirements may include estab-lishing patient registration and eligibility testing, triage, appointment scheduling, im-munizations tracking and updating, cashiers, and third-party billing. Another health service may need all of these plus a master patient index and health records tracking and purging system, staff scheduling, tracking of codes (e.g., ICD9-CM, CPT4, APG), scanning of forms and bar-codes, an accounting system (e.g., budget, payables, receiv-ables), applying administrative "hold credits," inventory management, ancillary ser-vices system(s) (laboratory, radiology, pharmacy), and more. With the state of current technology, computer information systems can be as sophisticated (and costly) as a budget allows.

Selecting a Software System

For college health administrators there is always pressure to "pick something off the shelf and just install it." This may be a good solution for some few, usually small, college health services which have few policies and procedures in place and look for direction to the software vendor. But for most health services, a major effort is required in the selection of a software package. Customarily, the formal process includes the development of a "request for proposal" (RFP) for distribution to potential vendors. In the authors' opinion, an RFP is preferred to a bid request in this context. Typically, a "bid" requires that the lowest offer is the one selected while an RFP allows one to take into account factors other than the "bottom line." Thus, while a "bid" may work well for computer hardware, an RFP is preferable for software. In any case, many institutions may require the use and expertise of the institution's information technology division and the purchasing department.

Policies and Procedures

Written policy and procedures are essential for smooth operation of a college health service. Institutional policies and procedures should generally be available in both hard copy and via the campus computer network. Additionally, health services should have an internal policy and procedures manual which may be segmented into clinical and non-clinical functional areas. Organizing such a manual to follow the table of contents of one of the national accrediting associations' "standards" is wise. In that way, the manual is as complete as possible relative to the organization's scope and level of services, while preparing the health service for accreditation at some future time.

RISK MANAGEMENT

Risk management has played an increasingly important role in administration in recent years. In November 1999 the Institute of Medicine released a report titled, "To Err Is Human: Building A Safer Health System." [23] The abstract of the report states, "Experts estimate that as many as 98,000 people die in any given year from medical errors that occur in hospitals. That's more than die from motor vehicle accidents, breast cancer, or AIDS—three causes that receive far more public attention. Indeed, more people die annually from medication errors than from workplace injuries. Add the financial cost to the human tragedy, and medical error easily rises to the top ranks of urgent, widespread public problems."[23,p.27] While these hospital statistics may not be directly comparable to a health service operation, there is no question that as a result of this report, risk management will become increasingly important in the coming years. Any health care organization, including a student health service, must develop and maintain a program of risk management that is "designed to protect the life and welfare of an organization's patients and employees"[23,p.4] and visitors. It is critical to identify and manage risks instead of reacting to problems after the fact.

The purpose of risk management in college health is to provide assessment and surveillance of issues and events which could adversely affect the service, quality of care, reputation, and fiscal integrity of the health service and the institution. This is accomplished by monitoring and implementing appropriate policies and procedures.

The following components are most likely to impact a college health service and therefore most necessary to be considered in a risk management program:

- Some areas are required by law (OSHA), which include but are not limited to: facilities and management issues (tornado drills, fire drills, emergency disaster plan, safety and security issues), bloodborne pathogens, hazardous communication, employee training, hepatitis B vaccination, and TB testing.
- Some areas are regulated by accrediting agencies as a part of a quality management and improvement program. Compliance issues include but are not limited to: tracking occurrences (trends noted and corrective actions such as prescription labeling errors), credentialing, confidentiality issues, patient/customer complaints, aspects of quality of care, including outcome studies, satisfaction surveys, liability issues.
- Fiscal integrity; that is, honest and ethical stewardship of financial and other resources.
- Humanitarian concerns; providing a safe and secure place of employment, particularly through new employee orientation and training.

STAKEHOLDER INVOLVEMENT

Stakeholders are those persons, groups, or organized entities impacted by, and/or who influence, the organization in question. For a college health service, stakeholders include students, parents, college/university administrators, faculty and staff, local medical group(s), community hospitals, and others. A key to a successful student health service is identifying and meeting the reasonable expectations and concerns of stakeholders. If poor service is provided, students will complain and seek health care elsewhere, leading to a decrease in utilization and ultimately to a critical lack of student support. Similarly, institutional officers expect an efficiently operated organization. If a health service is constantly plagued by student complaints, high staff turnover, and continued operating problems, the director is not meeting the expectations of the administrative official who is also a stakeholder. The importance of listening to and understanding stakeholders cannot be overestimated.

Stakeholders may, at times, have conflicting and sometimes unreasonable demands. For example, students and their parents want the best quality service possible and they usually want it "now." Fulfilling their needs implies a "richly staffed" organization that is able to respond immediately to all demands for service. However, when vice-presidents, presidents, and boards of trustees balance total institutional needs and affordability, the health service does not rank first in priority. The health service director is therefore faced with balancing the needs of the students/parents and the institution.

In developing a strategic plan (such as described earlier) it is essential that stakeholders be identified, their expectations be listed, and the strategy used by health service staff meet their needs. For students, one approach employed by many health services is to establish a student health advisory committee (SHAC) to provide input into programs, budget requests, insurance benefits, discuss student needs/complaints, customer service expectations, and more. "Guidelines for a College Health Program," published by the American College Health Association (ACHA), identifies possible relationships between health service staff and students.[24]

Parents are stakeholders whose concerns focus on being assured that if their students are injured or become ill, the health service staff will accommodate their children in a timely and high-quality manner. Considering employees as stakeholders requires management to invite employees to identify their concerns and ideas, to respond to their questions, involve them in the decision-making process, and praise them for their work.

Administrators as stakeholders can be powerful advocates for the health service to other members of the college/university, parents, and the larger community. If a health service operates efficiently and is known to offer high quality of care, senior administrators will have an easier time in expressing their confidence about the services and continuing their support for the services provided.

In short, stakeholders can generate a broad base of support, which is invaluable to the success of the health service and the quality of care provided.

ASSESSMENT, EVALUATION, AND COMPARISON

Assessment and evaluation are critical elements in the management process. Without informal and formal feedback regarding program operations, health services have neither information about the effectiveness of services, overall quality, patient satisfaction, and adequacy of programs nor an objective basis on which to make needed program changes. Assessment of a health care organization is related to many factors including, for example, patient, professional, and societal expectations; activities; outcomes; accreditation; and benchmarking. (Since the assessment of health services is such a complex topic, chapter 4 in this text is devoted entirely to accreditation and quality assurance, and this discussion will not be repeated in detail here.)

Evaluation of a student health service also includes certain basic factors:

- How many students are utilizing the services?
- Are students satisfied with the services received?
- Are the program objectives being accomplished?
- Are the objectives being accomplished in the most cost-efficient manner?

Utilization is a measure of activity. While such activity measures are basic, it is essential that evaluation does not stop with how many students are using the services provided. Quality is as important as quantity; thus administrators must know the outcome or impact of a service, and evaluation must include all four measures to evaluate overall performance.

In developing an evaluation process it is useful to follow certain basic principles of data acquisition. For example, when considering activity measures the data must be available, economical, and timely. For outcome measures, consideration should be given to what services should be measured, the validity and reliability of survey questions, and answering basic questions, such as who will receive the results and what will be done with the information.

Knowing utilization trends can help validate whether services are meeting the needs of the population. Typical utilization measures may include the total number of annual visits; visits by gender, by class, by place of residence, or by number of ancillary services provided (lab, x-ray, pharmacy); reason for the visit (procedure or diagnosis); total number and percentage of individual students using the program; and others. It is important to know the demographics of the student body (e.g., enrollment by class, race, age, gender, number of international students), to compare this data with health service utilization. Such comparisons will help determine if the students receiving care are representative of the total students enrolled.

Consumer satisfaction is an important (perhaps the most important) outcome measure used to assess the quality of service, because it is positively correlated with patient compliance and subsequent care-seeking behavior. Patient satisfaction surveys can assess many different aspects of the patient's encounter with the health service, ranging from meeting needs and expectations to complex questionnaires which ask about availability, accessibility, interpersonal aspects of care, financial issues, and resolution of the health problem.

Internal Reports

Ongoing internal reports periodically distributed (e.g., monthly or quarterly) to staff can be an invaluable source of assistance and feedback. Information on the number of patient visits by area (women's health, general medicine, urgent care), major diagnoses, and scheduled events, such as a flu shot clinic, are helpful in making management decisions. A major benefit is that staff become aware of what is happening within the organization and can make comparative judgments themselves. A staff's performance and commitment can be improved when they understand the overall impact of their work.

Marketing Surveys

Marketing surveys (as discussed in the section on strategic planning) focus on identifying and measuring the needs of the customers/students. Student health service staff are involved in marketing whether or not they are aware of it. Awareness of, and adoption of, marketing principles helps health services be more effective in achieving their objectives. Obviously, most student health service staff do not have formal training or experience in marketing. However, many campuses have an institutional research department or an academic marketing department, usually in a school/college of business, that has expertise in the development and administration of marketing surveys. Health service administrators are urged to request assistance in the development, implementation, and utilization of such surveys. Understanding the expectations and desires of students assists the organization in its efforts to improve patient satisfaction.

Benchmarking and Networking

Benchmarking is a comparative process which compares a series of internal processes or resources used in the provision of care with the same processes or resources used by similar institutions. Benchmark examples can include the number or percent of eligible students who use the health service, visits per FTE provider, number of providers per 1,000 enrollees, number of support staff per physician, number of tests ordered, productivity, size of facility, or the cost per visit. This performance information is shared among peer health services to determine "best practices" in key performance areas. In recent years the American College Health Association has developed a benchmarking instrument that is used by health services throughout the country. As a result, it is likely that an increased emphasis will be placed on benchmarking by higher education institutions.

Networking is the sharing of information, formally and informally (problems, solutions, new approaches), among persons who have similar interests. The best example of networking among college health professionals is the Student Health Service's listserv. This electronic mailing list currently links over 1,500 persons across the country, all of whom work in areas of college health. The speed of this medium assures that a person who asks a question can expect to receive several answers within a day or two. This person can then contact responding individuals directly for further clarification or discussion.

Opportunities for face-to-face networking occur through attendance at the American College Health Association's annual national meeting as well as at the regional/affiliate meetings that occur throughout the year. Many student health services within a state or region often have their own meetings once or twice a year where health service staff can meet and discuss common problems/issues. These meetings can be especially meaningful, since many of the same problems may be impacting all the programs. Examples of such networking efforts include the Big 10 Health Services, Big 12 Conference, Sunbelt Directors, California State Schools, Illinois and Wisconsin Consortium of Student Health Programs, the Kentucky College Health group, and the Student Health Services at Academic Medical Centers group.

Financial Audits, Relicensing Reviews, Annual Reports

Other approaches to assess and evaluate a student health service include financial audits, review of compliance with licensure requirements, and annual reports. Financial audits document where funds were spent and if financial policies and procedures were followed. Audits show what dollars were expended for selected budget categories (i.e., personnel, commodities, contractual, equipment, travel) and/or programs (i.e., clinic, ancillary services, health promotion) and provide a comparison with the budgeted amounts. Audits typically report expenditures for the last three years. This presentation of historical trends, especially when combined with a projected budget, provides additional insight for making forecasts.

Every student health service has staff (physicians, nurses, etc.) and/or programs that are required to be licensed. Establishment of a "tickler list" that prompts the director to request proof of license renewals is one procedure to assure that staff are in compliance with applicable state and federal laws. After the renewal license has been received and verified by the director (or his/her designee), copies of the licenses should be retained in a credential book, as should proof of having met the requirements for renewal, such as continuing education certificates. Staff who do not renew licenses before the expiration date must cease working until the renewal has been accomplished.

Annual reports are an important management tool. Such reports provide a comprehensive overview of the student health service's operations and finances by: [25]

- documenting the effectiveness of the services provided;
- keeping upper management informed;
- relating functions to the institutional mission;
- presenting data/ information that can be used in making decisions/policy;
- creating a favorable impression;
- highlighting important trends or unusual activities, situations, or occurrences.

In short, it is an evaluation and assessment of the organization's progress in achieving its mission, goals, and objectives. The report usually includes a financial narrative, which elaborates on the importance of specific changes in financial data and unusual situations. The non-financial narrative documents a summary of activity, growth, and comparison to previous years; history; and employee accomplishments, such as productivity and development. Further, a well-done annual report is an excellent public relations tool for distribution to stakeholders.

Use of Consultants

External consultation is sometimes a useful management tool. Consultants can add objectivity and credibility to an evaluation process. They may "think out of the box," because their broad exposure to numerous clients has kept them abreast of new concepts and practices and they are not vested in the outcome of their evaluations. Some consultants are hired to resolve difficult situations and can take the "political heat" where there is intense conflict.

When contracting with an external consultant, it is essential to define the expectations of the consultation—explaining the problem (or opportunity), how long it has existed, who is involved, what the consultant is expected to do (onsite visit, interview staff, review background data), what is expected in the report, to whom the report is to be delivered, and how much it will cost. Consultants should be asked to submit a written response to the above, list his/her qualifications (education and experience), and provide a list of references. The American College Health Association also has a consultation program, which evaluates health services and provides written recommendations to the contracting institution. According to ACHA's website, the focus of a consultation can be:[24]

- reexamining the health service's scope and quality of service
- consideration of options such as privatizing the health service
- preparing for accreditation
- addressing issues such as staffing and leadership

A Word About Outsourcing

No discussion about assessment and evaluation would be complete without some mention of outsourcing or privatization. In the past few years, outsourcing portions or all of a student health service has been the subject of some controversy. Much of the concern has been based on a belief that a for-profit company cannot provide the same quality as a not-for-profit health service. Other responses have derived from an emotional perspective motivated by the perception that some outsourcing companies were using marketing tactics that bypassed the health service administration and by a fear that some (or all) health service staff might lose their employment. Without question, outsourcing decisions have been made by college/university administrations without regard to how well the health service was performing in delivering services to students. In these cases the higher administration believed (rightly or wrongly) that economic or service improvements would result from outsourcing. Or, in some cases, higher administration simply wanted to (admittedly) relieve themselves of the responsibility of overseeing a health service operation.

There are, in many cases, positive results from outsourcing, particularly ancillary services. For example, many health services outsource laboratory and radiology. In these instances, appropriate outsourcing often extends the capability and quality of services at a lower cost than performing them in the health service.

When consideration is given to outsourcing the entire program, Wertz suggested (in 1996) that the primary reasons for outsourcing are:[26]

- Cost savings and budgetary constraints
- Improve quality of services
- Contractor expertise, professional management, or better technology

The challenge to any health service program is to remain competitive and improve services in the face of declining resources. Thus, the bottom-line question for health service administration is the extent to which a change adds value (i.e., increases quality and economy).

In a 1996 presentation entitled "Why Consider Outsourcing for Student Health Services," Ericson, Mills, and Wirag reviewed a series of questions that an institution needs to ask of health service directors.[27] A full response to these questions may help a health service remain a viable entity within an institution such that the chances of outsourcing may be reduced or unlikely. These questions are:

- What am I doing to prepare for the future?
- Am I aware of the changing environments?

- Do I understand the potential impact of these changes on the student health service?
- How do I assure the student health service contributes to the institutional mission?
- Do I continually assess our own programs?
- Am I taking advantage of the opportunities, which may present themselves in the broader health care marketplace?
- Have I assessed the needs of students?
- How have I demonstrated that the health service is meeting the needs of students?
- How have I demonstrated that the health service is providing quality care?
- How have I demonstrated that the health service is competitive and cost effective?
- How have I shown consumer satisfaction?
- Have I been able to get above my own job security and look at the broader picture?

When an institution is considering outsourcing, a director has options. He or she can ignore the situation or present "self-serving" reasons not to proceed or, conversely, may participate in the review about the inclination/possibility of outsourcing the health service. The latter approach represents an opportunity for opening a dialogue with senior administrators and may help steer the process to a successful conclusion.

FINANCIAL APPROACHES AND STRUCTURES [28,29]

Assumptions Regarding College Health Financing

- The health service is a financial entity—to provide effective services year after year, there must be a continuous source of funds that is clearly defined and accepted by central administration. One of the guiding assumptions stated at the beginning of this chapter is that the institution wants to make available a set of needed services. To do this requires a physical facility, sufficient numbers of qualified personnel, equipment and supplies, and adequate financing. Thus, the health service is a self-contained financial entity within the institution that must have reliable and permanent sources of funds.
- Financing must exhibit links to plans/goals/objectives—budgeting and financing is viewed as a systematic plan for using resources (personnel, facilities, equipment) to achieve these goals and objectives.
- Funding must be adequate to support quality programs—health services are routinely compared to the standard of care in the community. If a student health service cannot meet the community standard or expectations of its stakeholders, then it may be underutilized, quality will suffer, and students will not support the program. Financing must be adequate to ensure excellence in performance. If this means postponement of some aspects of a program, so be it. It will be difficult, if not impossible, to provide a quality program of services if the funding is not adequate to support needed numbers of personnel, provide adequate space, or have available appropriate equipment/supplies.
- Agreement must exist between scope of programs and services—problems regarding the inadequacy of student health service budgets are common. Health service staff may believe that upper administration is unsympathetic in its response for more money, while

administrators believe the health service staff are being unrealistic in their demands. Often, the source of the problem may be attributed to the health service staff narrowly interpreting the purpose of their existence as only the care of sick and injured students. They must comprehend the "big picture" and how the program contributes to the overall institutional mission. The administration may, on the other hand, be operating from a belief that an adequate program already exists and any expansion will create an additional fiscal burden or liability to the college/university, and thereby may fail to perceive how the health service can positively impact the institutional community beyond direct clinical care.

Sources of Funding (Pros and Cons)

One of the most important questions in financing a health program is how the program is to be funded. The purpose of this section is to identify several options and discuss the pros and cons of each. The approach utilized may vary from campus to campus and from time to time depending upon:

- the philosophy and commitment of the administration;
- the ability of the college/university to provide the funds needed from the existing budget to maintain a quality program;
- the competition from other services who depend upon the same fund source to operate their program;
- the fee recommended by a fee committee composed of students and perhaps faculty and staff;
- the willingness of the institution to look at non-tuition revenue sources.

Prepaid Health Fee[29, p.28]

Prepayment is defined as payment in advance by a designated group (for example, full-time students) for a specified set of services for a definite time period. The fees are established according to the number of students expected to be eligible for services and the projected expenditures for the next year. A designated (segregated) health fee is identified as a separate cost item for tuition and fees. Fees are collected by the institution, and the funds remain on-campus for use by the health service. In this instance they may be considered auxiliary fees; administrators of these funds typically have more administrative control and managerial flexibility than with tuition dollars. Because designated fees are separate from the general tuition fund, they are not in direct competition with academic areas for operating dollars.

Pros
- The burden of health care is borne by the entire group at a cost less than if paid individually.
- The funding of the program is predictable and stable, which allows for more accurate financial projections.
- Fee-for-service collection mechanisms and resulting logistical problems and costs are eliminated.

- Pooling of fees increases the purchasing power of the health service.
- Through prepayment, students are able to budget for the cost of their health care.
- Institutional loans or scholarships often cover the fee.
- Funds are typically available for those activities of the health service which are not related to direct clinical care (e.g., public health responsibilities, health education and preventive services).

Cons

- Students who never use the program are paying a fee for which they will receive no clinical benefit.
- In times of declining enrollment the revenue will decrease.
- The program is "at risk" to provide care for each student seeking help.

Tuition or General Revenue

In this arrangement, funds for operating the health program come from the college/university tuition or general fund. They are prepaid but not segregated and not separate from academic general budgets. In public institutions the funds may come directly from tuition dollars reallocated back to the institution by the state or may be combined with a general (or non-instructional) fee.

Pros

- Confirms the institution's commitment to provide health services to students.
- The burden is borne by the entire group.
- Institutional loans or scholarships often cover the fee (as an "unidentified" portion of tuition).

Cons

- The health service is in direct competition with academic or other student service areas for financial support.
- The amount of funds may be decreased in times when the state reduces its support of the institution *or* when the institution reduces expenditures for nonacademic programs.
- The revenue will decrease when enrollment declines.
- Less flexibility and financial control by the health service.

Fee-for-Service

With fee-for-service financing, the student pays a fee each time he or she uses the health service. Though there are some health services which receive a majority of their funding from fee-for-service billing, the authors are aware of only a few which are currently financed wholly through a fee-for-service approach. Most often this method is used to supplement funds provided through one or more of the other financial approaches.

Pros

- In times of tight budgets or reduced budgets, it can provide additional income so that a constant level of service can be maintained.

- It educates the students about the realities of medical care and costs.
- It increases the student's valuation of services received.
- It decreases overutilization or unnecessary use of the health services.
- It decreases the cost to some individuals, i.e., non-users.
- It allows the student to avoid the health service and obtain his/her care elsewhere if he or she does not like the health service.

Cons

- Does not support financing for health service programs (such as public health activities) not involving direct clinical care.
- Students rarely budget for health care, so out-of-pocket costs are problematic.
- Underutilization may result, because students may not come in early in the course of their illness/disease because of having to pay a fee *or* some students may inappropriately delay or forgo care because of out-of-pocket costs.
- Underutilization will result because students will not take advantage of preventive programs.
- No way to finance health promotion programs.
- Financial consideration may outweigh medical decisions for both patients and practitioners at a time when students have no or few funds or other options available.
- Administrative costs of collection may increase.

Insurance

The major purpose of a third-party indemnity or self-insurance health plan is to supplement breadth of care by assuring financial access to services that are not practical to provide on campus. It is *not* a substitute for services which can be provided at the health service. Since all insurance premiums (including self-insured plans) have some overhead or administrative fee attached, students generally pay more for services provided at the health service through insurance than if the service were paid directly by a health fee. The general guidelines regarding what to provide in the on-campus health service are those services which are most commonly and predictably required and that have low unit costs, e.g., primary care, immunizations, allergy desensitization. Medical services to be *insured* should include those which are less predictably utilized and which have high unit costs; e.g., emergency room care or hospitalization. Many schools require some type of health insurance, either through a school plan (mandatory enrollment) or their own/family plan. Chapter 17 provides an in-depth review of insurance principles and practices at college and universities.

Pros

- Assures financial access to services such that the student will not have to interrupt his/her educational program to pay off large medical bills.
- Makes available a broader range of services than is feasible to be provided at the health service.

Cons

- Can be more costly to students if the insurance program is used as a substitute for services which can be more economically provided on campus.
- There may be "hidden barriers" to coverage (e.g., deductibles, co-pays, and scheduled benefits) that are not readily apparent.

Supplemental Sources

Some student health services are able to supplement their income by providing services to faculty/staff for on-the-job injuries, hepatitis B immunizations, OSHA physicals, providing bloodborne-pathogen control programs, or occupational health programs.

Further, many health services offer fee-for-service coverage to non-students, including students' families and less commonly, faculty/staff and their families. (See Chapter 20.) A second common source of supplemental income is by contracts (health science student exam and immunizations, provision of services to students attending other schools, billing for extra services to an athletic department, and others). Because of the intensive nature of these procedures, many student health services are able to assess a fee for the provision of such services. Other health services have contracted with nearby academic institutions that do not have a health service. Some health services have obtained grants or research funds which support portions of their program. In recent years many health services have obtained funds to aid in the development of drug and alcohol education and prevention programs and/or have contributed data for pharmaceutical research studies.

Pros

- Funds from the above sources can supplement the health service budget, thus reducing the need to ask for large increases in health fees.
- Involvement in activities that serve other portions of the college/university community can create a positive image of the program.
- Reliance by the university on the health service to perform these essential functions helps solidify the health service's role within the institution.

Cons

- Health service staff could become overly involved in the activities related to the above items at the expense of providing quality services to the students.
- "Soft" money for grants or research funds cannot be used to fund permanent programs.

Combinations of Funding Sources

In reality, most schools utilize a combination of the above funding mechanisms based on how the program is conceptualized by students and administration. For example, if students do not want to be "nickled-and-dimed" they will probably support a prepaid fee that pays for most, if not all, of the services provided and they will discourage use of fee-for-services charges. Administrators will probably support a designated prepaid fee if they want to assure that financial barriers are not a factor in seeking timely health care or if they want the health service to be out of the politics of the "academic funding arena." It is more than likely that whatever method is adopted, the philosophy of the major stakeholders and their views of the health service will be reflected.

By the pooling of finances, the cost of illness is borne by the entire group rather than by the sick/injured, and at a cost less than that available in the community. For the student and his/her parents, no new expense is involved, costs are less because of shared risks, and financial responsibility is still with the student. Thus, the funding of a health program is a way of meeting the need for health care from within the academic institution such that both student and institutional goals are facilitated.

TEN CHARACTERISTICS OF SUCCESSFUL COLLEGE HEALTH PROGRAMS

How Characteristics Were Determined

Together, two of the three authors of this chapter (WE, DM) have many years of service to the college health field and the health field in general. In each of their experiences it became increasingly apparent that there were factors that consistently determined program success, prompting collaboration on a study to determine the impact of Healthcare legislative and market reform on student health services. They identified and listed the characteristics and compared notes with their colleagues. The most successful programs tend to have most or all of these characteristics.

Brief Description and Discussion of the Ten Characteristics

1. Involvement of Stakeholders. A successful student health service is able to identify and connect with stakeholders, and to address their expectations and concerns.
2. Link to Institutional Mission. The SHS will more likely be viewed as an essential service when it is perceived as making a vital contribution to the success of the college or university.
3. Services Fulfill Need. The SHS staff understands the composition of the "student body" (number of students eligible for service, age, gender, race) and has access to historical data to determine the reasons for past use of services (incidence of diseases and injuries) and can therefore make predictions on what services are/will be needed.
4. Staff Committed to Service. Employees are concerned about customer service, care about students, and will respond to a crisis.
5. Service Efficiency and Productivity. To obtain efficiency and productivity, the resources are properly aligned and employees are working in positions for which they are trained and qualified and working at a pace commensurate with the setting. The use of benchmarking techniques is one way for an SHS administrator to review the efficiency and productivity of the service.
6. Appropriately Uses Technology. Successful programs have carefully defined the use and benefits of all software applications, selected appropriate programs, trained staff to take full advantage of program capability, maintained the hardware, evaluated programs, and followed a replacement schedule for programs and equipment. To *not* move forward in

this area can result in increased isolation of the health service from the larger healthcare community, inadequately prepared staff, and ultimately lesser-quality care and service.

7. Funding Keeps Pace with the Need. The budget is adjusted on a timely basis to respond to changes in technology and patient needs.

8. Minimal Uninsured Population. The institution takes the position that the number of uninsured students will be minimized by requiring some form of health insurance coverage, either through their parents, employer-group, purchase of a private health insurance policy, or through the college/university-sponsored plan.

9. Services Are Reviewed Periodically. An ongoing, systematic analysis of services is performed on a regularly recurring basis.

10. Adequate and Efficient Physical Facilities. The appearance and adequacy of the facility influences patients' perceptions and evaluation of the quality of services. This perception is influenced by the amount of space, operational efficiency, modern appearance, cleanliness, and lighting.

A FINAL WORD

One final thought is important regarding the administration and financing of a college health program; the program must be "connected" to the institution as well as the student body. The program must be woven into the fabric of the college/university environment such that everyone understands and appreciates the contribution that the health service makes to the students and institution. The program must be perceived to provide more than medical care, more than health promotion and education, and more than collaboration with others. It must be understood as a meaningful service, one that impacts the students throughout their lives and assures them the maximum number of productive years as contributing members of society.

The opportunities to which the health service can contribute will continue to change and evolve with the progress in the medical and behavioral sciences, higher education, and in the provision of health care. College health administrators must keep abreast of these changes and prepare the organization for the next step: They must be change agents by exploring ways in which the connections of the health service remain viable, not only with the institution, but within the larger community as well. The most significant role for an administrator is to be continually aware of his/her professional surroundings and trends and to develop a response that assures that the health service will remain a relevant contributor to the educational process.

NOTES

The original idea and draft of the "Ten Characteristics of Successful College Health Programs" was the result of consulting work with Stephen L. Beckley of Stephen L. Beckley and Associates, Inc. 1995–96.

For those interested in further discussion of strategic planning, the following sources may be useful.

Ginter, Peter M.; Swayne, Linda E.; & Duncan, W. Jack (1998). *Strategic Management of Health Care Organizations, 3d Ed.* Malden, Massachusetts: Blackwell Publishers, Inc.

Blair, J. & Fottler, M. (1998). *Strategic leadership for medical groups: Navigating your strategic web.* San Francisco, California: Jossey-Bass.

Fulk, J., & DeSanctis, G. (1999). *Shaping organizational form: Communication, connection, and community.* Thousand Oaks, California: Sage.

The references shown below offer additional detailed information on financial matters in health organizations:

Gapenski, Louis C. (1999). *Healthcare Finance: An Introduction to Accounting and Financial Management*, Chicago, Illinois: Health Administration Press.

Neumann, Bruce R.; Clement, Jan P.; & Cooper, Jean C. (1997). *Financial Management: Concepts and Applications for Health Care Organizations, 4th Ed.*, Dubuque, Iowa: Kendall/Hunt Publishing Company.

Prince, Thomas R. (1998). *Strategic Management for Health Care Entities: Creative Frameworks for Financial and Operational Analysis,* Chicago, Illinois: American Hospital Publishing, Inc.

REFERENCES

1. Microsoft® Word 97 SR-2. © 1983–97 Microsoft Corporation.

2. Yukl G. *Leadership in Organizations*, 3d Edition. Englewood Cliffs, NJ: Prentice Hall; 1994:43.

3. Fiedler FE. Research on leadership selection and training: One view of the future. *Administrative Science Quarterly.* 1996;41(2):242.

4. Chambers HE. The agencies of leadership. *Executive Excellence.* 1999;16(8):12.

5. Bass B. *Bass & Stogdill's Handbook of Leadership: Theory, Research, and Managerial Applications*, 3d Ed. New York: The Free Press; 1990.

6. Schein, EH. *The Corporate Culture Survival Guide: Sense and Nonsense About Culture Change.* San Francisco, CA: Jossey-Bass; 1999.

7. American College Health Association, Guidelines for a College Health Program. Standards Revision Work Group. Baltimore, MD; 1999:2–3.

8. Hudak RP, Brooke Jr. PP, Finstuen K, Trolinson J. Management competencies for medical practice executives: Skills, knowledge and abilities required for the future. *J Health Adm Ed.* 1999 Fall;15(4):219–39.

9. Accreditation Handbook for Ambulatory Health Care 2000. Accreditation Association for Ambulatory Health Care, Core Standards, p. 27.

10. Accreditation Manual for Ambulatory Health Care, Volume I, Standards. Oakbrook Terrace, IL: Joint Commission on Accreditation of Healthcare Organizations; 2000.

11. Daft RL, Lengel RH, Trevino LK. Message equivocality, media selection, and manager performance: Implications for information systems. *MIS Quarterly.* 1987;11(3):355–366.

12. Daft RL, Lengel RH. Organizational information requirements, media richness, and structural design. *Management Science.* 1986;22(5):554–571.

13. Mohr JJ, Sohi RS. Communication flows in distribution channels: Impact on assessments of communication quality and satisfaction. *Journal of Retailing.* 1995;71(4):393–417.

14. Rakich JS, Longest BB Jr., Darr K. *Managing Health Services Organizations: Strategic Planning and Marketing,* 3d Ed. Baltimore: Health Professions Press; 1992:320–321.

15. Likert R, Likert J, G. *New Ways of Managing Conflict.* New York: McGraw-Hill; 1976.

16. Tannenbaum R, Schmidt, WH. How to choose a leadership pattern. *Harvard Business Review.* May–June 1973;51:162–180.

17. Weed, LL. *Medical Records, Medical Education, and Patient Care; The Problem-Oriented Record as a Basic Tool.* Cleveland: Cleveland Press of Case Western Reserve University; 1971.

18. March JG, Weisinger-Baylon R. Ambiguity and Command: Organizational Perspectives on Military Decision Making. Boston: Pitman Publishing; 1986.

19. Takahashi N. A single garbage can model and the degree of anarchy in Japanese firms. *Human Relations.* 1997;50(1):91–109.

20. Pablo AL, Sitkin SB. Acquisition decision-making processes: The central role of risk. *Journal of Management.* 1996; 22(5):723–747.

21. Swanson DL. Neoclassical economic theory, executive control, and organizational outcomes. *Human Relations.* 1996; 496:735–757.

22. Health Insurance Portability and Accounting (HIPAA). HR. 1941. Introduced in the 106th Congress in the House by Rep. Gary A. Condit (18th District, California) and with sixty-eight co-sponsors on May 25, 1999.

23. Institute of Medicine report entitled, "To Err Is Human: Building A Safer Health System." November 1999.

24. ACHA Website: http://www.acha.org/prg-service/csp.htm

25. Schneiter P. *The Annual Report: Indispensable Management Tool.* College Health Executive Development Series. Edited by E. D. Lovett. Provo, UT: Brigham Young University. 1973:111–119.

26. Wertz R. Outsourcing Survey of 938 Schools. Published by National Association of College Auxiliary Services, Charlottesville, VA. 1997.

27. Ericson W, Mills DJ, Wirag RJ. Why Consider Outsourcing for Student Health Services? Presentation to the Mid-America College Health Association, 1996.

28. Edison GR. Prepayment versus fee for service. *J Am Coll Health Assoc.* 1970;18:325–329.

29. Osborne MM. Financing the health program. In A.S. Knowles (Ed.), *Handbook of College and University Administration,* Vol. 2. New York: McGraw-Hill; 1970.

CHAPTER 4

QUALITY IMPROVEMENT AND ACCREDITATION ISSUES IN COLLEGE HEALTH

Betty Anne Johnson, MD, PhD, and Betty Reppert, PA-C, MPH

OVERVIEW

The mission of every student health service (SHS) is to provide high-quality health care in a cost-effective manner. Quality health care can be defined in many different ways, however, and until recently, there was little agreement on how best to attain it. The Institute of Medicine defines quality of health care as "the degree to which health care services for individuals and populations increases the likelihood of desired health outcomes and are consistent with current professional knowledge."[1] This definition reflects the growing consensus that the measurement of quality in health care should also include some assessment of outcomes of that care. As underscored by Chassin, it is important to understand that "quality is not the same as good outcomes. A patient may receive the best possible health care and still suffer a bad outcome, because medicine is a probabilistic phenomenon."[2]

At most, therefore, we should expect that high-quality health care will *increase the likelihood* of a good health outcome, and any attempt to measure overall quality in a health care system should involve assessment of both the health care processes and the outcomes of those processes. Further, most experts agree that quality health care should be provided at the lowest possible cost, using the appropriate level and amount of service. Formal quality improvement programs are designed to help health care organizations achieve all of these goals.

HISTORICAL PERSPECTIVE
(QUALITY ASSURANCE VERSUS QUALITY IMPROVEMENT)

Dr. W. Edwards Deming was an American statistician who developed a comprehensive theory for quality improvement. While serving as a consultant to the Japanese census after World War II, he educated Japanese scientists and engineers as to his quality improvement theory and created a total transformation in Japanese business, known today as the "Japanese Industrial Miracle." After witnessing this success in Japan, American industry also began implementing Deming's quality improvement theories.

In the health care industry, quality assurance (QA) programs had been in operation for years. These programs had traditionally involved a peer review process charged with distinguishing "bad" performers from "good" performers. The goal of QA was to maintain an acceptable level of performance by eliminating nonconforming outliers.[3] This "sort and shoot" mentality often resulted in a climate of defensiveness and lack of cooperation by medical staff. Quality improvement (QI), on the other hand, examines the entire work process to identify significant sources of variation that result in process breakdown. QI acknowledges that breakdowns in work processes are generally not the fault of the people doing their jobs; rather, they can be attributed to problems within the process itself. Therefore, assigning blame and responsibility to an individual perceived to be "at fault" will not fix the problem. QI also focuses on *improvement opportunities*, encouraging high achievers to influence the work process positively through implementation of "best practices."[3]

KEY CONCEPTS OF QUALITY IMPROVEMENT

The strength of the QI model as developed by Deming and expanded by others is derived from three key features.

Respect the needs of the "customer."

The needs of both "external customers" and "internal customers" must be understood and met. In the health care industry, "external customers" are usually the patients. Traditionally, health care providers have been reluctant to refer to patients as "customers" or "clients," yet this terminology reflects a growing sensitivity to both the clinical needs and the perceived needs of the health care consumer. College health providers have traditionally been more "customer-focused" than most other health care providers, possibly because of their unique patient base and because of pressures exerted by parents and university administration. Strategies for enhancing this service relationship with the "student customer" have been well described elsewhere.[4]

It is also important to understand that "student customers" may have different perceived needs than traditional patients. Students may be more interested in immediate access to service (same-day appointments or "walk-in" services) than continuity of care (seeing the same provider each visit). They may also be more interested in decreasing or eliminating "out-of-pocket" expenses (deductibles and co-pays). Further, their perceived health education needs may extend beyond learning how to manage their current illness or injury and include how to navigate the complex health care environment (health insurance, specialty referrals, and complex diagnostic testing).

Other "external customers" in the college health setting include payers (parents, health plans) and university administration. Parents and administration want assurance that the

SHS performs at least as well as community providers when quality is measured. In addition, these external customers are interested in keeping health care costs low for students.

QI theory defines "internal customers" as the employees within the SHS, and other teams or departments within the larger college/university organization (e.g., Division of Student Affairs; the main referral laboratory or the ED at the teaching hospital). In this context, QI encourages each worker to do his or her best for the next person within the organization and to expect the best from others as well. Process quality is strongly influenced by how staff members relate to one another. QI emphasizes understanding workers' needs as well as customer needs.

Process inefficiency results from process variation.

Most inefficiencies in work processes are the result of measurable variations within the process itself. QI requires that work processes be studied using solid statistical methods and that formal problem-solving approaches be used to decrease variation in those processes. The focus, therefore, is shifted away from individual workers and onto the work process itself. For example, when walk-in patients experience long waits to be seen, rather than blaming individual providers for inadequate productivity, a quality improvement approach would collect data on all factors that influence the wait-time (e.g., difficulties predicting walk-in volume throughout the day, inadequate staffing, inefficient triage of more complex patients, and similar problems). Problem-solving, then, is directed at mechanisms to decrease the variation in the wait-time and more closely approach an acceptable standard.

A team approach is the best approach.

A team approach is the most effective means of identifying problems in work processes and of generating solutions. QI is an organization-wide effort, involving workers in every department and at every professional level, clinical and non-clinical. Fundamental to QI theory is respect for employees and their knowledge, which is demonstrated by encouraging their active involvement in process improvement. Leaders must be willing to listen to the workers who actually perform the process and who are the real experts on what works and what doesn't. QI fosters communication and breaks down hierarchical barriers that are often present in health care organizations.

BENEFITS AND CAVEATS OF A QUALITY IMPROVEMENT PROGRAM

Although health care organizations may initiate QI programs to satisfy accreditation or regulatory requirements, other benefits become obvious over time. Some of these benefits include increased patient and employee satisfaction, improved efficiency and internal communication, increased consistency in work processes, and decreased costs. More recently, HMOs have begun publishing measures of clinical performance as a means of strengthening market share. College health services, too, may use QI to enhance visibility and assure students, parents, and administration of the quality of their organization.

Some caveats should be considered prior to initiating a QI program. First, QI requires a long-term commitment to continuous change. QI is not a "quick-fix." The leadership, in particular, must not only be knowledgeable about QI theory and techniques, but must also endorse QI, be willing to commit time, staff, and resources to the program, and be prepared to meet resistance. As pointed out by Balestracci and Barlow, "Mysterious resistance is often encountered even when implementing a change that is obviously beneficial to a specific area."[3] Staff may already feel overwhelmed handling the daily workload of patients and feel that any attempt at QI activities will only make a difficult day unbearable. Involving as many employees as possible in the change-planning process will improve its chances of success. Participation leads to ownership and ownership engenders enthusiasm.

QUALITY IMPROVEMENT VERSUS OUTCOMES ASSESSMENT

Improvement in work processes has been readily demonstrated by the use of QI programming. Curiously, it has been more difficult to prove that QI programs directly increase the likelihood of good health outcomes for patient populations.[5] One possible explanation for this phenomenon is that outcomes of care are influenced by many factors outside the health care organization's control (e.g., social and environmental factors, comorbidities, patient behavior). Furthermore, when assessing health outcomes, it is important to choose valid quality measures. Such outcome measures must be closely related to processes of care which were manipulated to attempt to improve that outcome.[2]

Outcomes which are important to students, parents, and university administration may differ from those traditionally thought important by health care providers. Whereas health care providers and insurance companies may concentrate on outcomes such as decreased ED and hospitalization rates, students may feel that improved psychosocial functioning, in addition to a sense of physical well-being, is more important. Decreased class absenteeism from illness may be important to students, parents, and faculty. University administration will be interested in improving retention rates for students with medical diagnoses such as mood disorders, attention deficit hyperactivity disorder, and learning disabilities. If the SHS embarks on a QI project to improve any of these outcomes, it is important to carefully design the program to maximally effect these outcomes and to choose valid quality measures when collecting the data.

INITIATING A QUALITY IMPROVEMENT PROGRAM*

QIP Advisory Body

The first step in developing a QIP is to organize a team of interdisciplinary-practice staff to design, implement, monitor, and assess change in the health care processes within the SHS. This QIP Advisory Body should consist of representatives from all units within the SHS and should reflect all layers of professional staff.

---

* A glossary of terms defining the terminology used in the QIP is shown in Appendix 1.

The interdisciplinary composition of the QIP Advisory Body is critical to its success, enhancing communication and giving ownership to the people who are responsible for the health care process under study. These individuals study the process, design changes to the process, carry out the process, and will ultimately be affected by any changes to the process. The QIP Advisory Body should meet on a regular basis throughout the year and review the information gathered during the previous review cycle.

QIP Coordinator

The QIP Coordinator should have superior organizational and communication skills, and ideally, formal training in QI, through workshops or seminars. Although the coordinator does not have to be a clinician, a highly respected clinician may be more persuasive in convincing other clinicians, particularly physicians, to endorse QI. The QIP Coordinator is charged with the overall operation of the quality improvement program, including:

- prioritizing studies
- data collection, storage, and analysis
- development and reporting of preliminary action plans
- implementation and monitoring of final action plans
- communication of QIP activities with leadership and staff

Choosing a Methodology

Of the various QI methodologies described in the literature,[6] two specific models are of particular interest to college health service managers. The first model has been proposed by the Accreditation Association for Ambulatory Health Care (AAAHC)[7] and endorsed by the American College Health Association in its "Guidelines for a College Health Program."[8] This five-step program, "closing the QI loop," includes the following:

- identification of important problems in the care of patients
- evaluation of the frequency, severity, and source of suspected problems
- implementation of measures to resolve suspected problems
- reevaluation to assure that corrective action achieved and sustained the desired outcome; if problems persist, an alternative action plan is implemented
- communication to staff as well as leadership about all aspects of the quality improvement activities

In addition, the AAAHC has developed an Institute of Quality Improvement (IQI) that offers consulting services and provides education and research on clinical performance improvement in the ambulatory setting. An SHS can choose to participate in this QI program and can submit data from its own institution. The data is then analyzed by the IQI and reported graphically, thereby allowing the SHS to compare its performance to its peers.

The second methodology is used by the Joint Commission on Accreditation of Healthcare Organizations (JCAHO), and is detailed in this chapter. JCAHO offers several resources on this topic including two manuals, *Performance Improvement in Ambulatory Care*[9] and *Using Performance Improvement Tools in Ambulatory Care.*[10] Additionally, JCAHO offers several workshops and seminars dedicated to accreditation standards and performance improvement in ambulatory care.

Design-Measure-Assess-Improve

JCAHO utilizes the Design-Measure-Assess-Improve process improvement model. This model is outlined as follows:[9]

Design

Determine data needed to monitor the improvement in the process.
Determine tests for the improvement monitoring plan.

Measure

Collect and analyze data on improvement in the process

Assess

Establish decision/review points to determine the effectiveness of changes
Assess the effects of improvements
Analyze the improvement results

Improve

Team meets on a regular basis to determine what was learned
Tests or actions are repeated, if necessary, to ensure improvement in the process
Generalized improvements

IMPLEMENTING A QUALITY IMPROVEMENT PROGRAM

Design

The planning phase of the QIP may involve design of a new health care process for the SHS (such as adding a travel clinic) or redesign of an existing process to improve outcomes (e.g., decrease class absenteeism for asthmatics by changing the asthma management protocol to reflect National Heart, Lung and Blood Institute guidelines).[11] The following six principles are helpful in designing QIP activities:

QIP activities should be driven by the strategic priorities of the SHS.

Many SHSs have mission statements and strategic plans which are intermeshed with the strategic plan of the university. As an example, at many universities, the SHS administratively reports to the division of student affairs. One common goal of a division of student affairs is to monitor and report on the quality of the student experience. Therefore, one of the objectives in an SHS strategic plan should be to quantitatively determine student satisfaction with the SHS. To accomplish this objective, an annual patient satisfaction survey can be performed by sampling a set of users of the SHS stratified by age, sex, and race. The results are analyzed and compared with results from previous years to identify trends, and these trends, if any, are reported to the QIP Advisory Body for consideration. A new QI project may be designed on the basis of these results.

QIP activities should address both patient-focused and organization-focused functions.

As defined by JCAHO, patient-focused functions (patient rights and organization ethics, assessment of patients, care of patients, education of patients and family, and continuity of care) involve direct and indirect care of the patient, including assessment, treatment, and education of patients. Organization functions (improving organization performance, leadership, management of the environment of care, management of human resources, management of information, and surveillance, prevention, and control of infection) have no direct patient-care involvement but enable patient-care activities to take place through governance, facility safety, adequate staffing, and technical support. Table 1 gives examples of both patient-focused and organization-focused functions that have been sources of QIP projects at the authors' SHS.

Priority should be given to those aspects of patient care that are high-volume, high-risk, and/or problem-prone.

Health care processes that affect a large percentage of patients should be chosen for study. In college health, possibilities might include appropriate antibiotic usage for respiratory infections, management of asthma exacerbations, or notification of patients of abnormal Pap smear results. Certain diagnoses might be selected for study because they are high risk (e.g., anorexia nervosa, pelvic inflammatory disease, pyelonephritis); certain health care processes might be selected for study because they are high risk (e.g., medication dispensing errors). Problem-prone areas might include waiting times for walk-in patients or timely referrals for medication evaluation for students with depression.

Patient outcomes and satisfaction should be emphasized in the QIP.

In addition to surveys of patient satisfaction, specific patient outcomes should be monitored. Here it is important that valid quality measures are selected. First, the health care outcome should be meaningful in the college health setting. Current literature contains many citations defining and measuring quality of care for diabetic, hypertensive, and asthmatic patients.[12,13,14,15] However, the approach that is used for these patients may not be so useful for college health. Patients with diabetes and hypertension represent a relatively small proportion of the total number of patients seen in an SHS. Furthermore, they may be followed primarily by specialists outside the SHS; therefore, a quality measure such as the level of glycosylated hemoglobin may not be valid, as the SHS may have little impact on this parameter. Although the incidences of diabetic retinopathy or stroke are important long-term outcomes of these chronic diseases, they are unlikely to be measurable over the period of time that most students spend in college. For asthmatic patients, the health outcomes that are frequently cited in the literature include ED utilization

Table 1. Virginia Commonwealth University Quality Improvement Project

PATIENT-FOCUSED
1. Patient Rights and Organization Ethics
    Informed Consent
2. Assessment of Patient
    Laboratory Services
        Quality Control
        Patient notification of abnormal Pap smear results
    Completion of health history form by third visit
    Diagnosis Reviews
    Practitioner Reviews
3. Care of Patient
    Pharmacy Services
        Adverse drug reactions
        Prescription pad security
        Documentation of current medications/allergies
        Sample medications
    Diagnosis Reviews
    Practitioner Reviews
4. Education of Patients and Family
    Documentation of education/prevention on diagnosis reviews
5. Continuity of Care
    Timely receipt of information for referrals, ER visits, etc.
    Diagnosis Reviews
    Practitioner Reviews

ORGANIZATION-FOCUSED
1. Environment of Care
    Biohazardous waste handling
    Sharps box security/safety
    Staff fire extinguisher training
2. Infection Control
    Post-procedure complications
    Staff hepatitis B and PPD log
3. Human Resources
    Credentialing of licensed independent practitioners
4. Information Manangement
    Timely completion of charting
    Receipt of information from referrals
5. Leadership
    Patient satisfaction survey
    Staff satisfaction survey
6. Quality or Performance Improvement

and hospitalizations. It may be more appropriate in a college health setting to target (as important outcomes) a decrease in class absenteeism, ability to participate in sports activities, psychosocial functioning, or quality-of-life issues.

Second, if a particular health care outcome is chosen for study, it should be closely linked to processes of care that can be manipulated to improve that outcome.[2] For example, education about emergency contraception and its provision might be an excellent quality measure, because these processes of care have been shown to reduce the unintended pregnancy rate.[16] It would be unlikely, however, that a SHS could show a reduction in the number of cases of cervical cancer in users of their women's health clinic by decreasing the number of Pap smears with "no endocervical cells."

The individual workers who perform the health care processes on a daily basis are often the best source for identifying both problems and solutions for the QIP.

Fundamental to QI theory is a profound respect for the "worker." The worker may have the best appreciation for the inefficiencies in existing processes. Berwick poses five questions for workers:[17]

- Do you ever waste time waiting, when you should not have to?
- Do you ever redo your work because something failed the first time?
- Do the procedures you use waste steps, duplicate efforts, or frustrate you through their unpredictability?
- Is information that you need ever lost?
- Does communication ever fail?

Respect for employees and their knowledge and soliciting their ideas for solutions to problems such as these help enlist their active involvement in the improvement process and decrease resistance to change.

QIP activities should draw upon knowledge from expert sources.

In the design of a new health care process or in redesigning an existing one, a wealth of information is available in the literature, on websites and electronic mailing lists, and through consultation with other SHSs. Clinical guidelines for prevention and management of many diseases have been published. The QI Advisory Body should assure that all of the health care processes in the SHS clinic are based upon up-to-date information.

Measure

This phase of QIP implementation involves collection and analysis of data about the health care process or the outcome being studied. Appropriately collected, valid, baseline data are essential for initially understanding the process, for decision-making about improvements, and for determining if any changes actually occurred because of planned interventions. Measurements can also be used to determine if a critical process (for example, handling of narcotics) is "in control" (within acceptable limits of variation).

Many useful internal databases may already exist within the SHS. Some SHSs may use a medical information system which links appointment scheduling, patient registration, cash collections, and billing with ancillary services such as laboratory, pharmacy, and radiology. These relational databases can be used to study such diverse areas as practitioner productivity, prescribing and test-ordering patterns, time to next available appointment by provider/type of appointment/length of appointment, diagnosis frequency, surveillance of infectious diseases, and others. Relational databases can eliminate the need for chart review; for example, urine culture data and pharmacy records could be linked to determine if appropriate antibiotics were given for urinary tract infection.[18] Another approach to data collection for a QI program is to plan the data collection as part of the charting and documentation for a care process—for example, charting nursing care by protocol on preprinted forms, thus assuring standardization of care, decreased charting time, and easy data retrieval for QI review.[19]

Patient satisfaction should be surveyed on a regular basis, using valid statistical methods. A rich literature exists about assessing patient satisfaction,[20,21,22] including information on how to write a survey specific to an SHS.[23]

In addition to collecting data for other purposes, the QIP Advisory Body should collect data specific to the health care process being studied. Therefore, the Advisory Body needs to establish *indicators*, i.e., measures that are quantitative (can be expressed in units of measurement), valid (identify events that warrant review), and reliable (accurately and completely identify occurrences; yield the same result when repeated by the same observer on multiple occasions or when multiple observers measure a single event).[9] Indicators may be measures of the process itself or measures of the outcomes of that process.

Indicators may be of two types: sentinel-event indicators or aggregate-data indicators. Sentinel-event indicators capture data about an event or occurrence that is of such significance that it requires investigation each time such an indicator is identified. In the SHS setting, an example of sentinel-event indicators might be an unscheduled hospital admission within 24 hours for the same complaint expressed at the clinic visit. Other examples include a missed diagnosis or a misdiagnosis resulting in a serious delay in treatment or a medication error resulting in student injury or death. Sentinel-event indicators should signal a mandatory investigation, but these indicators are rare and therefore should not be the sole measure of quality in the SHS.

Aggregate-data indicators are more useful measures of quality because they quantify processes or outcomes that may be related to many causes. These events may occur frequently. Aggregate data indicators consist of two types: rate-based indicators and continuous-variable indicators. Rate-based indicators are proportions or ratios. For example:

$$\frac{\text{\# of patients with abnormal Pap smear results who were notified}}{\text{\# of patients with abnormal Pap smear results}}$$

$$\frac{\text{\# of sharps box containers} > 3/4 \text{ full}}{\text{\# of sharps box containers in the clinic}}$$

$$\frac{\text{\# of clinical staff recveiving the influenza vaccine}}{\text{\# of eligible clinical staff}}$$

$$\frac{\text{\# of patients receiving a quinolone for UTI}}{\text{\# of patients with UTIs}}$$

Continuous-variable indicators are aggregate-data indicators whose values may fall anywhere along a continuous scale. Examples of continuous-variable indicators are the number of no-show appointments by day of week, the number of students diagnosed with sexually transmitted infections, or the number of prescriptions dispensed.

Indicators are often chosen from one of the nine dimensions of performance or quality.[9] These nine dimensions are listed and defined in Appendix 2. By scrutiny of these nine dimensions of performance, an SHS can not only determine the efficacy and appropriateness of a health care process ("Are we doing the right thing?"), but also assess this process for its availability, timeliness, effectiveness, continuity, safety, and efficiency, as well as the respect and caring with which the process is performed ("Are we doing the right thing well?"). The advantage to this approach is that each dimension can be measured and, therefore, improved. Appendix 3 gives a detailed look at a QIP project demonstrating the use of these types of measures.

Assess

To be useful, the data collected in the "Measure" phase must be analyzed and interpreted. Then the leaders can make judgments, formulate action plans, and implement improvements of existing processes. Additionally, assessment is particularly important if the SHS has developed a new process, (e.g., adding a travel clinic.) Performance of this new process should be compared to expectations, with patient satisfaction assessed as an outcome.

Assessment requires comparing data with some point of reference. Reference points may be of four types:[9]

- historical patterns within the SHS (e.g., comparison with a longitudinal internal database)
- aggregate external reference databases and benchmarking
- practice guidelines or clinical protocols
- desired performance targets or thresholds

Historical Patterns

After an SHS has collected data over time, current performance can be compared with past performance, allowing the organization to act as its own control group. If the format of many of the questions has been essentially unchanged over time, it is possible to compare results with previous years' performance.

Historical data comparison allows analysis of variation in the process. There are two types of causes for variation in a process: common-cause variation and special-cause variation. Common-cause variation results from random variation; a process that varies only because of common causes is said to be stable. This type of stable process can be improved. For example:

Patient satisfaction with clinic appointment availability has been collected for many years.

The percentage of patients responding either neutrally or favorably to this question varies between 80-85% over the past five years. Analysis of "reason for appointment" reveals that 15% of patient appointment visits could be potentially handled over the phone with an appropriate level of professional consultation. Based on this information, the SHS decides to institute a triage mechanism for appointment scheduling. The resulting decrease in demand for clinic appointments results in shorter waits for appointments. When patient satisfaction with appointment availability is assessed the following year, the rate of satisfaction has increased to 90%.

The other type of variation, special-cause variation, results from special circumstances that may be difficult to predict. This type of cause results in a marked variation in the process. Addressing special-cause variation eliminates aberrant performance but does not improve the overall level of performance. For example:

A provider resigns with short notice in the middle of the influenza season. Patient satisfaction with clinic appointment availability drops significantly for that year. Hiring replacement staff for the following year results in a return to "baseline" for patient satisfaction on this aspect of care.

Aggregate External Reference Databases and Benchmarking

Comparisons between and among SHSs are useful performance measurements. ACHA regularly carries out national benchmarking projects and health-risk behaviors projects. Additionally, ACHA collects information on immunization practices at its member colleges and universities, allowing an SHS to compare its immunization program with programs at other institutions.

The Institute for Quality Improvement (IQI) of the AAAHC, in collaboration with ACHA, has developed a prospective, inexpensive, clinical performance measurement program designed to assist SHSs in examining their compliance with the asthma management standards issued by the National Heart, Lung, and Blood Institute. Data collected by an SHS is submitted to the IQI, which then analyzes and reports the results graphically to participating institutions. The SHS can then view its performance on these standards relative to that of its peers.

Practice Guidelines or Clinical Protocols

Practice guidelines are increasingly being promoted by governmental agencies, professional societies, and managed care corporations. One prominent example is the National Committee for Quality Assurance (NCQA), which assesses and reports on the quality of managed care plans through such measures as HEDIS (Health Plan Employer Data and Information Set), which defines a set of performance measurements. These practice guidelines can provide useful comparative reference points. ACHA has immunization guidelines and guidelines for tuberculosis screening on campuses. The Agency for Healthcare Research and Quality (AHRQ) has clinical practice guidelines available, many of which may be of interest to college health services. Preventive health guidelines are also available from the American College of Physicians and the U.S. Preventive Services Task

Force. Practice guidelines for asthma have been prepared by the National Heart, Lung and Blood Institute and promoted by drug companies and health insurance companies.[11]

Desired Performance Targets (Thresholds)

The SHS can also determine its own targets or thresholds for evaluation. For example, abnormal Pap smear results may be considered high-risk, high-volume as well as problem-prone. Therefore, leadership may decide that it is essential that 100 percent of patients with abnormal Pap smears be notified. On the other hand, a threshold of 80 percent may be adequate when determining the acceptable level of staff training on fire extinguisher use, since there will be an excellent chance that at least one trained staff member is present at any given time.

Assessment Tools

There are many different statistical tools that can assist the QIP Advisory Body in transforming data into meaningful information. Sophisticated training in statistics is not necessary to use these simple tools. Four such tools are run charts, Pareto charts, flowcharts, and cause-and-effect diagrams. A detailed presentation of these, and other useful statistical tools, is given in JCAHO's manual *Performance Improvement in Ambulatory Care.*[9] A model QI project, improvement in "stat" laboratory turnaround time, has been described, demonstrating the use of the flowchart and the Pareto chart.[24]

Improve

Once the assessment has been completed, the next step is to determine specific goals for improvement. Examples might include: decreasing the percentage of "no endocervical cells" on Pap smears to 5 percent; decreasing the waiting time for walk-ins to less than 30 minutes; or increasing the steroid inhaler use of patients diagnosed with chronic, persistent asthma by 20 percent. With specific performance goals set, it is possible to assess the overall degree of success of the intervention.

After a specific important goal is established, a preliminary action plan should be designed, based on data collected and analyzed during the measure and assessment phases. The preliminary action plan should be piloted before full-scale implementation. For example: "The clinic autoclave needs to be repaired or replaced. A cost-benefit analysis suggests that switching from metal to plastic specula may be worthwhile. Before investing in a year's supply of plastic specula, however, it would be advisable to purchase only a month's supply of the plastic specula to assure that the product is acceptable to patients and staff."

Once the preliminary action plan has been implemented and data on its performance collected and analyzed, adjustments are made, if necessary, and a final action plan is implemented. The improvement cycle does not stop here, however, as the effectiveness of the change needs to monitored and assessed in the future to assure that improvement not only occurs but is maintained. Once the improvement has become part of standard operating procedure and is functioning suitably, the process may be dropped from the regular QIP agenda. Spot checks may be performed at regular intervals to assure that the process continues to maintain acceptable quality.

SUMMARY

Application of quality improvement methods to health care processes in an SHS increases patient and employee satisfaction, improves efficiency and internal communication, increases consistency in work processes, decreases costs, and may increase the likelihood of good health outcomes for the patients served. The QIP Advisory Body should be interdisciplinary, with representatives from all units within the SHS. The QIP Coordinator should have superior organizational and communication skills and should obtain formal training in quality improvement theory and techniques. A rich literature exists detailing QI methodologies. All involve several phases, including self-inspection to identify problems, planning and implementing improvements, and measuring change. QI requires a long-term commitment to continuous change, and the SHS leadership, in particular, must be willing to commit time, staff, and resources to develop and maintain an effective program.

ACCREDITATION

Overview

The choice by an SHS to become accredited is purely voluntary. However, increasing numbers of SHSs are seeking formal accreditation for a variety of reasons. First, university administration, parents, and students seek assurance that their student health fee dollars support a high-quality service. Accreditation provides objective evidence of quality and allows comparison of the SHS with other similar centers. Second, accreditation assures that health care processes within the SHS are "in control" through continuous self-inspection. These quality improvement, safety, and risk management programs decrease costs, increase efficiency, and may decrease the legal liability of the SHS. All of these are attractive to the university administration. Third, accreditation permits sharing of service roles for those SHSs that are providers for their university's managed care product or for those SHSs integrated into their academic medical center. These SHSs may provide primary care services for faculty, staff, students, and dependents and may also provide employee or workers' compensation services. Fourth, the accreditation process often promotes internal communication and team-building, motivating staff members in a positive way. Finally, accreditation enhances the visibility of the SHS and may well make it more competitive internally for university financial support and space.

ACHA Guidelines for a College Health Program

For SHSs interested in improving the quality of their programs without undergoing formal accreditation, the ACHA has published a monograph entitled "Guidelines for a College Health Program."[8] Many of the standards in this monograph are similar to the accreditation standards of both AAAHC and JCAHO. In fact, the standards in the monograph are cross-referenced by number with the AAAHC standards, although the ACHA guidelines may differ in some details. If an SHS is interested in formal accreditation, however, this monograph should not substitute for the accreditation manuals published by each of the accrediting bodies.

Choices of Accrediting Bodies

Ambulatory care clinics can be accredited through two different nonprofit agencies: the Accreditation Association of Ambulatory Health Care (AAAHC, Wilmette, Illinois) or the Joint Commission on Accreditation of Healthcare Organizations (JCAHO, Oakbrook Terrace, Illinois). As of February 2000, 126 of the estimated 1,500 college and university SHSs in the United States were accredited as free-standing ambulatory clinics; 99 through AAAHC and 27 through JCAHO. There is also an additional group of 20 SHSs which are accredited through their academic medical center, with 19 of the 20 (95 percent) being accredited through JCAHO.[25]

When free from outside constraints, most SHSs choose AAAHC as their accrediting body. There are several explanations for this. First, AAAHC standards are less prescriptive than JCAHO standards. Second, AAAHC accreditation is far less expensive than accreditation through JCAHO and thus more within the financial scope of most SHS budgets. Third, AAAHC since its inception has been involved with college health and may be more visible as an accrediting body. Finally, AAAHC's Institute for Quality Improvement offers clinical performance measurement opportunities that may be helpful for small SHSs which lack sufficient staff to conduct such programs in-house.

On the other hand, the majority of SHSs at academic medical centers (30/47; 64 percent) choose JCAHO as their accrediting body, most likely reflecting the accreditation choice of their parent institution.[25]

Similarities and Differences in the Accrediting Bodies

AAAHC, since its inception in 1979, has always concentrated exclusively on ambulatory care. Currently, over 1,200 organizations are accredited nationwide through AAAHC, including ambulatory surgery facilities, college and university health centers, single and multispecialty group practices, and health networks. A major recent contribution to quality health care nationwide has been AAAHC's involvement in review of health maintenance organizations (HMOs), resulting in its adoption in 1997 of special adjunct standards for managed care organizations. AAAHC, like JCAHO, now requires that health care organizations provide data to compare themselves with other similar organizations on key indicators. AAAHC's Institute for Quality Improvement provides clinical performance benchmarking opportunities that measure patient-physician interaction, utilize real-time data collection (no burdensome chart review), and provide "at-a-glance" reporting so that participating institutions can understand their performance relative to that of their peers.

AAAHC surveyors are volunteers who are actively practicing professionals. Throughout the accreditation process, these surveyors place emphasis on "constructive consultation and education, not finding fault."[26] AAAHC standards have been developed, reviewed, and revised by these surveyors and other health care professionals over the years. The AAAHC core standards include the following major categories:

- Rights of Patients
- Governance
- Administration
- Quality of Care
- Quality Management and Improvement
- Clinical Records
- Professional Improvement
- Facilities and Environment

JCAHO, a much larger organization than AAAHC, began as a hospital-accrediting agency but in 1975 began surveying ambulatory care centers as well. Currently, JCAHO evaluates and accredits nearly 20,000 health care organizations in the U.S., including hospitals, health care networks, managed care organizations, and facilities providing home care, long-term care, and behavioral health care, as well as laboratory and ambulatory care services.

Joint commission standards have been developed in consultation with experts in health care and measurement, health care providers, purchasers, and consumers. As mentioned, the JCAHO standards tend to be more detailed and explicit than the AAAHC standards. JCAHO standards are divided into two groups:

Patient-focused standards
- Patient Rights and Organization Ethics
- Assessment of Patient
- Care of Patient
- Education of Patients and Family
- Continuity of Care

Organization-focused standards
- Environment of Care
- Surveillance, Prevention and Control of Infection
- Human Resources
- Information Management
- Leadership
- Performance Improvement

Unlike AAAHC surveyors, JCAHO surveyors are paid and include such diverse categories of professionals as physicians, nurses, health care administrators, medical technologists, psychologists, respiratory therapists, pharmacists, durable medical equipment providers, and social workers. In addition, the JCAHO central office employs over 500 individuals.

Cost of Accreditation

One of the major differences between the two accrediting bodies is cost. Because AAAHC is a smaller organization with volunteer surveyors, its cost of accreditation is far less than JCAHO's. As an example, direct fees for accreditation with AAAHC in 1998 were calculated to be $3,500 for one medium-sized school in the South. For the same school, the direct fees for accreditation through JCAHO were $13,688. Indirect costs added substantially to the expense and totaled $30,135. (Many of these costs were one-time only, driven by safety requirements to bring the facility into compliance with Environment of Care standards. Other costs were related to initial survey expenses and included costs of sending staff members to JCAHO seminars and payment for a "mock" survey [$7,800]. Some of the indirect costs were optional and included $11,200 to purchase defibrillators and $1,900 to cover staff training in advanced cardiac life support. JCAHO standards do not require this level of emergency preparedness in college health centers.)

Laboratory Accreditation

Many SHSs operate their own in-house laboratory. These laboratories may range in complexity from simple units providing only rapid screening tests ("kit" tests) to full-scale diagnostic laboratories.

Laboratory accreditation is complicated because of the various layers of regulation involved. An excellent guide to understanding the intricacies of laboratory regulation as well as how the various inspection and accrediting bodies interrelate can be found in Laessig and Ehrmeyer's "The New Poor Man's (Person's) Guide to the Regulations (CLIA '88, JCAHO, CAP & COLA)."[27] All SHS laboratories must be "certified," whether the clinic chooses to become accredited. All laboratory testing, including point-of-care testing, is regulated according to the Clinical Laboratory Improvement Amendment of 1988 (CLIA '88). Approved laboratories receive a CLIA certificate after inspection. (Point-of-care testing [POCT] refers to any analytical testing that is performed at sites outside the traditional laboratory environment, generally within or near where health care is delivered to patients. Therefore, by definition, many "in-house" SHS laboratories perform POCT.) CLIA '88 establishes the minimum regulations which govern laboratory testing; however, all laboratories, including POCT sites, can choose to follow The Centers for Medicare and Medicaid Services' (CMS's) CLIA regulations or the requirements established by "deemed" organizations. CMS has judged three deemed organizations to meet or exceed the CLIA requirements:

- Commission on Office Laboratory Accreditation (COLA): a nonprofit physician-directed, national laboratory accrediting organization
- Laboratory Accreditation Program of the College of American Pathologists (LAP-CAP): a program administered by the CAP, in which all participants are required to serve as inspectors of other sites
- JCAHO: laboratory accreditation surveys take place separately from clinic surveys

Therefore, SHS laboratories, in general, have four choices of inspection agencies, but ultimately, the inspection must result in a CLIA certificate. The choice of inspection agencies is typically determined at the institutional level if the SHS laboratory is part of a larger, hospital-based laboratory. The first question, then, that needs to be answered regarding accreditation of the SHS laboratory is "Who holds the CLIA '88 certificate?"[29] If the SHS is on a campus with an academic medical center, then the central hospital laboratory may hold a single CLIA '88 certificate which covers all hospital laboratory testing as well as all POCT. In this case, the central laboratory is responsible for the overall quality control for the main laboratory as well as the satellite testing sites.

Another scenario is that various testing sites, including the SHS laboratory, may hold separate CLIA '88 certificates. In this case, the SHS laboratory is viewed by CMS as an independent laboratory and is responsible for meeting all regulatory requirements. The second question regarding accreditation of the SHS laboratory is "What accrediting agency will inspect the SHS clinic?" AAAHC does not do formal laboratory inspection but accepts CLIA, COLA, LAP-CAP, or JCAHO laboratory inspections. JCAHO, on the other hand, accepts only LAP-CAP or COLA laboratory inspection as a substitute for its own. If the SHS laboratory chooses to be inspected by JCAHO, the laboratory survey takes place separately from the clinic survey. To prepare for this survey, the SHS must use the JCAHO laboratory manual, which is almost as detailed as the clinic manual.[28] In compliance with CLIA regulations, laboratory inspections for all of the regulatory agencies occur every two years, whereas clinics are surveyed every three years.

The final question regarding accreditation of the SHS laboratory is "What level of complexity of testing is being performed?" CLIA '88 regulations divide testing into four categories: waived, provider-performed microscopy (PPM), moderate complexity, and high complexity. Many of the procedures done in an SHS laboratory are categorized as waived or moderate-complexity tests. It is important to define the level of complexity of each test, as each level has different regulatory requirements for qualifications of testing personnel, quality control methods, and proficiency testing. Moderate-or high-complexity testing generally requires external proficiency testing. *CMS and COLA regulations do not require inspection of POCT sites if the site performs only waived testing and/or PPM* (see definitions below). JCAHO and CAP, on the other hand, have specific standards for all categories of tests, including waived tests and PPM, and both of these agencies inspect for compliance with these standards.

The list of waived tests is maintained by the Centers for Disease Control (CDC). Reagent or test-kit manufacturers also maintain current information on the classification of their products. Commonly used waived tests include urine dipstick and pregnancy tests, tests for fecal occult blood, and rapid tests for group A streptococcus and infectious mononucleosis. Not all reagents or products of a single group are considered waived; therefore, the manufacturer or the CDC list must be consulted for each test.

The PPM category is limited to nine specific types of tests which must be performed by physicians or midlevel practitioners as part of their practice of medicine. The microscope is the primary instrument used to perform all of these tests. PPM includes:

- Direct wet mount preparations (suspended in saline or water) examined for the presence or absence of bacteria, fungi, parasites, and human cellular elements
- Potassium hydroxide (KOH) preparations
- Pinworm examinations
- Fern tests
- Postcoital direct qualitative examinations of vaginal or cervical mucus
- Urine dipsticks and sediment examinations

- Nasal smears for granulocytes
- Fecal leukocyte examinations
- Qualitative semen analysis (limited to the presence or absence of sperm and detection of motility)

A description of the regulatory standards for COLA, LAP-CAP, and JCAHO is beyond the scope of this chapter. The interested reader should contact these organizations for specific publications detailing these standards. A practical approach to establishing a CLIA-certified laboratory in a student health service has been described in a paper by Nash and Ross.[29]

Pre-survey Processes

For organizations interested in pursuing accreditation for the first time, it is prudent to send the accreditation team leader and key staff to one of the AAAHC or JCAHO training seminars. In addition, JCAHO, in particular, publishes many resources to assist with the accreditation process, including detailed manuals on quality improvement programming. The ACHA also has a Consultation Service, which will visit SHSs and give an in-depth analysis of the program. This consultative visit should be scheduled well in advance of the actual survey, as it can take four to six weeks to receive a report from the consultant. A mock survey by an actual JCAHO surveyor may be extremely helpful, although costly. One resource which might be useful to an SHS preparing for accreditation is the article by Johnson and Reppert.[30]

It may be useful to contact a facility that has been recently surveyed to determine the most troublesome aspects of their survey. Survey teams tend to focus on similar issues during any given cycle. For AAAHC, an inadequate quality improvement program is the most common reason cited for organizations failing to receive a full three-year accreditation. Appropriate credentialing of licensed independent practitioners is also a common problem. JCAHO publishes many manuals dealing with the standards that organizations find most troublesome and giving detailed information about how to satisfy those standards.

The accreditation process for both AAAHC and JCAHO involves several steps. The first step is to submit a completed application form along with a nonrefundable deposit. For JCAHO, the application should be filed 12 months before the anticipated visit; AAAHC suggests submitting the application four to five months ahead of time. The application contains a presurvey questionnaire and instructions on how to advertise the public information interview. Other documents may be required at the time of application as well. Once the application has been received and reviewed, the survey dates are scheduled. If so desired, a surveyor with a background in college health may be requested at the time of application.

Both AAAHC and JCAHO require that a notice be posted prominently in the clinic at least four weeks in advance of the survey. This posting invites anyone with either positive comments or valid quality-of-care concerns about the SHS to participate in an interview with surveyors on the day of the survey. JCAHO also requires that this notice be posted in the local newspaper.

A few weeks before the survey, a member of the survey team will contact the SHS and review information on the presurvey questionnaire. The surveyor may request additional information or documents to review prior to the survey. The agenda for the survey is determined, and any special needs of the survey team can then be clarified.

Survey Fees

Survey fees are based on information submitted in the application and presurvey documents. Fees for both organizations are based on the size of the SHS and the number of geographic sites that must be surveyed. Other factors influencing the survey fee include the type and range of services offered, the number of surveyors, and the number of days assigned for the survey.

Surveyors

Surveyors for AAAHC are peers who are actively practicing in their field at the time of the survey. The number of surveyors depends upon the size of the SHS. For JCAHO, usually two surveyors will be assigned: an administrative surveyor and a physician surveyor. The physician surveyor reviews the medical records and addresses the patient-focused standards, whereas the administrative surveyor reviews the organization-focused standards. Both surveyors evaluate the quality control mechanisms in place in the clinic.

The Accreditation Decision

AAAHC has five categories of accreditation decisions:

1. Three-year accreditation: awarded when the organization is in substantial compliance with the standards.
2. One-year accreditation: awarded when part of the organization is in substantial compliance, but other areas need improvement. In this case, the organization must have a second survey within ten months of the initial survey.
3. Deferred accreditation decision: the organization does not meet standards but demonstrates the desire and the ability to do so given further time. In this case, and within three months of the notification of the deferral accreditation decision, the organization must request another on-site survey, which will take place within six months of the original survey.
4. Provisional six-month accreditation decision: the organization is in compliance but has not been operational long enough or has not demonstrated the ability to continue to comply with standards. Again, within three months of the notification of the provisional accreditation decision, another on-site survey must be requested, and this re-survey must take place within six months of the original survey.
5. Denial or revocation of an accreditation decision.

JCAHO also has five categories of accreditation decisions:

1. Accreditation with or without Type I recommendations: Type I recommendations must be resolved within a specified period of time, or the accreditation may be revoked.
2. Conditional Accreditation: substantial deficits are present and must be corrected by the time of the follow-up survey.
3. Provisional Accreditation: substantial compliance has been demonstrated, but a second survey is required within 6 months to demonstrate continued compliance.
4. Preliminary Non-accreditation: a plan of correction must be submitted and approved by JCAHO; then sufficient compliance must be demonstrated at a six month follow-up survey.
5. Not Accredited: substantial compliance has not been demonstrated. This status may also be conferred when an organization withdraws from JCAHO or when the organization withdraws from the accreditation process.

Summary

Accreditation of the SHS through AAAHC or JCAHO can be expensive and time-consuming, and often requires one and a half to two years of planning and work. However, there are many benefits. Accreditation provides objective evidence of quality and allows comparison of the SHS with other similar centers. Accreditation assures that health care processes within the SHS are "in control," and, through quality improvement, safety, and risk management programs, may decrease the legal liability of the SHS. Accreditation permits sharing of service roles for those SHSs that are providers for their university's managed care product or for those SHSs integrated into their academic medical center. Finally, the accreditation process promotes internal communication and team-building, and serves to enhance the visibility of the SHS within the university community.

APPENDIX 1—GLOSSARY OF TERMS

Asssessment Tools: graphical or other methods for converting performance data into useful information. Four specific examples include:
1. Run Chart: a graph illustrating performance over time
2. Pareto Chart: A chart that shows, in descending order, the frequency of problems in a process. The "Pareto Principle" states that the majority of errors derive from but a few of the causes. Managers should focus on the "vital few" rather than the "useful many" contributing causes to a problem, thereby effecting the greatest change most efficiently.
3. Cause-and-Effect (Fishbone or Ishikawa) Diagram: a graphic tool used to organize possible contributing causes to a problem
4. Flowchart: a graphic that shows the actual steps in a process

Benchmarking: comparing a characteristic in your organization against a standard derived from other organizations known for their quality

Customer (Internal and External): A customer is someone who is impacted by the product. In the case of health care, the product is "health care services" and the *external customer* is generally the patient. Other external customers may be parents (in the case of an SHS), payers, or health plans. *Internal customers* may be employees, teams, or departments (including the university administration) within the organization, all of which are impacted by the production of "health care services" as well.

Design-Measure-Assess-Improve: cycle of planning, collecting data, analyzing data and instituting change to improve a process

Functions and Processes: *Processes* are linked, goal-directed activities designed to accomplish a *function*. A *function* is a group of processes with a common goal. As an example: screening for cervical cancer is a *function,* whereas routine gynecologic appointment scheduling, health education activities targeted at women using the clinic for routine gynecologic care, Pap specimen collection and interpretation, and notification of the patient of an abnormal Pap result are all *processes* which serve to accomplish the *function* of cervical cancer screening.

Indicator: a valid and reliable quantitative measure related to a dimension of performance. As an example: when examining the "availability" (*dimension of performance*) of appointments for routine gynecologic care, one *indicator* would be the number of days until next available appointment.

Quality Improvement (QI): a methodology for improving the quality of health care processes in an organization on an ongoing basis. Synonymous terms include performance improvement (PI), continuous improvement (CI), total quality management (TQM), and total quality control (TQC).

Thresholds: a performance level that signifies a need for further study and action. For example, the QI Advisory Body may determine that 100 percent of patient visits for psychotropic medication evaluation should contain documentation of whether suicidal ideation is present. If diagnosis review of selected medical records shows that only 80 percent show documentation about suicidal ideation, then the threshold has not been met and more intensive special assessment by the QI Advisory Body is triggered.

APPENDIX 2—NINE DIMENSIONS OF PERFORMANCE

Doing the Right Thing

1. The efficacy of the procedure or treatment in relation to the patient's condition.

The degree to which the care of the patient has been shown to accomplish the desired or projected outcome(s).

2. The appropriateness of a specific test, procedure, or service to meet the patient's needs.

The degree to which the care provided is relevant to the patient's clinical needs, given the current state of knowledge.

Doing the Right Thing Well

3. The availability of a needed test, procedure, treatment, or service to the patient who needs it.

The degree to which appropriate care is available to meet patients' needs.

4. The timeliness with which a needed test, procedure, treatment, or service is provided to the patient.

The degree to which care is provided to the patient at the most beneficial or necessary time

5. The effectiveness with which tests, procedures, treatments, and services are provided.

The degree to which the care is provided in the correct manner, given the current state of knowledge, to achieve the desired or projected outcome(s) for the patient

6. The continuity of the services provided to the patient with respect to other services, practitioners, and providers, and over time.

The degree to which the care for the patient is coordinated among practitioners, among organizations, and over time.

7. The safety of the patient (and others) to whom the services are provided.

The degree to which the risk of an intervention and the risk in the care environment are reduced for the patient and others, including the health care provider.

8. The efficiency with which services are provided.

The relationship between the outcomes (results of care) and the resources used to deliver patient care.

9. The respect and caring with which services are provided.

The degree to which the patient or a designee is involved in his or her own care decisions and to which those providing services do so with sensitivity and respect for the patient's needs, expectations, and individual differences.

APPENDIX 3—DETAIL OF A QIP PROJECT

Aspect of Care

Documentation of medications and allergies

Rationale

To assure the safety of patients being prescribed medication

Type of Measure

Process

Dimension of Performance

Efficacy	No
Appropriateness	Yes
Availability	No
Timeliness	No
Effectiveness	Yes
Continuity	Yes
Safety	Yes
Efficiency	No
Respect and Caring	No

Data Collection

Every six months the QIP Coordinator will designate a staff member to retrospectively review medical records of patients who have received medications during office visits within the previous six months. Pharmacy records will be used to identify these patients. Two percent of records will be reviewed.

Numerator Description

Indicators (rate-based aggregate-data indicators): Number of medical records with documentation of the following within the progress note for the office visit in which the medication was prescribed:

- Allergies
- Last menstrual period and/or unprotected intercourse for all female patients
- Prescription medication dose, interval, and duration of medication
- All current medications being taken by the patient
- Chronic medications (recorded on the health history form by the third patient visit)

Denominator Description

Number of medical records reviewed

REFERENCES

1. Lohr KN (ed.). Medicare: a strategy for quality assurance. Vol 1. Institute of Medicine. Washington, DC; National Academy Press 1990, p. 21.

2. Chassin MR. Quality improvement nearing the 21st century: Prospects and perils. Am J of Med Qual 1996;11:S4–7.

3. Balestracci D, Barlow JL. Quality Improvement: Practical Applications for Medical Group Practice. Englewood, CO: Center for Research in Ambulatory Health Care Administration, 1996.

4. Delene LM. Relationship marketing and service quality. J Am Coll Health 1992;40:265–269.

5. Shortell SM, Bennet CL, Byck GR. Assessing the impact of continuous quality improvement on clinical practice: What it will take to accelerate progress. Milbank Q 1998;76:593–624.

6. Bender AD, and Krasnick C. Quality practice management: How to apply the principles of total quality management to a medical practice. Swarthmore, PA: Thayer Press, 1993.

7. Accreditation Handbook for Ambulatory Health Care. Skokie, IL: Accreditation Association for Ambulatory Health Care, 2000.

8. American College Health Association, Standards Revision Work Group; Guidelines for a College Health Program. Baltimore: American College Health Association, 1999.

9. Performance Improvement in Ambulatory Care. Oakbrook Terrace, IL: Joint Commission on Accreditation of Healthcare Organizations, 1997.

10. Using Performance Improvement Tools in Ambulatory Care. Oakbrook Terrace, IL: Joint Commission on Accreditation of Health Care Organizations, 1998.

11. The Expert Panel II: Guidelines for the Diagnosis and Management of Asthma. Bethesda, MD: National Heart, Lung, and Blood Institute, National Institutes of Health; 1997.

12. Blonde L, Dey J, Testa MA, Guthrie RD. Defining and measuring quality of diabetes care. Primary Care 1999;26:841–855.

13. Marshall CL, Bluestein M, Chapin C, Davis T, Gersten J, Harris C, Hodgin A, Larsen W, Rigberg H, Krishnaswami V, Darling B. Outpatient management of diabetes mellitus in five Arizona Medicare managed care plans. Am J Med Qual 1996;11:87–93.

14. Weber M. Guidelines for assessing outcomes of antihypertensive treatment. Am J Cardiol 1999;84(2A):2K–4K

15. Rosen AK, Mayer-Oakes A. Developing a tool for analyzing medical care utilization of adult asthma patients in indemnity and managed care plans: Can an episodes of care framework be used? Am J of Med Qual 1998;13:203–212.

16. Glasier A, Baird D. The effects of self-administering emergency contraception. NEJM 1998;339:1–4.

17. Berwick DM. Sounding board: continuous improvement as an ideal in health care. NEJM 1989;320:53–56.

18. Miller ST, Flanagan E. The transition from quality assurance to continuous quality improvement in ambulatory care. QRB 1993;19:62–65.

19. Nice R, Steed M. Building a nursing quality management program on preprinted charting forms. J Am Coll Health 1999;48:41–43.

20. Isenberg SF, Stewart MG. Utilizing patient satisfaction data to assess quality improvement in community-based medical practices. Am J Med Qual 1998;13:188–194.

21. Andrzejewski N, Lagua RT. Use of a customer satisfaction survey by health care regulators: A tool for total quality management. Public Health Reports 1997;112:206–211.

22. Jatulis DE, Bundek NI, Legorreta AP. Identifying predictors of satisfaction with access to medical care and quality of care. Am J Med Qual 1997;12:11–18.

23. Epstein KR, Laine C, Farber NJ, Nelson EC, Davidoff F. Patients' perceptions of office medical practice: Judging quality through the patients' eyes. Am J. Med Qual 1996;11:73–80.

24. Bluth EI, Lambert DJ, Lohmann TP, Franklin DN, Bourgeois M, Kardinal CG, Dalovisio JR, Williams, MM, Becker AS. Improvement in "stat" laboratory turnaround time: A model continuous quality improvement project. Arch Intern Med 1992;152:837–840.

25. Johnson BA. The accreditation status of student health services at academic medical centers. Jt Comm J Qual Improv 2000;26:160–165.

26. "Why AAAHC?" www.aaahc.org, 2000.

27. Laessig RH, Ehrmeyer S. The new poor man's (person's) guide to the regulations (CLIA '88, JCAHO, CAP & COLA). R & S Consultants, 629 Chatham Terrace, Madison, WI 53711, Feb. 2000.

28. Joint Commission on Accreditation of Health Care Organizations, 2000-2001 Comprehensive Accreditation Manual for Pathology and Clinical Laboratory Services, Oakbrook Terrace, IL: Joint Commission on Accreditation of Health Care Organizations; 2000.

29. Nash KA, Ross A. Setting up a CLIA-certified laboratory in a student health services clinic. J Am Coll Health 1999;48:138–140.

30. Johnson BA, Reppert BR. Achieving JCAHO accreditation in a university student health center. Clin Perform and Qual Health Care 1998;6:114–128.

CHAPTER 5

PRIMARY CARE ISSUES IN COLLEGE HEALTH

John M. Dorman, MD, and William A. Christmas, MD

HISTORICAL PERSPECTIVE

As American colleges and universities proliferated in the nineteenth century, concerns developed on the part of college administrations that the health status of college students (to the extent that it interfered with the pursuit of their studies) was an issue deserving attention. The expectation was, in this pre-antibiotic era, that optimizing health through education about nutrition, exercise, and mental health would render the individual less susceptible to communicable and other diseases, thereby leading to a more vigorous and satisfying life (and by extension, to a more effective learning environment). Thus it is not surprising that the early college health services focused on physical activity and studies of hygiene as the benchmarks of a health program. However, the occurrence of epidemic infectious diseases on campuses also caused a major concern for the health of students, at the same time disrupting the operation of the educational institution. One of the most effective means of limiting the spread of epidemic diseases was thought to be the practice of quarantine. Quarantines were most effectively carried out in colleges by placing ill students in an infirmary. Vassar and Wellesley colleges were pioneers in establishing infirmaries for the care and isolation of sick women students; Princeton University and the College of William and Mary were among the first institutions to open infirmaries for men. During the first half of the 20th century, infirmary care was the cornerstone of health services on residential campuses, with "sick call" (ambulatory care) relegated to a secondary role. With the development of vaccines to prevent many common infectious diseases and with the advent of the antibiotic era in the 1940s, quarantine as a means of controlling disease became less important and the need for infirmaries began to wane. As a result, during the latter half of the 20th century, many colleges and universities phased out their infirmaries entirely and redirected resources to primary and/or multispecialty ambulatory care programs and health promotion and outreach. Thus, in the past 50 years, the medical services provided by college and university health services have become the new cornerstone on which a comprehensive health program is built.

THE DELIVERY OF MEDICAL SERVICES

Standard local medical practices or emergency rooms near a college or university have, through time, generally proved unsatisfactory as the sole providers of health services for the college population. For traditional-aged undergraduates, going to college is usually their first attempt at independent living away from home. Many of their visits to a medical practice are for apparently trivial problems, which while seen as "nuisance visits" in private practice, may be appreciated by college health providers as "teachable moments." Also, knowledge of developmental goals of this age group is important, and the student affairs division at a college is particularly cognizant of these goals; consequently, that division is, most often, the natural organizational home for health services.[2]

In order to respond to student needs and, indeed, to expectations of parents and the college/university administration, "a well organized and adequately funded college health center should strive to meet the following goals through its medical services activities: 1) accessible medical services; 2) reasonable cost to the student for these services; 3) emphasis on preventive and health education services; 4) integration with (other) student affairs departments (i.e., residential life, counseling center, and international educational services) and 5) confidentiality of medical information preserved."[2, p. 521]

Medical care activities of health services are typically divided into four areas: primary clinical care, urgent care, emergency care, and increasingly less common, infirmary care.[2] "Primary Care is first-contact, longitudinal care that is comprehensive and person-centered rather than disease or organ-system specific."[3] This description defines well the role of college health providers. Not unlike any primary care office, there is also the ongoing challenge of not missing the occasional very serious ailment among a sea of relatively minor complaints. However, the delivery of primary care to the student population differs significantly from care of other populations in at least one very important way, since there is a substantial annual turnover of members of the group. For example, at one large California university, fully one-third of the students are new each year, interfering with extended continuity of care and creating a never ending need to educate the student population about health matters and the use of the health care system (Stanford, the SHS of author John Dorman).

Provision of emergency and urgent care services requires 24-hour on-site operation at the student health service or, when the health center is closed, student access to an alternative site, for example, an urgent treatment center or hospital emergency room. Accessibility to medical assistance and advice can be enhanced by provision of a 24-hour on-call system using an answering service and beeper (or cellular phone). Traditionally aged undergraduate college students tend to overuse emergency medical services for reasons of convenience and lack of knowledge about economical and appropriate use of the health care system. The use of an on-call system for health-related questions substantially reduces after-hours visits to emergency facilities.

As mentioned, infirmary care has rapidly become outmoded on many campuses.

This is due to low utilization, advances in technology, and liability/licensing concerns regarding non-ambulatory care. Further, 24-hour-per-day infirmary care is very expensive. Scarce resources are better used in enhancing ambulatory care as well as primary and secondary prevention programs.

The expertise and training of college health physicians varies, since at the present time there is no specific residency training program for college health. Those physicians trained in pediatrics, particularly with an adolescent medicine fellowship, are especially attuned to the developmental challenges faced by the undergraduate college population. However, pediatricians may feel uncomfortable dealing with gynecological problems or with older graduate and professional students. Internists may feel very comfortable with the latter group, but may be at something of a loss in considering such chief complaints as chondromalacia or infections from a navel piercing. Many family practice programs, particularly those with a sports medicine emphasis, have recently provided excellent training for the college health physician. Other disciplines, such as preventive medicine, emergency medicine, and gynecology, may also be found among college health primary care practitioners. Perhaps the best physician staff, particularly in large clinics, is a mix of clinicians with varied training and backgrounds to best handle the myriad of clinical and public health issues faced by a large, modern college health service.

In addition to physicians, a variety of clinical providers from other disciplines participate in college health (e.g., mid-level providers such as nurse practitioners and physician assistants, registered and licensed practical nurses, and medical assistants). In fact, one of the strengths of college health has always been its interdisciplinary approach to health care delivery. Nurse practitioners were active in the college health field long before they had widespread acceptance in the remainder of the medical community. Now, it is not uncommon for some smaller college health services to be *directed* by nurse practitioners, physician assistants, social workers, or health educators.

Services other than primary clinical care are also an important part of a college health service's responsibilities. It is often possible to contract, either on-site or off-site, with local specialists for such services as orthopedics, dermatology, gynecology, and allergy. Administration of allergy shots may be a useful and convenient service for those students on immunotherapy regimens prescribed by an allergist. Some facilities may be able to provide complete health assessments, often for a fee, for those students requiring medical evaluations for jobs, graduate schools, and scholarships. Laboratory, radiology, pharmacy, and physical therapy services should be available to students, whether on-site or readily available at a nearby facility.

Given the numbers of international students attending U.S. colleges and universities and the frequent travel of many domestic students to foreign countries, many health services now provide travel medicine services, including malaria prophylaxis, recommended immunizations, and special advice for such situations as travelers' diarrhea and altitude sickness.

Athletic medicine remains a special concern of college health services. While athletes may receive care either from a physician trained in primary care who has a special interest in sports medicine, by an orthopedic consultant, or by both, the best interests of the student-athlete are served if medical care of the athlete is managed under the umbrella of the student health service, regardless of who performs direct clinical care. However, in practice this situation is often the exception rather than the rule, particularly at most NCAA Division I schools.[2]

Student health services routinely struggle with the pros and cons of seeing patients by an appointment system as opposed to a walk-in service. An appointment system decreases waiting time and more closely simulates traditional practice settings which students encounter in the "real world." Such a system requires that provision be made for emergent and urgent problems by such mechanisms as an urgent care clinician or team with a same-day appointment schedule, and/or nurse triage of patients to fill blocks of provider time held open for urgent problems. Clearly, an appointment system distributes workload evenly throughout the day and makes the most efficient use of resources. Also, students may more easily see the provider of their choice on an appointment basis, rather than the one who is on urgent duty, thereby enhancing continuity of care. However, a full appointment system increases the administrative duties of the nursing and appointment desk staff. Although many students prefer a walk-in service with "no waiting" at any hour which is convenient for them, including evenings, nights and weekends, this level of service is rarely achievable because the resources of health services are typically modest and do not permit institutions to staff for the peaks of this spectrum of coverage.

Confidentiality of medical information in dealing with student patients cannot be overemphasized. Records that are maintained in the course of the patient-physician relationship with a student are excluded from the Buckley Amendment and from the Family Educational Rights to Privacy Act (FERPA), which refer exclusively to educational records; therefore, a student's medical records cannot be disclosed to academic personnel without the student's consent. This nondisclosure policy also applies to friends of the patient, family members and therapists, or physicians not involved in the patient's immediate care. While an exception to this policy applies to students under the age of 18 (whose parents may request medical information), many states specifically exclude certain types of information from being shared with parents and guardians without the minor's permission. Contraception and treatment for sexually transmitted diseases or mental health visits are commonly included in this category.

THE ISSUE OF PREADMISSION REQUIREMENTS

From the outset, admission history and physical examinations (sometimes including certain laboratory tests such as complete blood counts and urinalyses) were typically required for incoming college students, whether these were accomplished prior to coming to campus or upon arrival. Presently, the focus is on an abbreviated health history and recommended institutional prematriculation immunizations (RIPIs, formerly prematriculation immunization requirements, or PIRs), rather than a full medical evaluation. RIPIs currently recommended by ACHA include two measles-mumps-rubella (MMR), tetanus-diphtheria (TD) within 10 years, a primary polio series, a hepatitis B series, and tuberculosis screening, primarily for international students from high-risk areas.[4] Health science students may also be required to provide proof of varicella immunity and tuberculosis screening.[5]

COMMON MEDICAL PROBLEMS

There is a common misconception among the medical community that those ailments seen in a college health service consist of little more than "runny noses, sore throats, and sprained ankles." In today's large, modern college health service, with an age range of patients from 16 to 60, the variety of diagnoses is comparable to that of any primary care practice which serves a young adult population, with a special emphasis on gynecological and mental health services (both of which are included in many college health programs). This section discusses briefly several of the most common problems and dilemmas seen in college health services, some of which are unique to the college campus; however, it is not intended to be a textbook on medicine. Those seeking specific help in diagnosis and treatment should consult any good clinical text.

Table 1 lists the 50 most common diagnoses, by frequency, encountered in the treatment of both men and women (excluding immunizations) at one large college health service (University of Kentucky Student Health Service, 1998) during a one-year period in the late 1990s. Table 2 lists the 50 most frequent diagnoses for women, and Table 3 gives similar data for male patients in the same year. (Tables 2 and 3 include all encounters, i.e., primary care, gynecology services, mental health services, allergy shots, and immunizations.) During the year studied, approximately 56% of visits to the primary care clinic were made by women, while 44 percent were made by males. When gynecology clinic visits are added, approximately 70 percent of visits for primary care were by women.[6] This particular campus has an enrollment of approximately 55 percent women and 45 percent men.

DERMATOLOGY

Acne, urticaria, viral warts, and contact dermatitis (such as poison oak or ivy) are commonly seen, as are a variety of viral, bacterial, and fungal infections such as tinea pedis and cruris, the latter perhaps more common because of the close quarters and (sometimes) poor hygiene in some collegiate settings. Less frequent, but not uncommon, are such conditions as pityriasis rosea, herpes zoster, fungal infections of the toenails, and dysplastic nevi.

ENT/RESPIRATORY

Upper respiratory infections (colds) and allergies account for more visits to primary care medical facilities than any other acute illness; college health centers are no exception. While most students are aware that there is no specific treatment for viral upper respiratory infections, many are concerned that they may have strep throat, sinusitis, otitis media, bronchitis, or pneumonia (or "hope" they do, so they may receive antibiotic treatment). Obviously, since most do not have a serious illness, two major challenges exist in dealing with the student: first, differentiating the significant illness from the minor one; and, second, explaining to them why viral infections do not need antibiotic treatment. Many providers, unfortunately, find it easier to give patients antibiotics. Not surprisingly, such treatment ensures that the student will return for the next "cold" as well.

Bronchitis manifested by a cough, which can persist for several weeks, is a common and perplexing problem. Most infectious disease experts disdain the use of antibiotics for bronchitis, because most of the etiologic agents (respiratory viruses, pertussis, and TWAR strains of chlamydia) are thought to cause only self-limited disease.[7] Asthma associated with allergies is a common complaint, and must be differentiated from an infectious bronchitis. It is not uncommon for a respiratory infection to trigger broncho-spasm in those so predisposed, thus complicating the etiology of a cough. Most of these problems can be treated by the primary care provider, but occasionally specialist inter-vention may be necessary. Spontaneous pneumothorax, while not common, must be con-sidered in any student with sudden onset of cough, chest pain, and shortness of breath.

CARDIOVASCULAR

"In most college student populations, sedentary life style and high blood cholesterol will be the most prevalent modifiable risk factors, followed by smoking and hypertension."[8p. 743] However, since none of these initially cause symptoms or observable illness, students rarely present to a health service with related complaints (perhaps nowhere else is the value of a well-run primary prevention/health education program so well demonstrated). The most common cardiac symptom is probably an irregular cardiac rhythm, which usually is benign. Chest pain in the average college age group usually is not cardiac in origin. Systolic heart murmurs may sometimes be found during routine physical exams, especially in athletes, and a decision must be made about further evaluations, e.g., echocardiography. Visits for "cardiac" symptoms or concerns, however, may be used as an opportunity to review other cardiovascular risk factors with the student patient.

GASTROENTEROLOGY

Gastroenteritis, usually viral and usually self-limited, is often caused by Norwalk-like viruses and among students is a common intestinal complaint, with nausea, vomiting, and diarrhea. If symptoms are severe and accompanied by fever and hematochezia, a bacterial etiology should be considered. Given the international travel exposure by many students, parasitic causes of gastroenteritis need consideration. With their frequent epi-sodes of stress, irregular hours, and unusual diets, many students have intestinal distress they fear may be peptic in nature. While this is, in fact, not unusual, most symptoms will respond to a reduction of gastric irritants and a more regular lifestyle, even without antacids. Inflammatory bowel disease, such as Crohn's disease or ulcerative colitis, is also seen with some frequency in this population. Fortunately, many symptoms which may initially suggest these more serious diagnoses result from irritable bowel syndrome, which may respond to some of the previously mentioned lifestyle modifications.

Hepatitis is uncommon in the student population. Hepatitis A is usually, but not always, travel-related, and is now vaccine-preventable. Hepatitis B is usually seen as a chronic infection, diagnosed on a random blood test; it is also vaccine-preventable. The vaccination is recommended as part of the RIPI. Hepatitis C is seen even less frequently than "A" or "B" and is most commonly associated with parenteral drug abuse, or transfusion or organ transplantation prior to 1990. Sexual transmission may occur, but the virus is not commonly spread in this manner.[9]

Urological Conditions

Acute bacterial cystitis in sexually active women is a common diagnosis in college students. It is easily treated with a short course of antibiotics. Pyelonephritis is less common and may appear without urinary symptoms. Urethritis is more commonly seen in men, and is usually sexually transmitted; Chlamydia is the most common cause. Epididymitis and prostatitis are occasionally seen, and may or may not be sexually transmitted. Genital warts and herpes simplex may be seen in men and women and are probably far more widespread in sexually active individuals than is commonly believed.

Gynecologic Conditions

Vaginitis is the most common gynecologic diagnosis, and in this population may be caused by yeast, bacteria, or rarely, trichomonas. The differential diagnosis of abdominal pain in women must always include the intestinal, urologic, and gynecologic systems, for example, appendicitis, pyelonephritis, and pelvic inflammatory disease, as well as ectopic pregnancy or a ruptured ovarian cyst. The Pap smear remains an important method by which to diagnose cervical HPV infection and dysplasia. (The reader is referred to Chapter 8 in this text for a more detailed exposition of gynecologic issues in college women.)

Neurological Conditions

Headaches, both muscular tension and migraine, are quite common in the student population. Occasionally, neurologic consultation is necessary for problematic cases. Oral contraceptive use and stress may complicate the diagnosis. Viral encephalomeningitis is not common in the college age group but must be considered in any differential diagnosis of headache. Meningococcal meningitis is a very rare event on the campus, important to mention principally because of its catastrophic nature and the public anxiety associated with a single case. Recent recommendations from the Advisory Committee on Immunization Practices suggest that health care providers for college freshmen who plan to live in dormitories should "inform these students and their parents about meningococcal disease and the benefits of vaccination."[10, p.15] Multiple sclerosis is also rare but overwhelming in its discovery and is usually first diagnosed in the young adult age group.

Musculoskeletal

Sprains and minor injuries are to be expected and, indeed, are very common in an active young population. Most will respond to conservative treatment; some will require physical therapy. The application of the Ottawa criteria to determine the need for X-rays in ankle sprains has been very reliable in reducing unnecessary X-rays.[11] Fractures, dislocations, ruptured lumbar discs, and major knee injuries may require orthopedic assistance. Rheumatologic problems are less common than injury, but are, unfortunately, not rare in college students and need consideration in a diagnostic evaluation.

MISCELLANEOUS

Infectious mononucleosis is probably seen more in college students than in any other population. The infection in younger age groups is relatively mild, common, and often not recognized, particularly in lower socioeconomic classes. However, in college-age students, it is one of the most impressive infectious diseases commonly seen, and lasts longer than most other viral infections. Antibiotics are of no benefit; prednisone has been used in some severe cases, but controlled studies that prove benefit are lacking.

Lyme disease is much feared but infrequently seen, especially in western parts of the country. Only deer ticks carry and transmit the infection, and they must be attached to the skin for at least one to two days to transmit the disease. Antibiotics may be used after tick bites if there is a high frequency of infected ticks in the area and attachment is greater than one to two days.[12]

A diagnosis of malaria must be considered if a student who has recently traveled to an endemic area presents with fever, especially if he or she has not taken malaria prophylaxis properly.

Fatigue is a common presenting complaint of the overworked, overstressed student. It is rare that a physical cause can be found for fatigue, either on physical examination or by laboratory studies; however, anemia, hypothyroidism, and metabolic derangements should be considered in the differential diagnosis. The diagnosis of chronic fatigue syndrome is one of exclusion and must satisfy the National Institute for Health criteria to be labeled as such.[13] Depression may be an underlying cause, and the provider must consider whether he or she is comfortable prescribing antidepressant medications, or whether a referral to mental health services is appropriate (and acceptable to the student). Stress and psychosomatic issues must always be distinguished from physical ailments. Often both present together, requiring a medical provider and mental health counselor to work collaboratively.

Eating disorders, anorexia and bulimia, are diagnoses that also require intense medical/psychological coordination, often with help of a nutritional therapist as well.

UNUSUAL DIAGNOSES IN COLLEGE HEALTH

Many of the above problems may seem routine, but a high index of suspicion is essential when dealing with college students. Their lifestyles, their international travel, their tendency to not make personal health a priority, all predispose to unusual problems. A few unusual diagnoses seen by one author of this chapter (John Dorman) in the last year include glandular cell carcinoma of the endometrium requiring hysterectomy, visceral larva migrans with tropical eosinophilia, typhoid fever, non-Hodgkins lymphoma, toxic megacolon exacerbating ulcerative proctitis, requiring emergency colectomy, pulmonary embolism, and a pituitary tumor complicated by a cerebrovascular accident.

THE ISSUE OF PERIODIC EXAMINATIONS

Depending upon resources, health services may or may not be able to provide routine health maintenance examinations for students. Annual physical examinations are no longer recommended by most authorities. In 1996, the United States Preventive Services Task Force advised, instead, periodic health maintenance evaluations.[14] In the college age group, little in the way of actual physical examination is recommended during this evaluation: height, weight, blood pressure, and for women, a Pap test and chlamydia screen. Other health maintenance considerations which are much more important for college students include dealing with issues of high-risk behavior; alcohol and other drug abuse; use of seat belts, helmets, and smoke detectors; gun safety; tobacco use; consideration/ screening for sexually transmitted diseases (STDs), with discussion of abstinence/condom use/contraception; diet (including calcium intake for women, and folic acid for women contemplating pregnancy); exercise; cholesterol screening; dental care, including flossing and fluoride; and immunizations (which are covered by the college RIPIs). High-risk students should be further considered for other STD screening (chlamydia, gonorrhea, HIV), melanoma screening, and other immunizations such as influenza, pneumococcal, varicella, and hepatitis A vaccines.

SPECULATION ON THE FUTURE

In recent years some of the most dramatic changes in medical practice have been in the technologic areas—so-called medical informatics. The availability of email and Internet access to nearly all college students made it inevitable that computers will have a major impact on the delivery of health services to students. A student patient may come to the clinician having already researched a presumed diagnosis on the Internet, where he or she may, or may not, have used reliable sources.

Students have always been difficult to contact, but advances in recent years, such as voice mail and email, have made the process much easier, as the provider can leave messages for the student to read and reply to at leisure. Making (and canceling) appointments by email or through the Internet is technically quite possible and is being done at some SHSs. However, these new advances raise confidentiality questions never considered by a previous generation of clinicians, particularly considering the apparent indestructibility of email messages.[15]

Health maintenance organizations (HMOs) are already entrenched in the medical marketplace and have been incorporated into the college health environment as well. However, students with HMO coverage based "at home," which may be a long distance from where they are attending college, may find themselves with no coverage for nonemergent care. Dealing with this problem may require action on the national level, either by an organization such as ACHA or by the federal government.

In an era of escalating costs, outsourcing, that is, a college or university contracting with outside providers to provide medical care for the student body, is increasing. Indeed, in recent years, for-profit organizations have been formed which purport to have special expertise in operating student health services. These firms offer their services to colleges for a contracted fee, and will "come onto the campus" to run the health service. It remains to be seen whether this development will ultimately benefit the overall health of the college student population (and fulfill the public health and collaborative missions of the traditional, institutionally run health service) or whether the outsourcing movement will even continue.

Table 1. Fifty Most Common Diagnoses for Men and Women, 1997-98[6] (excluding immunizations)

CPT Code	Diagnosis	Number
V72.3	GYN Exam	4901
465.9	Acute URI	4090
V65.40	Counseling NOS	3491 (1)
V25.41	Contraceptive Pill Surveillance	3306
V82.9	Screening Condition NOS	2648 (2)
311.	Depressive Disorder NEC	2061
V68.89	Administrative Encounters NEC	1914 (3)
848.9	Sprain NOS	1571
595.9	Cystitis	1033
477.9	Allergic Rhinitis	1004
461.9	Acute Sinusitis NOS	973
078.	Viral Warts NOS, NEC	936
462	Acute Pharyngitis	912
300.00	Anxiety State NOS	696
998.2	Acc. OP Laceration	696
V70.3	Med. Exam NEC Admin.	656 (4)
795.0	Abnormal Pap Smear—Cervix	646
466.0	Acute Bronchitis	591
112.1	Candidal Vulvovaginitis	567
924.9	Contusion NOS	519
616.10	Vaginitis NOS	488
314.9	Hyperkinetic Syndrome NOS	481
V74.5	Screen for VD	465
692.9	Dermatitis NOS	461
493.90	Asthma W/O Status	454
382.9	Otitis Media NOS	419
784.0	Headache	410
034.0	Strep Sore Throat	405
009.0	Infectious Enteritis NOS	416
078.11	Condyloma Acuminatum	412
706.1	Acne NEC	403
463.	Acute Tonsillitis	394
296.80	Bi-Polar NOS	380

**Table 1. Fifty Most Common Diagnoses for Men and Women, 1997-98[6]
(excluding immunizations)** *(continued)*

CPT Code	Diagnosis	Number
372.30	Conjunctivitis NOS	365
789.09	Abdominal Pain Site NEC	345
079.99	Viral Infection NOS	328
216.9	Benign Neoplasm Skin NOS	312
300.3	OBC Disorder	307
309.81	Prolong Post Traumatic Stress	288
V68.1	Issue Repeat Prescript	288
V62.89	Psychological Stress NEC	274
879.9	Open Wound Site NOS	268
780.7	Malaise & Fatigue	267
E920.5	Acc—Hypodermic Needle	264
682.9	Cellulitis	264
309.9	Adjustment Reaction, NOS	241
785.6	Enlargement Lymph Nodes	237
117.9	Mycoses	231
V72.4	Preg. Exam—Preg. Unconfirmed	226
V25.40	Contracept. Surveillance	221

Notes
(1) V65.40—Counseling, health education, review lab studies
(2) V82.9—Special screening for unspecified conditions
(3) V68.89—Encounters for administrative purposes
(4) V70.3—Physical examinations (athletic, school, insurance, travel)

**Table 2. Most Frequent Diagnosis by Encounters[6]
(Report lists the top 50 diagnoses for women)**

ICD9 Code	DescriptionW/Diag	Number
V74.1	Screening-Pulmonary TB	8153
V72.3	Gynecologic Examination	4901
V25.41	Contracep Pill Surveillance	3304
V65.40	Counseling NOS	3225
465.9	Acute URI NOS	2654
V14.7	HX-Vaccine Allergy	2366
V82.9	Screen Cond NOS	1784
311	Depressive Disorder NEC	1576
V06.4	Vac-Measle-Mumps-Rubella	1276
V68.89	Admin Encounter NEC	1228
V05.3	Vac for Viral Hepatitis	1124
595.9	Cystitis NOS	998

Table 2. Most Frequent Diagnosis by Encounters[6]
(Report lists the top 50 diagnoses for women) *(continued)*

ICD9 Code	DescriptionW/Diag	Number
848.9	Sprain NOS	829
461.9	Acute Sinusitis NOS	742
477.9	Allergic Rhinitis NOS	662
795.0	Abn Pap Smear—Cervix	646
112.1	Candidal Vulvovaginitis	567
462	Acute Pharyngitis	543
998.2	Accidental OP Laceration	510
300.00	Anxiety State NOS	498
616.10	Vaginitis NOS	488
466.0	Acute Bronchitis	379
V74.5	Screen for VD	370
078.10	Viral Warts NOS	314
493.90	Asthma W/O Status Asth	311
784.0	Headache	308
924.9	Contusion NOS	301
692.9	Dermatitis NOS	299
706.1	Acne NEC	299
078.11	Condyloma Acuminatum	294
309.81	Prolong Posttraum Stress	288
034.0	Strep Sore Throat	272
789.09	Abdominal Pain—Site NEC	259
009.0	Infectious Enteritis NOS	258
382.9	Otitis Media NOS	256
V70.3	Med Exam NEC-Admin	255
296.80	Bi-Polar NOS	240
463	Acute tonsillitis	227
V72.4	Preg Exam—Preg Uncomfirm	226
V25.40	Contracep Surveil NOS	221
300.0	OBC Disorder	220
372.30	Conjunctivitis NOS	216
V62.89	Psychological Stress NEC	214
079.99	Viral Infection NOS	203
216.9	Benign Neoplasm Skin NOS	202
780.7	Malaise and Fatigue	197
616.9	Female Genit Inflam NOS	189
E920.5	ACC—Hypodermic Needle	189
307.50	Eating Disorder NOS	185
626.0	Absence of Menstruation	185

Table 3. Most Used Diagnoses by Encounters[6]
(Report lists the top 50 diagnoses for men)

ICD9 Code	Description W/Diag	Number
V74.1	Screening—Pulmonary TB	3924
465.9	Acute URI NOS	1431
V14.7	HX-Vaccine Allergy	964
V82.9	Screen Cond NOS	847
848.9	Sprain NOS	729
V05.3	Vacc for Viral Hepatitis	588
V06.4	Vac-Measle-Mumps-Rubella	579
V68.89	Admin Encounter NEC	564
311	Depressive Disorder NEC	473
V70.3	Med Exam NEC-Admin	400
078.10	Viral Warts NOS	380
462	Acute Pharyngitis	369
477.9	Allergic Rhinitis NOS	342
314.9	Hyperkinetic Synd NOS	297
V65.40	Counseling NOS	262
461.9	Acute Sinusitis NOS	230
924.9	Contusion NOS	216
466.0	Acute Bronchitis	212
300.00	Anxiety State NOS	198
V68.1	Issue Repeat Prescript	190
998.2	Accidental OP Laceration	184
382.9	Otitis Media NOS	163
692.9	Dermatitis NOS	162
009.0	Infectious Enteritis NOS	158
879.8	Open Wound Site NOS	158
463	Acute Tonsillitis	153
372.30	Conjunctivitis NOS	149
493.90	Asthma W/O Status Asth	143
296.80	Manic-Depressive NOS	140
034.0	Strep Sore Throat	133
V58.3	Atten-Surg Dressing/Sut	128
079.99	Viral Infection NOS	123
V06.5	Vacc-Tetanus & Diptheria	121
078.11	Condyloma Acuminatum	118
117.9	Mycoses NEC & NOS	111
216.9	Benign Neoplasm Skin NOS	110
401.9	Hypertension NOS	105
706.1	Acne NEC	104
829.0	Fracture NOS—Closed	103
784.0	Headache	102
309.9	Adjustment Reaction NOS	99
V74.5	Screen for VD	95

Table 3. Most Used Diagnoses by Encounters[6]
(Report lists the top 50 diagnoses for men) *(continued)*

ICD9 Code	Description W/Diag	Number
682.9	Cellulitis NOS	90
078.19	Viral Warts NEC	90
300.3	OBC Disorder	87
789.09	Abdominal Pain-Site NEC	86
099.40	NGU NOS	85
V70.0	Routine Medical Exam	84
785.6	Enlargement Lymph Nodes	83
724.2	Lumbago	78

REFERENCES

1. Christmas WA, Dorman JM. The Storey of college health hygiene. J Am Coll Health 1996;45:27–34.

2. Christmas, WA. Medical services for college health. In Wallace HM, Patrick K, Parcel GS, Igoe JB. Principles and Practices of Student Health. Oakland: Third Party Publishing Co.;1992:520–531.

3. Sim, I. What Is Primary Care? PC Teaching Module, Stanford University, June 24, 1996.

4. ACHA Vaccine-Preventable Diseases Task Force. Recommendations for institutional prematriculation immunizations. January 2000.

5. MMWR. Immunization of health-care workers. 1997;46:6,14.

6. University of Kentucky Student Health Service Statistics, 1998.

7. Gilbert DN, Moellering RC Jr., Sande MA. The Sanford Guide to Antimicrobial Therapy. 1998, 28th edition, p. 26.

8. Manchester R. Cholesterol and other CHD risk factors in the college population. In Wallace HM, Patrick K, Parcel GS, Igoe JB. Principles and Practices of Student Health. Oakland: Third Party Publishing Co.;1992:743.

9. MMWR. Recommendations for prevention and control of hepatitis C virus (HCV) infection and HCV-related chronic disease. 1998;47:7–8.

10. MMWR. Meningococcal Disease and College Students. Recommendations of the Advisory Committee on Immunization Practices. 2000;49:11–20.

11. Stiell IG, McKnight RD, Greenberg GH, et al. Implementation of the Ottawa ankle rules. JAMA 1994;271:827–832.

12. Behrman: Nelson Textbook of Pediatrics, Sixteenth Edition, 2000. WB Saunders Company, Chapter 219 by Shapiro ED.

13. Fukuda K, Straus SE, Hickie I, et al. The chronic fatigue syndrome: A comprehensive approach to its definition and study. Ann Intern Med 1994;121:953–958.

14. Office of Disease Prevention and Health Promotion, US Dept. of Health and Human Services, Public Health Service. Clinician's Handbook of Preventive Services. Washington DC, 1996, p. xix.

15. Christmas WA, Turner HS, and Crothers L. Should college health providers use email to communicate with their patients? Two points of view. J Am Coll Health. July 2000;49(1).

Chapter Six

Women's Health Issues and Contraception in College and University Health Services

Thomas Dale, MD, and Pamela Woodrum, ARNP

Historical Perspective

Gynecology services provided by college and university health programs evolved throughout the last century, with their development being closely intertwined with societal trends. The medical and social responses to the gynecological problems of previous generations of college women may seem almost quaint, and certainly inadequate, to women of the twenty-first century. Fledgling gynecologic programs within college and university health services matured because of the requests, demands, and needs of college women. And, not surprisingly, these programs continue to be modified by community expectations and acceptance.

Until the 1960s most college women received their gynecologic care from their physicians at home. As the United States experienced the political and sexual revolution of that decade, college campuses were often the focal points that embraced change, creating a synthesis of increased expectations that reflected back to the extended community. As issues and services that had been ignored or hidden became more open and available, female students became more comfortable requesting gynecological services. Requests for the "new" oral contraceptive pills led to their becoming available through many health services.

This change in expectations continued into the seventies. Health service gynecologic personnel were presented with the challenge of evaluating and treating college women with structural abnormalities of the vagina, cervix, and uterus related to in utero exposure to synthetic estrogens (such as Diethylstilbestrol) given to their mothers in an attempt to prevent pregnancy loss. A legal shift in the availability of abortion enabled women of the seventies to arrive at campus health services requesting information about, and referral for, pregnancy terminations. The intrauterine device became a popular method of long-term and emergency contraception. The incidence of sexually transmitted diseases increased as oral contraceptive devices replaced barrier methods of birth control.

In the early eighties the appearance of the human immunodeficiency virus spurred promotion of condom use. Condom use, however, was not generally well accepted on college campuses and rates of infection with Chlamydia trachomatis, herpes simplex virus, and the human papillomavirus increased. With the increase in HPV came an increase in the number of Pap smears exhibiting cervical neoplasia. This problem and its sequelae became a major focus in college gynecologic care, necessitating access to colposcopy for many college women, either by referral or by inclusion of this capability within the health services. In some health services, computer-assisted tracking was instituted to assist in following the progress of the large numbers of abnormal Pap smears.

CURRENT STATUS

At present, gynecologic services vary from campus to campus. Each institution has unique resources that determine which problems can be addressed and the extent to which they can be evaluated and treated. Clinical staffing varies from a single provider with no ancillary services to entire departments composed of physicians, nurse practitioners, physician assistants and nurses, with laboratory and radiology facilities, and colposcopy and ultrasound capability.

While contemporary female college students range in age from 17 to 70 (with a diversity of cultural and ethnic backgrounds), most of the women who use on-campus health services are 17 to 27 years old. This age group is often medically nomadic, seeking medical care from their home physicians, the local public health department, Planned Parenthood, an emergency department, and urgent treatment centers, as well as their campus health services. Older students often continue to use their private long-term providers.

Students look to college health professionals for care of a wide range of medical problems. With the increasing open dialogue in women's health, campus health services have found the need to recruit clinicians who have been trained to respond to the unique needs of women in the university setting.

For most students, college is a time of transition. Major life-affecting choices are being made about relationships, commitments, sex, and pregnancy. Concerns develop about the balance of family and career. There may be unexpected and unwanted complications with their personal relationships. Students' encounters with the campus health service may be brief and transient, but volatile and dynamic, sometimes affecting their future. Their gynecological concerns often involve situations about which they do not want prior caregivers and family to be informed. Thus, they may choose a campus health service not only for convenience and cost, but for confidentiality as well.

If gynecological care is not available in the health service, provision for referrals should be made. If the clinician providing the care is uncomfortable discussing a particular health issue or is unable to discuss the issue without bias, referral should be made to a clinician (within or outside the health service) who can provide the health care. The gynecology clinician must combine the resources of medical technology and proper emotional support to assist each college woman in being a healthy unique individual.

PRIMARY PREVENTION IN WOMEN'S HEALTH

Data from the 1995 National College Health Risk Behavior Survey (United States) indicate that many college students engage in behaviors that place them at risk for serious health problems.[1] Some of these behaviors have particular significance to women's health in general and to gynecological health specifically.

Health Risk Behaviors

Tobacco

Women and Smoking: A Report of the Surgeon General makes it clear that smoking has become a woman's issue. The 2001 report summarizes health issues related to smoking by women.[2]

In 1987 lung cancer surpassed breast cancer as the leading cause of cancer deaths among women in the United States. Cigarette smoking is the major cause of lung, oropharyngeal, and bladder cancer in women. There is strong evidence for an increased risk of colorectal, liver, pancreatic, kidney, and cervical cancer in women smokers. Evidence is more limited but consistent with increased risks for laryngeal and esophageal cancer.[2] Smoking is a primary cause of chronic obstructive pulmonary disease. Women who smoke have a higher risk for coronary heart disease, stroke, subarachnoid hemorrhage, and peripheral vascular atherosclerosis, and an increased risk for death from ruptured abdominal aneurysm.[2]

Smoking in women is associated with delayed conception, primary and secondary infertility, ectopic pregnancy, spontaneous abortion, premature rupture of membranes, premature delivery, and low birth weight babies.[2] Women who smoke experience menopause earlier than nonsmokers. Postmenopausal women smokers have reduced bone mineral density of the hip and an increased risk for hip fracture compared with nonsmokers.[2]

The 1995 College Health Risk Behavior Survey reported that nearly three-fourths (74.8 percent) of U.S. college students had tried cigarette smoking; almost one-third (29.0 percent) were current smokers.[1] In the 1999 Harvard College Alcohol Survey nearly half (45.7 percent) of the respondents had used a tobacco product in the past year, and one-third (32.9 percent) currently used tobacco.[3] Cigarettes accounted for most of the tobacco use. In both studies, women smoked as frequently as men. Many college women acknowledge starting smoking to relieve stress, to control weight, or as a social activity while drinking alcohol with friends.

Alcohol

The College Health Risk Behavior Survey indicates that over one-third (34.5 percent) of college students reported episodic heavy drinking during the thirty days preceding the survey. Of the females who drank, 41.5 percent reported having drunk more than five alcoholic drinks on at least one occasion on more than one of the thirty days preceding the survey.[1]

Women metabolize and absorb alcohol differently from men, attaining higher levels of blood alcohol after drinking equivalent amounts of alcohol.[4] Research suggests that women are more vulnerable than men to alcohol-related problems. Women develop alcohol-induced liver disease after consuming less alcohol over a shorter period of time when compared with men.[5,6] Women are also more likely to develop alcoholic hepatitis and to die from cirrhosis than are men.[7]

Some studies support the premise that moderate to heavy use of alcohol increases the risk for breast cancer in women.[8] Alcohol consumption may interfere with the ability to conceive.[9,10] When compared with non-drinkers, women who consume alcohol during pregnancy have a higher risk of having babies with serious birth defects; fetal alcohol syndrome is the most devastating.[11,12]

Without question, alcohol intoxication is a significant contributing factor for sexual assault/acquaintance rape in the college population.[13–15]

Sexual Activity

The National College Health Risk Behavior Survey indicates that over three-fourths (86.1 percent) of U.S. college students have engaged in sexual intercourse during their lifetime. More than one-third (34.5 percent) have had sexual intercourse with six or more partners. More than two-thirds (68.2 percent) had engaged in sexual intercourse during the three months preceding the survey.[1]

High-risk sexual activity encompasses beginning sexual intercourse at an early age, having multiple sexual partners, and neglecting to use protection from pregnancy and sexually transmitted diseases. Sexually transmitted diseases, including human immunodeficiency virus (HIV), place the female student at risk for pelvic inflammatory disease, chronic pelvic pain, ectopic pregnancy, infertility, cervical neoplasia, liver pathology, and death.

Unplanned pregnancies in college women result in single parenting, marriage and parenting earlier than planned, adoption, or pregnancy termination. Pregnancy can delay the completion of studies and, for some young women, lowers any chance for earning a college degree. Pregnancy termination is not without medical or psychological risks.

Physical Activity and Nutrition

One particularly important health risk factor which requires consideration in college health is the female athlete triad which is seen in (young) women who train excessively or perform excess physical activity.

The triad is defined as a combination of disordered eating, amenorrhea, and osteoporosis. Disordered eating may encompass a wide range of harmful behaviors, from food restriction to binging and purging, all for the purpose of maintaining a thin physique (which coaches and/or judges of some events may find "desirable") or for the purpose of weight loss. The extreme of these eating disorders can be anorexia or bulimia.

Amenorrhea associated with extreme exercise or training appears to be caused by changes in hypothalamic function, with a resultant decrease in hormone level causing amenorrhea. Under such circumstances, amenorrhea can be classified as primary or secondary.[16] With primary amenorrhea, spontaneous uterine bleeding does not occur either by the age of 14 (without the development of secondary sexual characteristics) or by the age of 16 (with otherwise normal development). Secondary amenorrhea is defined as a six-month absence of menstrual bleeding in a woman who has previously had normal primary regular menses.

Osteoporosis is defined as the loss of bone mineral density and inadequate bone formation, both of which lead to increased bone fragility and therefore risk of fracture. For the athlete such loss of density creates a significant risk for stress fractures, as well as for more serious fractures of weight-bearing bones.

The prevalence of the female athlete triad is not certain, but various studies have reported eating disorders in 15 percent to 62 percent of female college athletes, and amenorrhea in 3.4 percent to 66 percent of female athletes, compared with only 2.5 percent of women in general populations.[16]

In addition to the female athlete triad, other considerations are important for the health of college women. Increasingly, it is clear that poor health habits of early life (lack of exercise, obesity, tobacco use) impact the development of cardiovascular disease, including coronary artery disease, in women as well as men. Further, it is clear that early bone health, associated particularly with regular exercise and adequate calcium intake, is important during young adulthood to lessen the severity of osteoporosis, which occurs with aging.

Interventions

The college or university health care provider can play an important role in health promotion and disease prevention by addressing health risk behaviors that affect women. The following suggestions may be useful for intervention. For a more detailed and current discussion of clinical preventive services, the reader should consult appropriate sources which are regularly updated. (An excellent reference is the U.S. Preventive Services Task Force [USPSTF], http://www.ahcpr.gov/clinic/uspstfix.htm.)

Tobacco
* Routinely assess the smoking status of every female student seeking gynecology services.
* Advise all smokers to quit.
* Provide information to explain the obstetric/gynecologic risks of smoking.
* Be prepared for referrals to a smoking-cessation counselor or a smoking-cessation program, preferably within the student health service. Nicotine replacement therapy and antidepressants should be available to assist in the cessation efforts, if needed.

Alcohol
* Question students engaging in risky sexual behavior about their alcohol use.
* Be alert for abusive relationships that may be secondary to alcohol consumption by the student or her partner.

- When alcohol abuse is suspected, assure confidentiality and discuss with the patient. Refer for appropriate counseling when needed.

Sexual Activity

- Include sexual history to help assess the student's risk of sexually transmitted diseases and unwanted pregnancy.
- Provide contraceptive counseling, including information about emergency contraception.
- Provide information about prevention of sexually transmitted diseases.
- Offer hepatitis B vaccine to all students.

Female Athlete Triad

- Recognition of risk factors is essential to making the diagnosis. Athletic endeavors that emphasize low body weight and lean physique—gymnastics, ballet, distance running— should be particularly monitored.
- Prevention through education is crucial. Coaches and athletes must be aware of the risks of the triad.
- Screening at the time of the preseason preparticipation physical examination should include a careful menstrual history, dietary history, and exercise history to identify the female at risk.
- Once the diagnosis is made, treatment is essential. This may involve lifestyle changes. Specialist care, including psychiatrists or nutritionists, may be important. For intercollegiate athletics, involvement of coaches and athletic trainers is essential.
- While concerns about the effects of overexercise and excessive focus on diet and thinness are of concern (as discussed above), also of concern is the opposite; i.e., young women lacking regular exercise, with resultant poor physical conditioning and/or obesity. Correction of either of these by institution of a regular exercise program and by consultation in proper nutrition is an important intervention which can occur at the college age level to prevent later health problems (typically associated with aging) but having their origins in young adulthood.

Disease Screening

Breast Health

The National Cancer Institute reports that more than 180,000 American women are diagnosed with breast cancer each year.[17] Age is the most important factor in the risk for breast cancer, with increasing risk paralleling increasing age. Self-breast exam, exam by a health care professional, and mammography are the most effective measures for early detection of breast cancer.

The American Cancer Society guidelines for detection of breast cancer in asymptomatic women include:[18]

- Starting at age 20, breast self-exam every month
- From age 20 to 39, physical examination of the breast at least every three years by the woman's health care provider

- At age 40, physical examination of the breast every year by health care provider
- At age 40, an initial mammogram and then repeated annually

Mammography may be started before age 40 in women with a strong family history of breast cancer. Beginning annual exams by a health care provider prior to age 40 may also be appropriate for women at higher risk than the norm.

In a college or university health service, it is appropriate to do an annual breast exam in conjunction with the annual Pap smear. This is an excellent time to discuss individual breast cancer risk, teach breast self-exam, and reinforce monthly self-exam.

Cervical Health

Since 1955 the number of deaths from cervical cancer in American women has declined by 74 percent, due largely to the use of the Pap smear to detect early cellular changes. The Pap smear is used primarily to detect pre-invasive lesions that, when treated, can decrease the incidence of invasive cancer. Nonetheless, the American Cancer Society predicted that about 12,800 new cases of invasive cervical cancer would be diagnosed for 2000.[19]

The American College of Obstetricians and Gynecologists in the Committee on Gynecologic Practice states:

> Considering that cervical cancer has not been eradicated, that the incidence of cervical intraepithelial neoplasia appears to have increased over the past decade, that the Pap test has an appreciable false-negative rate, and that women tend to extend screening intervals, the proposed guidelines that recommend annual cervical cytologic screening for most women are prudent and warranted if early precursors to cervical cancer are to be detected and successfully treated.[20]

The increasing frequency of infection with the human papillomavirus supports the necessity for annual Pap smears in college women who have ever been sexually active. Routine screening with Pap smears is probably unnecessary for older women students who have undergone hysterectomy for benign gynecologic disease.[21]

Issues of Pregnancy

Female students visiting the health service may seek preconceptual advice, fertility assistance, pregnancy testing, pregnancy counseling, prenatal care, or pregnancy termination services. They may also arrive with physical complaints not immediately suggesting a pregnancy. Regardless of the patient's history, pregnancy should be included in the differential diagnosis in any student with amenorrhea, abdominal pain, or abnormal uterine bleeding. Not all students are ready to admit the possibility of pregnancy to themselves or to a health care provider. Depending on services offered in a particular health service, the clinician may either evaluate and provide care or evaluate and refer. College health clinicians evaluating students who are pregnant (planned or unplanned) must be able to provide care in an unbiased manner or, if unable to do so, refer to another clinician.

ISSUES RELATED TO CONTRACEPTION

A variety of contraceptive options are available, with each method having its own benefits and disadvantages. The student must decide which method is best for her in the context of her relationship, provided there is no medical risk or contraindication to her choice. Information provided about each method should be evidence based and sufficient to allow the student to make an informed decision. At the minimum, this information should include efficacy of the method, benefits and health risks, common side effects, correct usage, availability and cost, signs and symptoms indicating the need to return for evaluation, and return to fertility with discontinuation of contraception. Further, any discussion on contraception should include information as to whether or not that particular method is useful in helping to prevent sexually transmitted disease.

Table 1. Percentage of U.S. Women Experiencing Unintended Pregnancy during First Year of Use

Method	Typical Use[a]	Perfect Use[b]
Chance (no method)[c]	85	85
Spermicides[d]	26	6
Periodic abstinence	25	
Calendar		9
Ovulation method		3
Sympto-thermal[e]		2
Post-ovulation		1
Cap[f]		
Parous woman	40	26
Nulliparous woman	20	9
Diaphragm[f]	20	6
Withdrawal	19	4
Condom[g]		
Female (Reality®)	21	5
Male	14	3
Pill	5	
Progestin only		0.5
Combined		0.1
IUD		
ParaGard® (copper T 380A)	0.8	0.6
Progestasert®	2.0	1.5
Depo-Provera®	0.3	0.3
Norplant®	0.05	0.05
Female sterilization	0.5	0.5
Male sterilization	0.15	0.10

[a]Among *typical* couples who initiate use of a method (not necessarily for the first time), the percentage who experience an accidental pregnancy during the first year if they do not stop use for any other reason.

[b]Among couples who initiate use of a method (not necessarily for the first time) and who use it *perfectly* (both consistently and correctly), the percentage who experience an accidental pregnancy during the first year if they do not stop use for any other reason.

[c]The percentages in the second and third columns for becoming pregnant are based on data from populations where contraception is not used and from women who cease using contraception in order to become pregnant. Among such populations, about 89 percent become pregnant within one year. This estimate was lowered slightly (to 85 percent) to represent the percentages who would become pregnant within one year among women now relying on reversible methods of contraception if they abandoned contraception altogether.

[d]Foams, creams, gels, vaginal suppositories, and vaginal film.

[e]Cervical mucus (ovulation) method supplemented by calendar in the pre-ovulatory and basal body temperature in the post-ovulatory phases.

[f]With spermicidal cream or jelly.

[g]Without spermicides.

Adapted from contraceptive efficacy rates in Contraceptive Technology. *Seventeenth Revised Edition. Hatcher RA, et al., eds. New York: Ardent Media, Inc. 1998. With permission.*

Certain issues may be specifically important and directly relevant to teaching college women (many of whom may be planning contraception for the first time) about contraception in general, as well as relevant to their choice of a contraceptive method. A very brief discussion of a few important points which may need stressing follows. (Full discussions of contraceptive methods are readily available from many sources—see Suggested Resources—and therefore are not covered in detail in this text.)

Abstinence

Abstinence can mean refraining from all sexual behavior, refraining from any behavior involving genital contact, or refraining from penetrative sexual practices. A student's definition of abstinence determines her need for education about pregnancy and sexually transmitted disease prevention.

Coitus Interruptus (Withdrawal)

Coitus interruptus is withdrawing the penis from the vagina before male ejaculation occurs. While withdrawal can be used when no other method is available, or even in conjunction with another method, the risk of failure increases with repeated intercourse in a short time period, as some sperm may remain in the male's urethra after a prior ejaculation and be passed into the vagina with the pre-ejaculatory fluid.

Natural Family Planning (NFP)

Natural family planning is a "periodic abstinence" method of contraception that follows a woman's individual menstrual cycle to determine when intercourse is most likely (or least likely) to result in pregnancy. This method requires counseling the *couple*, not just the woman, and thus may present special difficulties for the unmarried college woman who is not in a long-term monogamous relationship. Counseling should be provided by a trained natural family planning instructor or by trained couples who have been educated by an organization such as the Couple to Couple League.

Mechanical barriers

Cervical cap

The cervical cap is a small rubber cup that is inserted into the vagina and placed over the cervix to block the entrance of sperm into the cervix. It covers the cervix completely and is held in place by suction. It must be fitted by a clinician and requires a prescription to obtain. Used with a spermicide, the cap must be inserted about 20 minutes before intercourse (before any penetration) and provides continuous protection for 48 hours. Additional spermicide is optional for repeated intercourse and is added with an applicator into the vagina without removing the cap. It must be left in place for at least eight hours after intercourse but should not remain on the cervix more than 48 hours. The "mechanics" and "planning" required to use this method may create obstacles to its proper (and therefore, effective) use in many college women.

Diaphragm

The diaphragm is a dome-shaped rubber cup with a flexible rim, which is inserted into the vagina so that the anterior rim fits snugly behind the pubic bone and the posterior rim sits in the posterior fornix behind the cervix. The diaphragm is a prescription device and must be fitted by a clinician. The diaphragm is used with a spermicide and can be inserted into the vagina up to six hours prior to intercourse; it must be left in place for at least six hours after intercourse. Additional spermicide is required for repeated intercourse. Thus, the same "mechanics" and "planning" issues related to the cervical cap are also concerns with the diaphragm.

Male Condom

The condom is a thin sheath placed over the glans and shaft of the penis to prevent sperm from entering the vagina and must be applied prior to any genital contact. A new condom must be used with each intercourse. While all condoms, whether latex, polyurethane, or lamb intestine (natural skin condoms), decrease the risk of pregnancy, only latex and polyurethane condoms have been documented to lower the risk of sexually transmitted diseases (STDs). Natural skin condoms do not offer similar protection and should be advised against if STD protection is needed. Oil-based products and some vaginal medications reduce latex integrity and increase the risk of leakage or breakage; thus, only water-based lubricants should be used with latex condoms.

Female Condom

The female condom is a loose-fitting plastic pouch that lines the vagina and prevents sperm from entering the vagina. It has two flexible rings, one inside at the closed end of the condom and the other around the open end. The inner ring serves as an insertion device and holds the condom in place in the vagina. The outer ring remains outside the vagina. The condom is pre-lubricated, does not require a prescription, and can be used only once. It can be inserted up to eight hours before sex, and should be removed after completion of intercourse. A male condom and the female condom should not be used together.

Spermicides

Spermicidal preparations (most containing nonoxynol-9) are available without a prescription in a variety of forms (foams, creams, jellies) and are inserted into the vagina prior to intercourse with an applicator or fingers, depending on the product. Each preparation has different directions for time of insertion and length of effectiveness and thus requires specific attention to details for use. All preparations should remain in the vagina for at least six hours after intercourse, with no douching and no tampon use during that time. Spermicides can be used alone, but effectiveness is increased with use of a male condom, a female condom, a diaphragm, or a cervical cap. Once again, the need to plan ahead and the required "mechanics" of use may present certain difficulties, particularly in the event of unplanned intercourse.

Intrauterine Devices (IUD)

IUDs can be a successful and safe contraceptive method for many women. However, they are best used in women who have had a child and who are in a stable, mutually monogamous relationship. Thus, the IUD may not be suitable for many college women. Additionally, the IUD should not be used in a woman with a history of pelvic inflammatory disease. Although debate still continues over the optimal time for insertion, an IUD can be inserted any time during the woman's menstrual cycle in the absence of pregnancy. If pregnancy occurs with an IUD in place, an ectopic pregnancy should always be considered.

Oral Contraceptive Pills (OCPs)

Combination OCPs

Most OCPs contain a combination of an estrogen and a progestin. OCPs containing less than 50 micrograms of estrogen are considered to be a safe, reliable method of contraception for most women. In addition, they have numerous non-contraceptive benefits which may be of importance to college women (e.g., improvement in acne). The primary mechanism of action is suppression of ovulation. Other possible mechanisms of action include alteration of the endometrium, making it unreceptive to ovum implantation, and thickening of cervical mucus so that sperm cannot enter the uterus.

All types of combination pills (with the exception of Mircette®) are taken for 21 days followed by 7 days free of active medication. The dosage of hormones may remain constant throughout the 21 active pills (monophasic) or may vary (multiphasic).

Estrogens currently used in OCPs in the United States are mestranol and ethinyl estradiol. All pills containing 35 or fewer micrograms of estrogen contain ethinyl estradiol. Progestins currently used are norethindrone, norethindrone acetate, norgestrel, levonorgestrel, ethynodiol diacetate, desogestrel, and norgestimate.

Most of the common side effects experienced with oral contraceptives (nausea, irregular or breakthrough bleeding or spotting, breast tenderness, moodiness, bloating) occur during the first two or three cycles of use and are self-limiting. Switching to a different pill formulation will usually benefit the student whose symptoms continue beyond the first three cycles.

Any student who chooses OCPs as a contraceptive method needs to be made aware of their risks. These include venous thromboembolism (VTE), acute myocardial infarction (AMI), and stroke, most notably in women who smoke. (There *is* a very small increase in absolute risks of VTE or ischemic stroke in healthy, nonsmoking women. The risk of MI or hemorrhagic stroke among these same women is even less and perhaps none at all.[22]) Carriers of the coagulation factor V Leiden mutation are clearly at increased risk for venous thrombosis.[23] According to the World Health Organization, the following list of conditions represents an unacceptable health risk if combination OCPs are used.

- Pregnancy
- Breastfeeding <6 weeks postpartum
- Age >35 years and smoking >20 cigarettes/day
- Hypertension >160/100 or with concomitant vascular disease
- Diabetes with complications
- Current or history of deep vein thrombosis
- Current or history of pulmonary embolism
- Major surgery with prolonged immobilization
- Current and history of ischemic heart disease
- History of cerebrovascular accident
- Complicated valvular heart disease
- Headaches with focal neurologic symptoms
- Current breast cancer
- Liver disease (active viral hepatitis, severe cirrhosis, liver tumors)

Progestin-Only Pills

Progestin-only pills, also known as "minipills," contain a small dose of norgestrel or norethindrone. A pill is taken at the same time every day, with no hormone-free interval between cycles. Because ovulation is not always suppressed with progestin-only pills, pregnancy prevention may be dependent on their effect on cervical mucus, the endometrium, and possibly on the fallopian tubes. However, other than in the breastfeeding woman, they are less effective than combined oral contraceptives. Progestin-only pills can be used in women for whom estrogen is contraindicated.

Levonorgestrel Contraceptive Implant

Norplant® is currently the only subdermal contraceptive used in the United States. This system consists of six flexible silastic rods, each containing 36 mg of levonorgestrel, inserted subdermally in the inner aspect of a woman's upper arm. This system provides five years of contraception. Insertion and removal of the implants are office procedures performed under local anesthesia. Insertion of Norplant ideally should occur within five days of the onset of menses to ensure the woman is not pregnant and prevent pregnancy during the first cycle of use, since adequate serum levels of the active hormone occur within 24 hours of insertion.[24] Mechanisms of action include inhibition of ovulation, thickening of cervical mucus, and endometrial atrophy. Irregular bleeding, acne, and headaches are the most common complaints in Norplant users. The daily release of progestin is undetectable within one week of removal.[25] Nonetheless, the relative "permanency"—five years of contraception and the difficulties sometimes involved in the insertion and removal of implants—make this an uncommon choice for college women.

Injectable Contraceptives

Depo-Provera® injection protects against pregnancy for three months (13 weeks). Initial dosing with Depo-Provera must be within the first five days of the menses in order to insure the absence of pregnancy and to inhibit ovulation during that first cycle. Lunelle protects against pregnancy for one month, and subsequent dosing is required every 20 to 30 days. Mechanisms of action of both include inhibition of ovulation and endometrial thinning. Complaints include irregular bleeding, weight gain, mood changes, and depression. With Depo-Provera approximately 50 to 75 percent of women become amenorrheic after one year of use; women may have a six- to twelve-month delay in fertility after discontinuation.[26] Although research published in the early 1990s indicated that use of Depo-Provera may be associated with decreased bone density,[27] more recent data indicate this impact on bone density may be a short-term or current-user effect.[28,29] The safety and side effects profile with Lunelle are similar to that of combination oral contraceptives. Return to fertility after discontinuation is generally one to three months.

While under specific circumstances injectable contraceptives may be useful in the college health setting, the need to visit the health service for regular injections may not be conducive to their frequent usage.

Emergency Contraception (EC)

EC, or postcoital contraception, is an option to prevent pregnancy in women who have had unprotected intercourse as a result of contraceptive failure, lack of planning, or rape. EC has been used in one form or another in university health services since the early 1970s, although it was not until 1998 that the FDA issued approval of any specific agent for this purpose. The three methods of emergency contraception currently available are discussed below.

Combination Emergency Contraception Pills (ECPs)

Most emergency contraceptive pills utilize a high dose of traditional oral contraceptives in a two-dose regimen. The original two-dose regimen was first described in 1974 by Professor Albert Yuzpe and was called the Yuzpe regimen in recognition of his research.[30] Since that time, additional OCP formulations have been utilized. However, it was not until February 1997 that the Food and Drug Administration (FDA) issued a statement that "certain combined oral contraceptives containing ethinyl estradiol and norgestrel or levonorgestrel are safe and effective for use as postcoital emergency contraception."[31] In 1998, Preven® became the first formulation specifically intended for EC approved by the FDA.

The first ECP dose is taken within 72 hours of unprotected intercourse; the second dose is taken 12 hours later. Because effectiveness decreases as the post-intercourse interval increases, treatment should begin as soon as possible.[32] Emergency contraception using combination pills reduces the risk of pregnancy by approximately 75 percent. The closer a woman is to ovulation at the time of unprotected intercourse, the less likely the method is to prevent pregnancy.[33] Because they are not as effective as consistent and correct use of precoital contraception, ECPs should not be used by a student as a routine method of contraception.

Students who take ECPs should be advised they may have nausea; some will experience vomiting. An anti-emetic taken one hour before each dose of hormones decreases nausea and vomiting. Less common side effects include headache, breast tenderness, and irregular bleeding. Menses may start several days early, on schedule, or several days late. A student who has not started her menses within three weeks after taking ECPs or within a few days after her expected date of menses should be screened for pregnancy. ECPs do not disrupt an established pregnancy (once implantation has occurred), and there is no evidence they have an adverse effect on a fetus.[34]

Progestin Only Emergency Contraceptive Pills

In July 1999, Plan B® became the first formulation of progestin-only pills approved by the FDA for emergency contraception. Ovrette® has been suggested for use in the past, but because of the number of pills required with each dose it has seldom been used. The progestin-only method can be used in a student for whom estrogen is contraindicated. The incidence of nausea and vomiting is less with this method than with the combination regimen.[32] Approximately 85 percent of the pregnancies that would have occurred without treatment are prevented, making this method more effective than combination ECPs.[32] The first dose of Ovrette is taken within 48 hours of unprotected intercourse, with a repeat dose 12 hours later. The first dose of Plan B® should be given within 72 hours and repeated in 12 hours.

Copper T Intrauterine Device

The copper T 380A (ParaGard®), can be inserted up to five days after unprotected intercourse. It can then be removed during the next menses or left in the uterus for ongoing contraception. Inserting the copper T IUD reduces the risk of pregnancy by more than 99 percent.[34] The most common side effects are the same as those with regular copper IUD use, i.e., increased menstrual bleeding and cramping. The IUD is not recommended for emergency contraception in women who are at increased risk of sexually transmitted diseases or in women who may have been infected with an STD secondary to rape. Due to higher risk-taking behavior by college women, most health service clinicians prefer oral regimens of emergency contraception.

SEXUAL ASSAULT

The 1995 National College Health Risk Behavior Survey reports that 13.1 percent of college students nationwide indicated they had been forced to have sexual intercourse against their will sometime during their lifetime.[1] Female students are significantly more likely than male students to be victims of sexual assault or rape. The National Institute of Justice estimates that annually in the United States one million women become victims of rape. Approximately 30 percent of rapes are reported to the police; 50 percent of rape victims tell no one of the assault.[35,36] Most victims know their attacker.[35] Acquaintance rape is frequently associated with alcohol use, by either the victim, the perpetrator, or both. Koss and Dinero found that alcohol use at the time of the assault was one of the four strongest predictors of the risk for rape.[38] Thus any program designed to reduce or prevent sexual assault *must* include a discussion of the association with the use and abuse of alcohol.

Drugs such as flunitrazepam (Rohypnol®) and gamma hydroxybutyrate (GHB) facilitate the crime of sexual assault. Although neither drug is approved for use in the United States, both are relatively easy to obtain. Usually administered without the intended victim's knowledge, often mixed in an alcoholic drink, these drugs can cause dizziness, drowsiness, memory loss, confusion, loss of consciousness, respiratory arrest, and death.

A college/university health service may provide acute rape evaluation and treatment or, if staff are not trained in appropriate protocol, they should refer immediately to an emergency department or a specified sexual assault center. Established protocols should be in place for the sexual assault exam, including those to follow in suspected drug-facilitated sexual assault. It is the responsibility of the health care provider to know the assault and rape laws in a particular state and to comply with all legal requirements. Many states have developed a sexual assault assessment kit that outlines the steps for gathering evidence. The following are basic guidelines for health services to follow:

- Provide prophylactic antibiotic therapy and immunization. (The *1998 Guidelines for Treatment of Sexually Transmitted Diseases* from the Centers for Disease Control and Prevention contains a section on the treatment of the sexual assault victim.[39])
- Provide therapy to prevent unwanted conception.
- Counsel the victim regarding the aspects of rape trauma syndrome, a group of symptoms experienced by victims of sexual assault. These symptoms can be acute or delayed.
- Encourage the victim to seek help from a professional counselor with expertise in working with victims of sexual assault. Referral to a rape crisis center is also appropriate. Not all victims will accept referral for counseling initially, but it is important to provide the victims with referral services for their use at such time as they might decide to seek assistance.
- Use future visits with the victim to reevaluate and reinforce the importance of counseling.

The reasons for postponement of care are numerous and include self-blame, embarrassment, fear, not knowing where to go for help, denial, or not realizing that what happened was sexual assault. The victim of a sexual assault may come to a health service months after the event with a complaint unrelated to the incident. There may be no mention of the past event, and physical exam may provide no clues. The health service clinician must be able to recognize the behavioral and psychologic sequelae and the physical health problems that may suggest a history of sexual assault.

FREQUENT GYNECOLOGICAL ISSUES IN CAMPUS HEALTH

Routine Well Patient Visits

The most frequent gynecologic visits to campus health centers are for preventive care. The exam should include a Pap smear and appropriate screening for sexually transmitted diseases (STDs), as well as evaluation for thyroid, breast, and pelvic disorders.

Visits for counseling are also frequent. Much of the counseling includes preventive information regarding the need for breast self-exam and Pap smear, the use of contraception, and prevention of sexually transmitted diseases. Counseling related to unwanted pregnancy and acquired STDs is often necessary, as well.

Visits for Common Infectious Medical Problems

The most frequent visits related to symptomatic infections are for vaginitis, urinary tract infections, and sexually transmitted diseases (STDs). Candida overgrowth and bacterial vaginosis are common, while allergic phenomena, trichomoniasis, nonspecific vaginitis, and nonspecific cervicitis are less commonly seen. Pharmaceutical marketing and convenience have influenced treatment of candida, with oral treatment now popular with many students. However, some students prefer vaginal gel as treatment, to avoid possible systemic side effects of oral medication.

Uncomplicated cystitis is the most common urinary tract infection seen in college health and typically responds well to treatment with short term antibiotics such as sulfamethoxazole/trimethoprim. Urinalysis is usually sufficient for diagnosis. Culture and sensitivity should be reserved for students with poor response to treatment or who have findings indicative of upper tract disease. Pyelonephritis can be serious but, fortunately, is infrequent in the college population. Urinary tract infections in the college female are often related to sexual activity. Education regarding the etiology, prevention, and treatment of this problem is a necessary component of the visit.

The most frequent STDs encountered in health services are human papillomaviruses (HPV), molluscum contagiosum, Chlamydia trachomatis, and herpes simplex virus (HSV). The incidence of HPV continues to increase, while chlamydia has been decreasing. HSV is a persistent problem. HPV and its sequelae have become an important health issue in campus gynecology. (The reader is referred to chapter 8 on STDs for a more complete discussion.)

Abnormal Pap Smears

Personnel, equipment, and the patient's insurance requirements often limit the evaluation of the abnormal Pap smear by health service clinicians. In addition to these factors, each center must decide at what point referral should be made. For those centers without a clinician skilled in colposcopy, biopsy, and treatment, early referral may be appropriate and necessary. Other institutions may have the resources needed for more complete evaluation and treatment. Most campus health services fall somewhere between these extremes. Before proceeding with biopsy and treatment, a discussion of the student's insurance coverage or financial situation is necessary to assure that the student does not become burdened with unexpected debts. At some point, the student may need referral to her primary provider or the specialist required by her family insurance. Because some students do not want parents to know of their abnormal Pap smears, they may prefer to make payments rather than use their insurance. Students without any insurance coverage may need education about options for financial assistance.

The nomenclature for categorizing Pap smears has changed several times over the last thirty years.

Table 2. Pap Smear Classification

Traditional Papanicolaou	World Health Organization	Richert and Barron	Bethesda
Class I	Normal	Class I	Within normal limits
Class II	Atypical	Class II Inflammatory atypia	ASC[c]
Class III	Mild dysplasia	CIN I[b]	Low grade SIL[d] (includes HPV)
	Moderate dysplasia	CIN II	High grade SIL
	Severe dysplasia/CIS[a]	CIN III	High grade SIL
Class IV	CIS	CIN III	High grade SIL
Class V			Squamous cell carcinoma

[a] carcinoma in situ; [b] Cervical intraepithelial neoplasia; [c] Atypical squamous cells; [d] Squamous intraepithelial lesion

Evaluation of the abnormal Pap smear has become a significant, and often troublesome, issue in college health. Most laboratories in the United States report Pap smear results according to the Bethesda System of classification introduced in 1988, revised in 1991, and in 2001.[40,41] The essence of this system is to provide the clinician with information regarding the adequacy of the specimen for evaluation, whether cells are normal or abnormal, and, if abnormal, whether "low grade" or "high grade." Categorization, descriptive diagnosis, and recommendations for further evaluation may be included in the pathological report of the smear.

In the current Bethesda System of classification the interpretation of the sample is reported as "satisfactory" or "unsatisfactory" for interpretation. If unsatisfactory, typically a request is made for repeat sampling after a proper cellular maturation time (usually about three months). If the specimen is satisfactory, it is reported as "normal" or "abnormal." If abnormal, the degree of abnormality is interpreted as low-grade squamous intraepithelial lesion (LGSIL) or high-grade squamous intraepithelial lesion (HGSIL). Often, no further information is provided, but at times the report may note a lack of cellularity limiting accurate evaluation or the presence of inflammation or reactive changes. Further subclassification of abnormalities may be related to the presence of squamous metaplasia, human papillomavirus, and glandular abnormalities.

Colposcopy for all squamous intraepithelial lesions (SIL) is advisable. If biopsy indicates LGSIL, many clinicians prefer to observe the patient with repeat Pap smears and colposcopy every three to four months, rather than advancing directly to treatment with laser, cryosurgery, or loop electrosurgical excision procedure (LEEP). In most younger females, improvement and/or resolution of the problem without further treatment is common. All women with HGSIL must be carefully evaluated and usually treated. AGC presents a more urgent dilemma, and evaluation should not be delayed, since glandular abnormalities may indicate the presence of an advanced lesion. Inconclusive diagnoses may be reported as atypical squamous cells (ASC) or atypical glandular cells (AGC).

Menstrual Irregularities

Menstrual irregularities and/or dysmenorrhea account for a large number of the complaints of college-age health women presenting to their health services. Requests for pain relief related to dysmenorrhea are frequent. Many women express a desire to start oral contraceptive pills to help control dysmenorrhea.

Secondary Amenorrhea

The most frequent cause of secondary amenorrhea seen in college health services is pregnancy. Hypothalamic hypofunction is not uncommon. Other causes are usually rare. Thus, evaluation of secondary amenorrhea in the college female must always begin with a pregnancy test. If the test is negative, a directed history and physical exam should follow. Hypothalamic hypofunction is suggested by extreme exercise, psychological stress, and decreased caloric intake from "dieting" or an eating disorder. Appropriate laboratory evaluation in this situation includes, at the minimum, serum prolactin, FSH, and TSH. Normal results would be expected in hypothalamic hypofunction. A progestin withdrawal test with 10 mg of medroxyprogesterone acetate administered daily for five days will determine the degree of associated hypoestrogenism. Withdrawal bleeding within ten days after completion of the medication indicates the woman has enough endogenous estrogen to produce endometrial growth. Absence of withdrawal bleeding indicates essentially no endogenous estrogen. Such low levels of estrogen may be associated with osteoporosis. Young women in this situation may be reluctant to increase weight or decrease exercise (for example, an athlete, particularly a long-distance runner), and may be hesitant to take hormone replacement or oral contraceptive pills as treatment. (For further discussion, see chapter 14 on Athletic Medicine.)

A rare cause of failure to have withdrawal bleeding following progestin stimulation is Asherman's syndrome—scarring of the endometrium with adhesions. In young college women this problem can sometimes follow dilatation and curettage or dilatation and evacuation.

Hyperandrogenism is suggested by hirsutism, acne, and body habitus with occasional truncal obesity. Serum testosterone may be elevated in these individuals. Polycystic ovarian syndrome may or may not present a similar picture with underlying insulin resistance.

Abnormal Vaginal Bleeding

While there are many causes of abnormal vaginal bleeding, the most troubling cause in college women is an abnormal pregnancy. Bleeding in early pregnancy, often before pregnancy has been confirmed, may be a complete, threatened, incomplete, or missed spontaneous abortion. With confirmation of pregnancy in a bleeding patient, the possibility of an ectopic pregnancy must be considered.

Diagnosis of the cause of abnormal vaginal bleeding requires a detailed history, which may reveal problems with contraception or bleeding secondary to trauma. In the absence of any of these general causes, dysfunctional uterine bleeding must be considered and requires a gynecologic endocrinology evaluation.

GYNECOLOGY AND THE MATURE WOMAN

Evaluation and treatment of problems common in the maturing woman is increasingly becoming the responsibility of college health clinicians, particularly in the realm of gynecological services. Menopause is defined as the permanent cessation of menses; a woman is considered to be menopausal when there has been no menses for one full year. This may occur as a result of retirement of ovarian function, removal of ovaries, or cessation of function as a result of chemotherapy or radiation. In the natural course of aging the average age of menopause is 51 years with a range of 45 to 55. The risk of pregnancy continues until a woman has not had a menstrual period for one year. Options for contraception are the same as for the younger contraceptive user, including male or female sterilization, as long as there is no medical contraindication.

While menstruation ceases abruptly with few systemic symptoms in some women, others become symptomatic months or even years prior to menopause. The transitional years leading up to menopause have been called the climacteric or perimenopause. Mood swings, muscle and joint pain, hot flushes, night sweats, irregular menstrual cycles, and sleep disturbances are not unusual during this time. The genitourinary system changes as a result of estrogen loss. Urinary tract infections, urinary incontinence, vaginal atrophy, vaginal dryness, dyspareunia, changes in libido, abnormal uterine bleeding, vulvar diseases, uterine prolapse, and gynecologic cancers can occur. When the production of estrogen ceases, the risks of cardiovascular disease, breast cancer, endometrial cancer, and osteoporosis increase.

College health clinicians must assist their older women patients in obtaining accurate information to make informed decisions about how best to deal with menopause-related effects, both short-term and long-term. A discussion of the benefits and risks of estrogen replacement therapy, the importance of adequate calcium and vitamin D intake, exercise, smoking cessation, and moderation of alcohol use is important at this time. Screening should include mammography, serum lipid evaluation, and thyroid function studies. The clinician should have knowledge of, or easy access to, information about herbal products and food supplements containing hormones, as many women seek remedies for menopausal symptoms outside the realm of established medical practice.

A FINAL NOTE

Medical advances continue to occur, and science continues to introduce new technology and new treatments. The media continue to bring medical information to the public, and Internet access has expanded the public's ability to research health issues. Not surprisingly, college women are increasingly informed about their own gynecologic health issues and expect more (and better) health care. It is therefore imperative that college and university health services stay abreast of advances in women's health issues and gynecological treatments and procedures. For most, that means the inclusion of gynecological care and counseling of the female student in their services, not only for young women, but increasingly for older women, as the demographics of students attending college undergo change in terms of age and in terms of the percentage of college students who are women.

SUGGESTED RESOURCES FOR THE GYN LIBRARY

Textbooks

Comprehensive Gynecology
Author: MISHELL, D
Publisher: Mosby-Yearbook, Published: 1997; Edition: 03

Contraceptive Technology
Author: HATCHER, R
Publisher: Ardent Media, Published: 1998; Edition: 17

Glass's Office Gynecology
Author: CURTIS, M
Publisher: Williams & Wilkins, Published: 1998; Edition: 05

Gynecology and Obstetrics (annual update)
Author: SCIARRA, J
Publisher: Lippincott-Raven

Scientific American Medicine (monthly update)
Author: DALE, D and FEDERMAN, D
Publisher: Healthcon/WebMD Corp.

Gynecology in Primary Care
Author: BARBIERI, RL et al.
Publisher: Scientific American Medicine, Inc.

Journals

American Family Physician
A journal of the American Academy of Family Physicians

Contraception
A journal of the Association of Reproductive Health Professionals

Journal of Lower Genital Tract Disease
A journal of the American Society for Colposcopy and Cervical Pathology

Monographs

ACOG Practice Bulletins: Clinical Practice Guidelines for Obstetricians-Gynecologists
American College of Obstetricians and Gynecologists

American Academy of Family Physicians (monthly series)
American Academy of Family Physicians

Guidelines for Treatment of Sexually Transmitted Diseases
Centers for Disease Control and Prevention (CDC)

MEETINGS

American Society for Colposcopy and Cervical Pathology
20 West Washington Street, Suite 1
Hagerstown, Maryland 21740

American College of Obstetricians and Gynecologists
Women's Health Care Physicians
409 12th Street, SW
PO Box 96920
Washington, DC 20090-6920

American Academy of Family Practice
8880 Ward Parkway
Kansas City, Missouri 64114-2797

REFERENCES

1. Centers for Disease Control and Prevention. National College Health Risk Behavior Survey—United States, 1995. MMWR 46 (SS-6): 1997.

2. Surgeon General's Report: Women and Smoking 2001. National Center for Chronic Disease and Prevention and Health Promotion, Centers for Disease Control and Prevention.

3. Rigotti et al. US college students' use of tobacco products. JAMA 284 (6): 699–705, 2000.

4. Frezza M., Di Padova C., Pozzato G, et al. High blood alcohol levels in women: The role of decreased gastric alcohol dehydrogenase activity and first-pass metabolism. N Eng J Med 322 (2): 95–99, 1990.

5. Tuyns, A.J, Pequignot, G. Greater risk of ascitic cirrhosis in females in relation to alcohol consumption. Int J Epidemiol 13 (1): 53–57, 1984.

6. Gavaler JS, and Arria AM. Increased susceptibility of women to alcoholic liver disease: Artifactual or real? In: Hall, P., ed. Alcoholic Liver Disease: Pathology and Pathogenesis. 2nd ed. London: Edward Arnold, 1995. pp. 123–133.

7. Hall PM. Factors influencing individual susceptibility to alcoholic liver disease. In Hall, PM., ed., Alcoholic Liver Disease: Pathology and Pathogenesis. 2nd ed. London: Edward Arnold, 1995. pp 299–316.

8. Smith-Warner SA., Spiegelman D, Yaun, SS, et al. Alcohol and breast cancer in women: A pooled analysis of cohort studies. JAMA 279 (7): 535–540, 1998.

9. Jensen, TK, et al. Does moderate alcohol consumption affect fertility? Follow up study among couples planning first pregnancy. BMJ 317: 505–510, 1998.

10. Hakim et al. Alcohol and caffeine consumption and decreased fertility. Fertil Steril 70: 632–637, 1998.

11. Prenatal exposure to alcohol. Alc, Res Hlth 24 (1): 32–41, 2000.

12. Fetal alcohol exposure and the brain. Alcohol Alert, no. 50, National Institute on Alcohol Abuse and Alcoholism, December 2000.

13. George WH, Gournic SJ, McAfee MP. Perceptions of post drinking female sexuality: Effects of gender, beverage choice, and drink payment. J Appl Soc Psychol 18: 1295–1317, 1988.

14. Abbey A. Acquaintance rape and alcohol consumption on college campuses: How are they linked? J Am Coll Health 39: 165–169, 1991.

15. Gross WC, Billingham RE. Alcohol consumption and sexual victimization among college women. Psychol Rep 82 (1): 80–82, 1998.

16. Hobart JA, Smucker DR. "The female athlete triad." American Family Physician. June 1, 2000. Taken from the website of The American Academy of Family Physicians on 8/25/00.

17. Feuer EJ, Wun LM. DEVCAN: Probability of developing or dying of cancer. Version 4.0. Bethesda MD: National Cancer Institute. 1999.

18. Summary of American Cancer Society recommendations for the early detection of cancer in asymptomatic people. American Cancer Society web site. Dec 2000.

19. Statistics. Uterine cervix. American Cancer Society web site. Dec 2000.

20. Routine cancer screening. ACOG committee opinion. Committee on Gynecologic Practice. 1993;128:1.

21. Pearce KF, Haefner HK, Sarwar SF, et al. Cytopathological findings on vaginal Papanicolaou smears after hysterectomy for benign gynecologic disease. N Eng J Med 335: 1559–62, 1996.

22. Meirik O. Cardiovascular safety and combined oral contraceptives. Contraception 1998; 57: 135–136.

23. Thorogood M. Stroke and steroid hormonal contraception. Contraception 1998; 57: 157–167.

24. Calvert J, et al. Contraception. AAFP Home Study Self-Assessment. Monograph 236. Feb 1999; 27.

25. Croxatto HB, Diaz S, Pavez M, et al. Clearance of levonorgestrel from the circulation following removal of Norplant subdermal implants. Contraception 1988; 38: 509.

26. Mishell DR. Pharmacokinetics of depot medroxyprogesterone acetate contraception. J Reprod Med (suppl); 1996; 41: 381–390.

27. Cundy T, Evans M, Roberts H, et al. Bone density in women receiving depot medroxyprogesterone acetate for contraception. BMJ 1991; 303: 13–16

28. Cundy T, Cornish J, Evans MC, et al. Recovery of bone density in women who stop using medroxyprogesterone acetate. BMJ 1994; 308: 247–248.

29. Petitti DB, Piaggio G, Mehta S, et al. Steroid hormone contraception and bone mineral density: A

cross-sectional study in an international population. The WHO Study of Hormonal Contraception and Bone Health. Obstet Gynecol 2000; 95: 736–744.

30. Yuzpe AA, Lancee WJ. Ethinylestradiol and dl-norgestrel as a postcoital contraceptive. Fertil Steril 1977; 28: 932–936.

31. Department of Health and Human Services. Prescription drug products; Certain combined oral contraceptives for use as postcoital emergency contraception; Notice. Federal Register. February 25, 1997; vol 62: no. 37: 8610–8612.

32. Task Force on Postovulatory Methods of Fertility Regulation: World Health Organization. Randomized controlled trial of levonorgestrel versus the Yuzpe regimen of combined oral contraceptives for emergency contraception. Lancet 1998; 352: 428–433.

33. Van Look P, Stewart F. Emergency contraception. In: Contraceptive Technology. Hatcher RA, et al. (eds.). New York: Ardent Media, Inc.; 1998; 277–295.

34. Glasier A. Emergency postcoital contraception. N Engl J Med 1997; 337: 1058–1064.

35. Bureau of Justice Statistics. Criminal victimization 1994. Washington, D.C.: U.S. Department of Justice, 1996; publication no. NCJ-158022.

36. Koss MP, Harvey MR. The rape victim: Clinical and community interventions. Newbury Park, California: Sage Publications, 1991.

37. Abbey A. Acquaintance rape and alcohol consumption on college campuses: How are they linked? J Am Coll Health 1991; 39:165–169.

38. Koss MP, Dinero TE. Discriminant analysis of risk factors for sexual victimization among a national sample of college women. J Consult Clin Psychol 1989; 57: 242–250.

39. Centers for Disease Control and Prevention. 1998 guidelines for treatment of sexually transmitted diseases. MMWR 1997; 47: No. RR-1.

40. Solomon D, Davey D, Kurman R et al. The 2001 Bethesda System Terminology for Reporting Results of Cervical Cytology. JAMA 287 (16): 2114–2119, 2002.

41. Wright T Jr, Cox JT, Messad LS et al. 2001 Consensus Guidelines for the Management of Women with Cervical Cytological Abnormalities. JAMA 287 (16): 2120–2129, 2002.

Chapter Seven

Nursing Issues in College Health

Nursing Practice
Karen M. Butler, RN, MSN

Issues for Nurse-Directed Health Services
Peggy Ingram Veeser, EdD, APRN, BC,
and Jean Benthien, MSN, RN-C

NURSING PRACTICE

Contemporary nursing, while the product of a rich evolution, has never deviated from its central core of caring for others. Beginning with Florence Nightingale in the 1800's and continuing with today's scholars and practitioners, nursing has had multiple definitions during the past 150 years. In 1860, Nightingale defined nursing as the noncurative practice in which the patient is put in the best condition possible for nature to act.[1] At midtwentieth century, Hildegarde Peplau described nursing as a significant therapeutic interpersonal process that functions in conjunction with other human processes to make health possible for individuals.[2] In 1966, Virginia Henderson stated that the unique function of the nurse is to assist individuals in regaining independence as quickly as possible by helping them, sick or well, to perform tasks contributing to health or its recovery (or peaceful death).[3] Dorothea Orem defined nursing, in 1980, as the provision of direct service to a client when he or she is unable to meet his or her self-care needs.[4] More recently, the American Nurses' Association (ANA) has defined nursing as "the diagnosis and treatment of human responses to actual or potential health problems." [5]

College health nursing incorporates elements from all these definitions. In the *Standards of College Health Nursing Practice,* published by the ANA in 1986, the college health nurse is defined as "a licensed professional nurse, prepared at the baccalaureate level, who has demonstrated expertise in college health nursing practice, interest in the health problems of young adults and the very diverse population in higher education. This nurse has a desire to become identified with the total institutional community."[6,p.23] It is upon this definition that college health nurses base their practice.

HISTORICAL PERSPECTIVES

The employment of nurses in college health was first documented in the late 1800s. They were utilized primarily to care for ill students in infirmary settings and, in some instances, to assist physicians. Culver Military Academy first involved nurses in ambulatory care settings, where a medical staff of one physician and two nurses took care of about 20 patients a day in the dispensary and made room visits as necessary.[7] However, as Johnson noted in 1935, "generally speaking, very little is heard of the nurse's part in the promotion of health in the colleges and universities of this country."[8,p.474]

That same year, Moorhouse conducted a study in which directors of college health services were interviewed to determine how nurses were being utilized and to determine what their educational preparation should be.[9] Her findings indicated that while nurses were involved in all aspects of care, from acute care to planning for (and providing) education and prevention programs, the extent of the responsibility was dependent on the level of physician involvement in the health service. She concluded that a college health nurse should, at least, have earned a bachelor's degree, and recommended that nurses be placed on the same level as other educators in their respective institutions in order to function as equals in the academic setting.

The first meeting of the American Student Health Association, later to become the American College Health Association (ACHA), was held in 1920, at which time college health was established as a specialty practice area.[10] Although nurses had been involved in college health for over 20 years, only physicians were present at this initial meeting; nurses were not formally included in ACHA until 1936 and first presented programming at that time. However, nursing was not recognized as a specific entity in ACHA until 1959, when the Nursing Section was established.[11]

College health nurses were granted the right to certification in 1990, thus acknowledging their unique body of knowledge. With the publication of the *Standards of College Health Nursing Practice,* representing a culmination of years of efforts among a few committed college health nurses and the ANA, college health nursing was now fully recognized as a specialty area in professional nursing practice; the first certification examination was held on October 5, 1991.[12]

SCOPE OF COLLEGE HEALTH NURSING PRACTICE

The mission of college health nursing "is directed toward enhancing the educational process by modifying or removing health-related barriers to learning, promoting optimal wellness, enabling individuals to make informed decisions about health-related concerns, and empowering students to be self-directed and well-informed consumers of health care."[13,p.2] This mission, supported by a set of beliefs and definitions, can be adjusted according to changes in societal and professional trends, with the operational framework being the nursing process. This set of beliefs includes but is not limited to the following:

- Education is the product of the college system, and promotion of good health throughout the college community is crucial to the educational process.

- College health is dynamic and reflects the lives of students and society in general.
- The health of students at every level of learning is important to the college health nurse; each individual is responsible for his or her own health.
- The role of the college health nurse is to promote health by providing information that assists the individual in making sound choices about health care.
- The student has developmental processes which he or she must achieve; they are often culturally dependent and may result in the student participating in risky behaviors.
- Confidentiality is of primary importance to the college health nurse.
- Specific services provided will depend upon available resources.[14]

Practice environments for the college health nurse vary greatly, from a single nurse-run operation to a complex, large academic medical center with a multidisciplinary staff. Each college community is also unique in terms of population, setting, program offerings, and faculty. The client population served varies from institution to institution, and often includes (in addition to students) faculty, staff, spouses, children, friends, and campus visitors.

The college health nurse plans for and carries out services within this diverse community. Major services may include:

- History taking with physical and mental health status assessment, and cultural assessment
- Emergent and acute illness and injury care, as well as chronic illness care
- Health education and promotion, disease prevention for individuals and groups, health restoration and rehabilitation
- Prioritization of services for individuals and groups, based on a logical system of assessment and triage
- Management and leadership for risk reduction, resource allocation, facilities
- and environment, personnel, program development, referral systems, continuous quality improvement, policy-making programs, information services, epidemiology and infection control, and environmental health and safety.[6]

Thus, the college health nurse may assume many roles and responsibilities, including direct nursing care, collaboration with other health care professionals, health education, professional development, research, management and leadership, consultation and client advocacy.[12]

STANDARDS OF COLLEGE HEALTH NURSING PRACTICE

The purpose of standards in college health nursing "is to bring to the attention of the nursing profession, the field of education, and consumers of college health services the specialty nature of college health nursing."[14,p.3] These standards represent agreed-upon levels of practice and are intended to assist nurses in describing, measuring, and providing guidance in the quest to achieve excellence in college health nursing care.

The standards of college health nursing practice are in accordance with ANA's definition of nursing, reflect current knowledge, are subject to testing and change, and are the accepted level of quality against which all nurses in college health nursing are measured.[12] In the standards, health is viewed as more than the absence of illness; it is living in the best possible functional state given one's particular life circumstances.[15]

The conceptual framework for the standards is the self-care theory; the operational framework is the nursing process. The following assumptions are important:[12]

- The majority of nurses in college health function as generalists with a specific patient population.
- College health clients are a generally healthy population; therefore, most of their health care should be concentrated in the area of self-care.
- As nursing knowledge is gained in the field of college health, the educational preparation of those nurses providing care must keep pace.
- Nurses who practice in college health abide by their respective state nurse practice acts.

Standards as included in the *College Health Nurse Resource and Study Guide* are:[12]

- Standard I (Organization of Nursing Services) identifies the need for college health nursing services to be planned, comprehensive units in which nurses assess, plan, implement and evaluate the nursing care they provide. It also speaks to the importance for the nursing administrator to have appropriate levels of education and experience to perform assigned responsibilities and calls for written policies and procedures upon which nurses are to base their practices.
- Standard II (Theory) describes nursing as an applied science, which uses theories and concepts from other disciplines, and calls for the need for nursing research to be conducted in college health settings.
- Standard III (Nursing Process) addresses the importance of the nursing process as well as its documentation.
- Standard IV (Interdisciplinary Collaboration) speaks to the importance of a team approach to college health with all disciplines, academic and/or clinical, working together to assist their clients in achieving the best level of health possible.
- Standard V (Research) states college health nurses should be willing, active participants in clinical research.
- Standard VI (Quality Assurance) speaks to the importance of peer review and evaluation of practice.
- Standard VII (Professional Development) discusses the need for college health nurses to become aware of new developments in the field on a timely basis, through attendance at continuing education programs, reading professional journals, networking with colleagues, and being active in professional organizations on local, state, regional, and national levels.
- Standard VIII (Community Health Systems) stresses the need for prevention planning and services in the college health community.

THEORETICAL BASIS FOR COLLEGE HEALTH NURSING

College health nursing is based on multiple theories, many of which focus on self-care, prevention, and wellness. Major theories include Maslow's Hierarchy of Needs, Growth and Development Theory, and Orem's Self-Care Deficit Theory.

Maslow's Hierarchy of Needs was developed in 1943. This theory proposes that each person has five categories of needs and that one cannot easily progress from one level to the next until the basic needs of the lower level are met. Those needs include physiological (basic needs for survival); safety (freedom from danger, disease, etc.); love (affection, acceptance, and recognition); esteem (self-respect); and self-actualization (self-fulfillment). Maslow contends that these needs serve as motivators for one to change in order to progress up the continuum.[12] Thus, one aspect of college health nursing is to assist students in the hierarchical progression.

Growth and Development Theory is based on the physical, sexual, psychological, and emotional changes experienced during adolescence, as well as tasks that must be accomplished in order for the adolescent to move to adulthood. Arnstein (1984)[16] and Medalie (1981),[17] have both examined stages of the mini-life-cycle occurring through four years of college.

In the freshman year, there is a transition from family life to individual life, during which students learn to make independent lifestyle decisions. The sophomore year is the time when students need to commit to their future plans in terms of careers, and may no longer feel comfortable with their changing role in their family. Many students have difficulty with this process, feeling out of place or without clear direction. During the junior year, students are usually learning about their chosen fields or careers, and therefore enjoy classes more. As they move closer to adult life, personal relationships become more important. The senior year generally brings anxiety about what life after college will be like. Often students try to accomplish remaining tasks quickly and without thinking though consequences. Both Arnstein and Medalie theorize that knowledge of this mini-life-cycle may enable health care providers to better assist clients seen at college health services.[16,17]

The Self-Care Theory, proposed by Dorothea Orem in 1971, states that individuals should be able to perform for themselves those tasks which maintain life and health and that only when individuals *cannot* perform these tasks should nurses intervene and assist in their implementation.[18] Orem describes three types of self-care demands: universal self-care requisites (such as food, air, and water); health-deviation self-care requisites (care required in the event of an injury or illness); and developmental self-care requisites (specialized requisites that are the result of a developmental process or particular life event). The theory suggests that whenever a deficit occurs in the ability to meet these self-care demands, there is a need for nursing. When providing care (in the context of this theory), the nurse uses a system that is compensatory or consultative in nature, to provide the education and the means for students to care for themselves whenever possible, and to empower them to do so.[19]

THE UNIQUE ENVIRONMENT OF COLLEGE HEALTH

Nursing practice in college health is unique in that the client population is generally healthy and already focused on the educational process. The population is diverse, including many races, cultures, ages, and values. Although there are many "traditional" college students (ages 17 to 24), who present with the typical developmental tasks of this age group, the number of nontraditional students is growing. Nontraditional students are usually older, may have families, often work full- or part-time, and generally come to campus only for classes. There are other special-needs groups on campus as well: athletes, health professions students, students with chronic illnesses and physical handicaps, international and minority students, and others. These groups require college health nurses to adapt traditional teachings and practices to the specific needs of the client with whom they are dealing at a given time. Many health services have responded to these unique needs by developing innovative health promotion programming, using both peer educators and health service personnel.[20]

Another factor contributing to the uniqueness of the college health environment is that it is influenced greatly by the academic calendar.[13] Heffern suggests that the highly structured academic schedule, and the demands it places on students acts as a significant source of stress.[11] Students have complicated, full schedules with classes, homework, extracurricular activities, social relationships, families, self-care needs, and, often, work. There is little time left over to be sick or to seek health care. Although many students come to college with their scholarly skills well formed, they typically have little knowledge of how to prevent or manage illness. Therefore, it is not necessarily a disease which causes a crisis but the response of the student to the disease. Heffern further suggests the college health nurse's role is to teach the process by which the body heals itself and to explain to students how to care for themselves. In this way, nurses have the opportunity to educate and care for students and to help them develop lifelong healthy behaviors. Every visit made by a student to a college health service should be seen as an educational opportunity for the nurse and a learning experience for the student. Additionally, nurses can educate students to become knowledgeable consumers of health care and responsible citizens who live healthy lifestyles.[21]

College health services may provide care for clients other than students, including faculty and staff (for both academic and medical settings), spouses, families, and campus visitors. Nurses are often in a unique position to influence employee health and infection control policies in their institutions and to educate clients in these areas. These clients may often be in the same older-adult age group as nontraditional students and may be interested in making healthy lifestyle changes which require educational and emotional support.[12]

HEALTH PROBLEMS OF COLLEGE STUDENTS

College students experience both acute and chronic illnesses, and suffer consequences of risky behavior. Grace observes that "college students risk some of the highest numbers of person years of life lost from illnesses and injuries that are largely preventable through alterations in their risky health behaviors."[22,p.242] He suggests it is possible that no other age group is so misunderstood and overlooked in planning, delivering, and financing their medical care.

Acute health problems seen in college students are similar to those seen in a general medical practice. These problems include musculoskeletal conditions, trauma, and minor infections.[23] Dermatological complaints are common. Infectious diseases, such as mononucleosis, rubeola, and varicella also occur, and the sequelae are often more severe than those experienced by children with the same infections. Serious medical conditions, such as appendicitis, endometriosis, ectopic pregnancy, and toxic shock syndrome, are not unusual. Sexual assault occurs not infrequently on college campuses.[24] Thus, college nurses must be astute in assessing signs and symptoms and not become complacent in their practices.[22] A nurse, using a focused history and physical assessment of the system(s) associated with the chief complaint, should evaluate every client who presents with an acute illness or injury and formulate a nursing diagnosis. The extent of the nursing plan of action will vary with the policies and procedures of the individual institution.[12]

Chronic medical problems, including asthma, diabetes, seizure disorders, migraine headaches, arthritis, and inflammatory bowel disease, are seen regularly.[25] In addition, particularly as the numbers of nontraditional students grow, more clients with hypertension and hyperlipidemia are diagnosed and treated at college health services. Most of these students are asymptomatic; problems are detected and diagnoses made only through regular medical screening.[22]

Cancer screening and early detection should be viewed as important responsibilities for college health nurses. Cancer is the fifth leading cause of death in people 15–24 years of age (following AIDS, accidents, homicide, and suicide).[22]

Other health problems encountered with some frequency include sexually transmitted diseases, such as hepatitis B, HIV, human papillomavirus, genital herpes simplex virus, chlamydia, and gonorrhea. Prevention programming for these diseases as a nursing intervention strategy is a must.

The incidence of eating disorders, including anorexia and bulimia, is increasing. Violence occurs on campus, just as it does in the society at large. More students with serious disabilities are attending college and require specialized care. Many mental health problems, including depression, anxiety, sexual problems, personality disorders, schizophrenia, and others, often first manifest themselves during the college years.[22] As is the case with any illness, the nurse dealing with these issues must perform an initial focused nursing history and physical assessment to be used in formulating a nursing diagnosis on which to base a plan of action.[12]

HEALTH PROMOTION AND PREVENTION

The greatest positive impact on students' current and future health can be made through health care promotion and prevention. Nursing actions directed towards health promotion include teaching, counseling, and motivating people to develop lifestyles that include the avoidance of risky behavior and good habits of self-care.[26] Risky behaviors often practiced by college students include abuse of alcohol, tobacco, and other drugs; risky sexual behaviors; suicide and stress; poor nutrition, including diet, weight, and body image; limited physical activity and fitness.[27] Substance abuse is particularly troubling, because it is so widespread; 85–95 percent of college students consume alcohol.[28]

Prevention in college health, as elsewhere, refers to activities directed toward protecting people from potential or actual threats to health and subsequent consequences. Prevention can be subdivided into three general categories: primary, secondary, and tertiary. Primary prevention involves specific measures taken to protect students from disease or injury before they occur. Nursing interventions include immunizations, programming aimed at the modification of risky behaviors (such as the use of alcohol, tobacco, and other drugs, as well as poor nutritional and exercise patterns), and programs to deal with sexually related problems, stress reduction, and injuries.

Secondary prevention includes early detection and rapid intervention to halt a (potential) disease process at an early stage. Examples of secondary prevention which may be used by college health nurses include tuberculosis screening, eye exams, diabetic screening, early detection cancer programs such as PAP smears and skin cancer clinics, screening for and treating contacts of persons with STDs, programming to teach breast and testicular self-examination, cholesterol screening, and blood pressure screening.

Tertiary prevention involves treatment of an existent disease process by performing activities that prevent or limit complications and disabilities and help restore the student to an optimal level of functioning. Ideally, this should begin in the early stages of recovery. The college nurse is well placed to assist in this process, if not directly, at the least by assisting the student in receiving necessary rehabilitation.

As students often delay treatment until a time that is convenient for them, college health nurses should actively participate in the planning of health services offered, so that prompt access and early intervention are available to students whenever possible.

ROLES OF THE COLLEGE HEALTH NURSE

Just as the definition of nursing has evolved over the years, so has the role of nurses. The *College Health Nurse Resource and Study Guide* defines "role" as "an organized set of expected behaviors for any given position."[12,p.2] These behaviors are outlined by multiple sources, including institutions, society, clients, peers, and colleagues, as well as by the individual practitioner. Roles identified as those essential to the practice of the college health nurse include advocacy, consultation, direct care, collaboration, research, education, and management/leadership.[12] Nurses often assume many of these roles simultaneously in their daily practices.

Client advocacy involves interpreting and defending the client's rights and opportunities in the health care system.[29] Examples include assisting clients with decisions about further care by providing information about other medical resources, or lobbying for a service that would promote good health, such as free vaccines. Nursing actions may include explaining to the client what other health care providers have done or said, as well as providing additional information necessary for good health care decisions.

Consultation involves helping to plan and set goals and functioning as a health information resource with clients. In this role, nurses may also provide information needed for the care of a client to his or her primary provider. Consultation may also occur on a much larger scale, e.g., serving as a public health consultant to the campus or community.

The direct care role involves use of the nursing process, viewing clients in a holistic manner, and the use of advanced knowledge and skills. Adherence to accepted standards of care is essential. Many institutions utilize protocols to be followed in the provision of clinical care. In addition, nurses should possess the necessary clinical knowledge and skills to care for a particular population. Continuing education and ongoing clinical practice strengthen this capability.

Collaboration involves the nurse, the client, and other health care providers working together and sharing information to reach a common goal. Teamwork is essential, and respect for others' thoughts and ideas is an inherent part of the process. Teamwork may also be extended to working with other departments on campus to formulate policies or to identify or meet needs.

College nurses should be actively involved in clinical research. Lach and Reifler have stated that college health professionals can make unique contributions to the body of scientific knowledge and, in fact, have an obligation to do so by participating in an active program of asking questions and seeking answers.[30] College nurses may become involved in research by initiating and performing formalized research projects; collaborating with other health professionals in formalized research, evaluating the effectiveness of nursing care; or using research findings of others in the provision of nursing care. Both qualitative and quantitative research can be performed in the college health setting.[12] Research is also a useful tool in program development, implementation, and evaluation.

Educational opportunities, as previously discussed, particularly in the areas of prevention and health promotion, are not limited to students but may extend to families of students, as well as to faculty or staff. Such education may occur incidentally or in a planned fashion.

All college health nurses have some responsibility in the areas of leadership and management. Management usually involves designated responsibilities within a job description. Key elements of the management role are planning, staffing, organizing, directing, and decision-making. Examples of areas that may require nursing management include time, budget, staff, and resources. Leadership involves functioning as a catalyst for change, whether in an assigned role or on an informal basis in the clinical setting.

TELEPHONE NURSING IN COLLEGE HEALTH

Telephone nursing is one of the fastest-growing areas of nursing specialization, and adapts well to the college health setting, where timing and opportunity are of utmost importance to the clients served. Telephone nurses must have excellent skills in communication, assessment, structured history-taking, and creative problem-solving, and must be able to accurately document these activities. A good telephone-nursing program can improve student access to the health service, be cost-effective, provide continuity of care, and increase patient and physician satisfaction.[31] Telephone nursing may be used in the areas of triage (the sorting and allocation of treatment to patients), health education and information, counseling, and intervention. Importantly, collaboration and clear communication with the clinical staff is essential to continuity of care as well as to the overall success of a telephone-nursing program.

Many institutions utilize formalized protocols on which to base telephone interactions. Commercial resources for telephone nursing protocols are readily available. The most common liability claims resulting from telephone nursing include failure to follow protocols and procedures, misdiagnosis of problems and/or symptoms, failure to follow up when indicated, failure to meet accepted standards of care, practicing outside the scope of nursing practice, and practicing across state lines.[31] Nurses must be cautious to limit their telephone interactions with clients to nursing actions consistent with their institution's policies, protocols, and procedures, as well as with nursing laws in their respective states.

USE OF PROTOCOLS IN COLLEGE HEALTH NURSING

Nursing protocols are contracts that spell out directives to the nurse for managing specific health problems.[32] They are not the same as standing orders, procedures, or guidelines. Protocols are written specifically for a designated symptom or diagnosis, and differ from standing orders in that they generally include specific information gathered from a client to be used in assessment and allow for decision-making by the nurse, whereas standing orders do not. The purpose for using protocols is twofold: to provide a methodical approach to care with the goal of improving health outcomes, and as a legal safeguard for the nurse with backup for nursing actions taken.[33] Protocols should be based on current best practices; their development requires a joint effort among the health care team. Physician input and collaboration is valuable, in both the development and implementation of protocols.

Standardized nursing protocols in college health should be based on nursing diagnoses.[34] After thorough assessment, the nurse implements nursing interventions designed to treat the client's response to illness (or threat of illness), not the illness itself. In addition, protocols used in college health should address the needs of the particular population to be served.[34] Protocols written in this manner allow nurses to function within their scope of practice as prescribed by the individual state nursing practice acts.

Protocols should not be viewed as a simple "cookbook" method of providing nursing care. The implementation of protocols requires a high level of professional sophistication and skill. If not followed carefully, protocols can be easily breached; to do so increases legal liability and is potentially dangerous to patients.[35] However, this is not to say that protocols should not have inherent flexibility when there is clear rationale for change in a particular situation agreed upon by the health care team and/or collaborating physician. Such changes should be carefully documented.[32]

Key areas for consideration in protocol development include definition of the target population to be served (i.e., college students); identification of the most commonly recurring health problems in the population; guidelines for providing patient care; and the goals of care, as well as the time frame for achieving the goal and documentation of how the goals were achieved, based on objective findings.[32] Other factors which need to be considered are specifics of the practice location and the educational preparation and experience of the nurse providers. Before protocols are implemented a plan should be developed for systematic evaluation so that the changing needs of the student population are addressed and the most current standard of care is always in place.[32]

CERTIFICATION OF COLLEGE HEALTH NURSES

College health is recognized as a separate nursing specialty, with certification having become available in 1991.[36] Certification is awarded to registered nurses who have met requirements outlined by the American Nurses Credentialing Center (ANCC), a subsidiary of the American Nurses Association. Through certification, a licensed, registered nurse is confirmed as having met predetermined standards established by the profession for specialty practice. The purpose of certification is to ensure an individual has mastered a body of knowledge and has acquired skills in that specialty. Certification provides the public with one way to identify competent people in a profession; it also aids the profession by encouraging and recognizing professional achievement.

In order to become certified, college health nurses must demonstrate specific areas of knowledge and skills essential to implement the *ANA Standards of College Health Nursing Practice* and meet the following requirements in order to be eligible to sit for the certification examination:

- Hold a current, active RN license in the United States
- Hold a baccalaureate or higher degree in nursing
- Have a minimum of 1,500 hours of practice as a licensed registered nurse in college health nursing within the past three years
- Currently practice at least 500 hours annually in college health nursing
- Have had thirty contact hours of continuing education applicable to college health within the past three years.[36]

Topics covered in the college health nursing certification examination include the foundations of college health, the environment of college health, client care, standards of professional performance, and issues and trends in college health. Certification is offered in collaboration with the American College Health Association; certified college health nurses participate in the design of test questions.

The practice requirement can be met if the nurse is engaged in either direct client care or direct clinical management, supervision, education, consultation, or direction of other persons to achieve or help achieve client goals. Certification renewal is required every five years and may be accomplished through continuing education, formal education, or retesting.

Certification has a profound impact on the personal, professional, and practice outcomes of certified nurses. Nurses in a Nursing Credentialing Research Coalition (NCRC) study stated certification enabled them to experience fewer untoward events and mistakes in providing clinical care than before they became certified.[37] They reported feeling more confident in their ability to assess early signs and symptoms of complications in their patients and to intervene earlier for these complications. The nurses also experienced more personal growth and job satisfaction, and believed they were viewed as more credible providers of care. Certification enabled nurses to become consultants within their job settings, increasing participation in leadership activities, and, in some cases, to receive increased financial benefits. The NCRC study also found certified nurses reporting high patient satisfaction ratings and better communication and collaboration with other health care providers; some certified nurses reported fewer disciplinary problems and work-related injuries than their colleagues.

In another study commissioned by the ANCC,[37] a consumer survey indicated 87 percent of consumers would be more confident about their health care if they knew their nurse was a certified specialist.

If college health is to be viewed as a specialty area of clinical practice, college health nurses should be certified. Through certification, not only are nurses better prepared to fulfill the designated roles of the college health nurse, but their advanced knowledge and skills improve health outcomes, thereby solidifying the importance of nursing in college health settings with clients, colleagues, and institutions.

THE ROLE OF ADVANCED PRACTICE NURSES IN COLLEGE HEALTH

College health services increasingly utilize the services of nurse practitioners and clinical nurse specialists. Nurse practitioners (NP) function by providing primary health care, including ordering and interpreting diagnostic tests, prescribing medications and other treatments, and teaching clients and their families. Many studies have documented that NPs provide high-quality, cost-effective care. Nichols estimates that if NPs were used to their full potential, the savings to the health care system in the United States would be between 6.4 and 8.75 billion dollars annually.[21] Indirect savings from improved access to health care, early detection, and increased preventive care are more difficult to measure, but would also result in significant monetary savings. Many college health services have clearly documented the legitimate and valuable role of the NP in the college/university setting, either individually or as part of a multidisciplinary team. A particularly important role for NPs is that of Nurse Director of Health Services (see part 2).

While clinical nurse specialists (CNS) do not have legal authority to independently provide primary care, they can make other significant contributions in a health service. The CNS is an adept clinician in his or her area of practice.[38] Roles that the CNS may fulfill in a college health setting include those of clinician, educator, researcher, and consultant, working with both students and with health services colleagues. The CNS can empower students to become knowledgeable consumers of health care and active participants in healthy lifestyles.[21]

FUTURE DIRECTIONS IN COLLEGE HEALTH NURSING PRACTICE

In order for nurses to continue to be viewed as valuable members of the college and university health care team, there must be a commitment to the mission of college health by nurses working in health services.[6] Fulfillment of this mission is important not only to the lives of individual students but to institutions' goals of graduating educated, responsible citizens. Aligning college health goals with those of the college and university is one way to help ensure that college health remains an integral part of higher education.

An emphasis on programming for health promotion, health education, and prevention must play a larger role in college health nursing in the future. This recommendation is in line with *Healthy People 2010: Understanding and Improving Health,* which speaks to the need to increase from 6 percent to 25 percent the proportion of college and university students who receive information from their institution on each of six priority health-risk behavior areas: injuries, tobacco use, alcohol and illicit drug use, sexual behavior resulting in undesirable consequences, poor dietary habits, and inadequate physical activity.[39]

It is no longer possible to provide the level and type of care appropriate for college students based purely on a biomedical model; college health professionals must function in a holistic manner. While it is typically assumed that college health services will care for clinical problems, the role of the health service in addressing larger issues, such as those pertaining to substance abuse, sexual health, and mental health, is not as often recognized or appreciated. Nurses who are proactive and participate in these activities are assisting students in maintaining the best health possible, enabling students to learn lifelong healthy behaviors, and increasing the awareness and importance of college health by responding to the needs of the larger university community.

Other issues that will play a role in the future of college health nursing are those related to the development of knowledge in the field. Active involvement in clinical research is crucial if nurses are to continue to make contributions to the body of scientific knowledge which makes college health unique. The result will be improved clinical practice as well as the identification of future research needs.

Nursing certification will become increasing significant as an indicator of advanced competency and specialization. In addition, nursing participation in national accreditation of college health facilities is vital. Accreditation is important in order to assure staff and students that their treatment regimens are as good as or better than the best the surrounding community has to offer.[40]

Quality assurance, utilizing the *Scope and Standards of College Health Nursing Practice* as the "gold standard," will become increasingly important as health services work to prove their worth to students and others at their institutions. A good quality-assurance program includes peer review of medical records, clinical practice, and preventive and educational programs, as well as a risk management program that reviews any incidents or untoward events and makes recommendations for intervention and correction.[41]

The mechanisms for the delivery of health care are evolving rapidly, and there are those who believe college health care can be adequately provided by health professionals who do not hold special education for, or interest in, college health. College health nurses must increase their understanding of the health issues that are important to those they serve. They must keep their services flexible and relevant and provide consistent high-quality services in a cost-effective manner. The use of advanced practice nurse practitioners will become increasingly important as health services work to provide a high quality of care while decreasing costs. Increasing involvement and collaboration with the institutional community, as well as with students, is essential to accomplishing the mission of college health nursing.

If college health nurses work with one another, as well as with other college health professionals, to pursue their mission, the future of college health nursing is assured. By assuming the roles described by the ANA—advocacy, consultation, direct care, collaboration, research, education, management/leadership—and by following the *Standards of Care for College Health Nursing* to assure high-quality care, college health nurses will continue to make a significant contribution to the health, well-being, and ultimate success of every individual fortunate enough to be a recipient of their care.

ISSUES FOR NURSE-DIRECTED COLLEGE HEALTH SERVICES

The Nurse-Directed Health Service is defined as a college or university health service which has as its primary administrative director a registered nurse (RN) or a nurse with a minimum of a master's degree in a specialty area of advanced practice nursing. The nurse director (ND) may be the solo clinical practitioner, share the practitioner roles with other staff, or provide only administrative oversight.

Nurse directors work primarily in small private institutions and community college systems. However, they may also serve in large state universities (particularly those with large commuter populations and relatively small health services) and associated satellite clinics.

The functions of the ND vary according to the size and resources of the health service. She/he may be the sole employee and have multiple responsibilities, including secretarial, administrative, academic, health promotion, case management, health care, and risk management functions. In larger settings, the ND may function primarily as an administrator and oversee a staff of several physicians, nurse practitioners, registered nurses, and other health care personnel. Less commonly, the ND may serve as a faculty member in an administrative role or as a member of nursing department faculty.

On some campuses, the administration may define the scope of practice or limitations for the college health service. Assigned responsibilities may range from the simplest of services, such as first aid and dispensing over the counter medication, to complex health care delivery that includes a full scope of medical, psychological, pharmacological, and educational services.

Regardless of the size of the institution or the specific scope of practice offered by the individual health service, the ND must still ensure provision of, or assist with, access to health care and health promotion services on the campus. Further, the ND may typically serve as coordinator or representative to campus health-related committees such as Student Health Advisory, Sexual Assault, Americans with Disabilities (ADA), Drug-Free Workplace, Infection Control, and Workers' Compensation Injuries.

SKILLS AND CREDENTIALS

Few specific nursing tracks are available which groom potential candidates for ND positions. Prior experience with adolescent health care, administration, and primary care is helpful, as is prior experience in college health nursing, including ANA certification. Most new NDs utilize other experts in college health to glean information regarding the operation of a college health service. Creative problem-solving skills as well as a sense of organizational management are helpful. The credentials of current NDs are varied and may range from registered nurses (RN) with advanced degrees in specialty areas, administration, or higher education to licensed practical/vocational nurses (LVN/LPN) in small community and private colleges. One pattern of hiring for small church affiliated institutions is to hire a nurse from the specific denomination or a nurse returning from an outreach mission to be the college nurse. These nurses are more likely to be in agreement with the mission of the institution.

While the minimum suggested educational preparation for college health nurses is the baccalaureate degree in nursing, the advanced practice nurse who has certification in college health (see part 1 of this chapter) and who is nationally board-certified by an appropriate nursing agency is the most logical choice for the nurse director role. Coupled with a master's degree, this educational preparation gives the APN the skills to relate to the student from a holistic perspective while providing direct patient care. The advanced practice preparation of the APN fosters communication among interdisciplinary team members, an understanding of community health needs, more advanced clinical knowledge, and the acquisition of skills which encourage creativity, initiative, and leadership.

STAFFING PATTERNS AND ADMINISTRATIVE CONSIDERATIONS

The ND, by virtue of the position, is usually responsible for employing staff for the health service necessitating skills in recruitment, hiring, writing job descriptions, scheduling, and salary negotiations. Typically, college health services are understaffed, and the ND must know how to access community and campus resources that complement and supplement available services. The ND also must prioritize services expected by the college administration while diplomatically setting limits based on staffing and quality control to avoid overextending.

Health services are most commonly administratively located in the reporting line of student services or student development. A few are under general campus services along with such departments as maintenance and public safety. Administrative control may also vary from a fairly autonomous operation to one that is bound by a rigid bureaucratic system. This is especially true in some community college systems and state-directed universities.

Just as administrative structure varies in higher education, so the reporting channel also varies. The ND may report to the dean of students, the business office, university services, residential life, a specific college, or directly to the president. Frequently these administrators have limited, if any, medical background and must rely on the clinical expertise and competency of the ND for guidance on health service activities and programs.

The ND may have a nine-month or academic appointment if the college or university is not in full session during the summer. Universities with summer school programs or an extensive program of summer camps and conferences may offer health services on a year-round basis. Often, the summer session is slower, allowing time for continuing education and program planning for the next academic year.

Activities and requirements related to accreditation may fall under the purview of the ND. Colleges and universities must maintain regional institutional and specialty accreditation to be eligible for federal financial aid for students. The accreditation process includes a section concerning student services, with particular attention to student health. College health services on campuses are important in helping to meet these standards. In addition, the health service often serves as a resource to assist in meeting the guidelines of the Americans with Disabilities Act (ADA).

CLINICAL SERVICES

Nurse directors must demonstrate expertise in meeting the health care needs of diverse client populations within the setting of higher education. This diversity is demonstrated (as previously discussed in Part I) by differences in age, culture, religion, economic and ethnic backgrounds, lifestyles, and purposes for joining the educational community. Further, in the context of the framework for college health nursing practice (health promotion, specific disease protection, case management, early diagnosis, prompt treatment to limit and or prevent disability, and rehabilitation), a variety of services must be provided or delegated by the ND.

The ND is usually the first line of health care on the educational campus which she/he serves. Triage and identification of those who can be seen and scheduled at the college health service is a universal responsibility. First aid for injuries and accidents is a common service as is appropriate referral for specialty or emergency care. Counseling, patient education, and advising regarding various health care needs are important functions. Case management for chronic illness and family care or coordination of care is necessary, especially for the student who is away from home for the first time. Scheduling patients for other providers such as a physician, nutritionist, or counselor also occurs in case management.

APN directors may provide direct primary care, especially in the area of women's health. Management of illness, in the form of episodic care and chronic diseases, and provision of screening exams and tests are included in the advanced practice management of patient care.

WELLNESS PROGRAMMING

Wellness programming is a vital part of student health care. For those small ND health services that have limited staff, creative use of community resources is essential. Some institutions successfully utilize a team approach for health promotion by joining with other areas that emphasize healthy living, such as athletics, human environmental science, nursing, sociology, and psychology. Health promotion can also involve programming that is planned, facilitated, and performed by peers such as Student Health Advisory Committee (SHAC) members, resident assistants, or other types of peer counselors.

Health fairs are an excellent way to market student health services and to encourage participation in health-related issues. Health themes such as smoking cessation, depression screening, and flu shots are examples of areas of focus for this type of event. Inviting community agencies to donate services and products also leads to improved awareness of local services.

STANDARDS OF CARE AND LEGAL ISSUES

NDs must have a working knowledge of the rules and regulations of their respective state Nurse Practice Acts, particularly the legal scope of practice for nursing and advanced practice. These rules and regulations may determine the scope of services that can be offered in a freestanding clinic and/or by a nurse director. All NDs should have standards of care on file in accordance with state law and quality assurance practices. States differ on requirements for physician supervision and for certain acts performed by nurses in advanced practice. States may require that such standards be developed jointly by a supervising physician and the nurse. These requirements vary but are required in most states when medications are prescribed, issued, or dispensed. If state law requires a supervising physician, the responsibilities of the physician should be outlined clearly for both parties.

NDs must have malpractice insurance provided either through the institution or by a private insurer. It is most appropriate for the institution to pay for this coverage. Only the ND can determine the scope of nursing practice and the appropriate roles for nurses in the college health service. The institution may make requests of the health service without understanding the legal ramifications of the request. The ND must be able to advise when requests for services are in conflict with relevant state law.

NETWORKING

Professional networking is particularly important to the ND role. There are a variety of avenues for networking; the new ND is encouraged to immediately begin to build communication bridges in institutional and community networks.

In institutional networking, the ND can make contact with other administrators in a variety of academic departments which interface with the health service. These might include nursing, kinesiology, athletic training, biology, education, and psychology, as well as any other health profession programs on or near campus. Other departments such as public safety, human resources, and physical plant have staff who can work in a consulting relationship with the ND.

For community networking, the ND can contact administrators and professionals in other health care-related agencies. Institutions within the community that are credible sources of networking partners include the local public health department and agencies such as the American Cancer Society, the American Red Cross, other colleges and universities, local physicians, and medical facilities.

ND alliances have been formed between NDs who are within a certain geographical area or who are working at similar types of institutions. Many of these groups meet on a regular basis and are available to each other by phone or e-mail correspondence. These alliances provide psychological support as well as informational resources.

Professional networking is encouraged within nursing organizations. The ND who is providing services for staff and faculty and charged with oversight of workers' compensation issues might find it helpful to join the Occupational Health Nurse Association. The American Nurses Association, its affiliates, and NP associations offer further networking and educational opportunities.

Perhaps the most important networking resource is the American College Health Association and its affiliates. ACHA provides continuing education opportunities, establishment of collegial networks, resources for standards of care, and many other positive benefits for all college health professionals. Within this organization, there are numerous opportunities to expand the knowledge base of the ND, to learn how to present educational activities, to participate in leadership roles, to learn current trends, and to grow as a specialist in college health care. Most importantly, ACHA has a specific section with focused programs for the Nurse-Directed Health Service. It is imperative that the ND of a college health service be actively involved with this professional organization.

Barriers to establishing networking systems most often are financial or minimal administrative support for these efforts. Strong arguments must be made for support of professional development and continuing education for the ND. These supports must include leave time, travel compensation, and conference budgeting. The ND who is encouraged to attend conferences and to participate in professional development will stay abreast of developments in the field and deliver the most appropriate nursing care to students.

SPECIAL ISSUES FOR THE NURSE DIRECTOR

The nurse director must be prepared for a significant change in role from "nurse as a caregiver" to "nurse as leader, politician, financial expert and community health advocate." It is the responsibility of the ND to take an active planning role in the institution concerning health-related issues as well as general student services. Budgetary constraints represent the most frequent challenge for the Nurse Director. Often this means creating a "clinic out of a closet" and establishing services where none have previously existed.

Most important, the ND must keep in mind a continued focus on the mission of the college health service and the key program stakeholders. With this sense of direction, the Nurse Director can lead the campus in creative health programs and a wellness-oriented environment for the institution of higher learning in which she or he is employed.

RESOURCES FOR THE COLLEGE HEALTH NURSE AND NURSE DIRECTOR

American Nurses Credentialing Center, *Board Certification Catalog*, 600 Maryland Ave. NW, Suite 100 West, Washington DC, 20024-2571, 800-284-CERT.

ACHA College Health Standards, ACHA Publications Department, PO Box 28937, Baltimore, MD 21240-8937, 410-859-1500.

ACHA Datashare III Survey Information. Order from ACHA. Cost is variable according to membership status.

ACHA Membership Directory, ACHA Publications Department, P.O. Box 28937, Baltimore, MD 21240-8937, 410-859-1500.

Adolescent Health Care: A Practical Guide, Third Edition, Lawrence Neinstein, MD, Williams and Wilkins, 351 West Camden Street, Baltimore, Maryland 21201-2436

The Blue Book—Program Development Guidelines for Nurse-Directed Health Services, ACHA Publications Department, PO Box 28937, Baltimore, MD 21240-8937.

Connections Quarterly, an online quarterly resource for nurse-directed health services. Maintained by Carol Mulvihill, University of Pittsburgh-Bradford, cjm6+@pitt.edu.

Health Services Procedures and Policy Manual for a Small School, Point Loma Nazarene University Health Services, 1999, Jean Benthien CRNP, MSN, available on line upon request at no charge, Jbenthie@ptloma.edu.

Nurse Practitioner Protocols, Sunbelt Medical Publishers, Matthew M. Cohen, MD, and Anni Lanigan, ARNP, PO Box 13512, Tallahassee, FL, 32317-3512.

Primary Care of Young Adults, Medical Examination Publishing Co., Katharine Reichert, MD, Excerpta Medica Company, 3003 New Hyde Park Road, New Hyde Park, New York.

Professional Organizations: ACHA and its affiliates, state organizations, i.e., California College Health Nurse Association Occupational Health Nurse Association; local, state, national nurse practitioner organizations; local networking.

Workbook on Establishing a Nurse-Managed Health Center, Pace University, Lienhard School of Nursing, 861 Bedford Road, Pleasantville, NY, 10570.

REFERENCES

1. Torres G. *Florence Nightingale, Nursing Theories*, p. 29. Englewood Cliffs, NJ: Prentice Hall. 1980.

2. Peplau H. *Interpersonal Relations in Nursing*, p. 16. New York: Putnam & Sons; 1952.

3. Henderson V. *The Nature of Nursing*, p. 15. New York: Macmillan Co. 1966.

4. Riehl JP, Roy SC. *The Orem Self-Care Nursing Model: Conceptual Models for Nursing Practice*. 2nd ed., p. 303. Norwalk, Conn.: Appleton-Century-Crofts. 1980.

5. *Nursing: A Social Policy Statement*, p. 18. Kansas City, Mo.: American Nurses Association. 1986.

6. *Scope and Standards of College Health Nursing Practice*, p. 2–23. Washington, D.C.: American Nurses Association. 1997.

7. Forsythe WE. Health services in American colleges and universities. *JAMA*. 1914;63(22):1926–1930.

8. Johnson LM. Student health and the college nurse. *Public Health Nurs*. 1935;27(9):474–476.

9. Moorhouse EL. The role of nurses in a college health program. *Public Health Nurs*. 1935;27(4):180–185.

10. Boynton RE. Historical development of college health services. *Student Medicine*. 1962;10(3):294–305.

11. Heffern MK. College health nursing: State of the art. *J Am Coll Health*. 1985;30:148–149.

12. *College Health Nurse Resource and Study Guide*, pp. 2–3. The Education Subcommittee of the College Health Nurse Certification Task Force. American College Health Association. 1994.

13. Congress on Nursing Practice (U.S.). *A Statement of the Scope of College Health Nursing Practice,* p. 2. Kansas City, Mo.: American Nurses Association. 1990.

14. American Nurses Association Task Force. *Standards of College Health Nursing,* p. 3. Kansas City, Mo.: American Nurses Association. 1986.

15. American Nurses Association. *Nursing: A Social Policy Statement,* p. 1. Kansas City, Mo.: American Nurses Association. 1980.

16. Arnstein RL. Developmental issues for college students. *Psychiatr Annals.* 1984;14(9):647–651.

17. Medalie J. The college years as a mini life cycle: Developmental tasks and adaptive options. *J Am Coll Health.* 1981;30:75–79.

18. Flynn JB, Heffron PB. *Nursing, from Concept to Practice,* p. 77. 2nd ed. Norwalk, Conn.: Appleton & Lange. 1988.

19. Runtz SE, Urtel JG. Evaluating your practice via a nursing model. *Nurse Pract.* 1983;3(3):39.

20. Flood L, Heaton M. The emerging role of the CNS in the college health setting. *Clin Nurse Specialist.* 1994;8(4):209.

21. Flood L, Heaton M. The emerging role of the CNS in the college health setting. *Clin Nurse Specialist.* 1994;8(4):212.

22. Grace TW. Health problems of college students. *J Am Coll Health.* 1997;45(5):243.

23. Fingar AR. Patient problems encountered at a student health service. *J Am Coll Health.* 1989;38:142–144.

24. Koss MP, Gidycz CA, Wisniewski N. The scope of rape incidence and prevalence of sexual aggression and victimization in a national sample of higher education students. *J Clin Consult Psychol.* 1987;55:162–170.

25. Patrick K, Grace T, Lovato C. Health issues for college students. *Ann Rev Public Health.* 1992;13:253–268.

26. Long BC. Medical-Surgical Nursing: A Nursing Process Approach, 2nd ed., p. 5. St. Louis: C.V. Mosby Co. 1989.

27. Zapka JG, Love MB. College health services: Setting for community, organizational, and individual change. *J Am Coll Health.* 1993;35:81–91.

28. Smith S, Smith C. *The College Student's Health Guide,* pp. 199–232. Los Altos, Calif.: Westchester Publishing Co. 1988.

29. Murray M. *Fundamentals of Nursing,* 2nd ed., p. 27. Englewood Cliffs, N.J.: Prentice Hall Inc. 1980.

30. Lach PA, Reifler CB. On doing research in a clinical setting. *J Am Coll Health.* 1980;29:154.

31. Hermann SB. Telephone triage in the college health setting. Presentation at Southern College Health Association. March, 1999.

32. Newman KD, Rozell BR, Farrell R. Protocols for college health nurses: Alive and well in the 1990s. *J Am Coll Health.* 1993;42:129.

33. Williamson G. Protocols for nursing practice. *Am Assoc Occup Health Nurses: Update series.* 1984;1(2):2–6.

34. Rutledge NL. Nursing diagnosis as a framework for college health nursing protocols. *J Am Coll Health.* 1994;24:175–176.

35. Moniz D. The legal danger of written protocols and standards of practice. *Nurse Pract.* 1992;17(9):58–60.

36. Nursing World's website for the American Nurses Credentialing Center. http://www.nursingworld.org June 2000.

37. American Nurses Credentialing Center, Board Certification Catalogue, 600 Maryland Avenue NW, Ste 100 West, Washington D.C. 20024-2571.

38. Clayton G. The clinical nurse specialist as leader. *Top Clin Nurs.* 1984;6(1):17–27.

39. U.S. Department of Health and Human Services, Public Health Service. *Healthy People 2010: Understanding and Improving Health,* 2nd ed. Washington, D.C.: U.S. Government Printing Office. November 2001.

40. DeArmond M. Designing the future of college health. *NASPA Journal.* 1990;27(4):278.

41. DeArmond M, Gridwell M, Cox J, McCutcheon M, Beauregard R, Charles K, Heffern M. College health toward the year 2000. *J Am Coll Health.* 1991;39:250.

CHAPTER EIGHT

SEXUALLY TRANSMITTED DISEASES AND COLLEGE HEALTH

Introduction and Prevention
H. Spencer Turner, MD, MS, FACPM

Risk Assessment and Management
Patricia R. Jennings, MHS, PA-C, and Alice C. Thornton, MD

INTRODUCTION AND PREVENTION

The diagnosis and treatment of sexually transmitted diseases (STDs) have been inextricably linked with the practice of college health—if not since its beginning—at least for the past 80 years. Dr. William F. Snow, who had previously been a director of the student health service at Stanford University, as the first director of the American Social Hygiene Association (ASHA) was assigned the responsibility of combating venereal diseases in the military, at the outset of World War I in 1918. The distribution of the funds appropriated by Congress to carry out that responsibility is of particular relevance to college health. A portion was distributed to state health departments, a portion to the U.S. Public Health Service to establish the first Division of Venereal Disease Control, and a portion to college health to assist in developing educational measures for venereal disease prevention. Dr. Thomas Storey (whose contributions to college health are chronicled in chapter 1) was named to the ASHA board responsible for distributing these funds. Storey was later to note that he believed the most important contribution of the board was the distribution of money to colleges and universities, since educating the future leaders of society on the concerns of venereal diseases might have lasting effects.[1]

Although congressional funding was discontinued following World War I, ASHA recognized the need to continue programs for venereal disease control on college campuses. As a direct result, in 1922, ASHA financed the formation and operation of the President's Committee of Fifty on College Hygiene, to stimulate the development and extension of instruction and training in hygiene in normal schools, colleges, and universities.[2,p.3] Through this committee, college presidents and those working in college health met together (for the first time) to collectively discuss issues related to health services on college campuses. Thus, while concerns about overall well-being and physical fitness may have been the impetus in the mid-nineteenth century for establishing college health, and the occurrence of epidemics on campuses in the early twentieth century was important for the development of "modern" health services, one could argue that the problem of STDs (or venereal disease) was an important factor behind the *continued* development and improvement of college and university health services.

With the onset of the Depression of the 1930s, funding for venereal disease control began to lessen. Fortunately, through the efforts of Dr. Thomas Parran, who had been Chief of the Venereal Disease Division of the Public Health Service, a public health campaign to increase the public's awareness of venereal diseases was begun. By the end of the 1930s, clinics had been formed in most of the larger cities of the United States and a central reporting and statistical system had been established, so that by the onset of World War II, the United States was better equipped to handle venereal disease problems than it had been at the outset of the previous war.

However, in a reflection of what had happened after World War I, federal funding for venereal disease eradication once again dropped very significantly following WWII. Thus, it is not surprising that in 1947 at the Third National Conference on Health in Colleges, the conference committee saw fit to recommend (1) blood tests for syphilis as part of college admission health examinations, (2) teaching of the essentials of venereal disease control (emphasizing that such control is a problem of conduct as well as of public health), and (3) immediate treatment by the student health service for students who contract a venereal disease.[3]

Nonetheless, with the availability of penicillin and the belief that treatment of venereal disease(s) was now simple, and with changes in many state laws (e.g., discontinuing requirements for a serology for syphilis prior to obtaining a marriage license, or no longer requiring a serology for a food handler's permit), by the 1970s, particularly following the era of "sexual freedom" of the 1960s, the prevalence of syphilis and gonorrhea again approached epidemic levels. The severity of the problem was such that in the early 1970s the National Commission on Venereal Disease was established, which ultimately resulted in the assignment of federal responsibility for venereal disease control to the Centers for Disease Control and Prevention (CDC) and creation of the Division of Sexually Transmitted Diseases.[4] Colleges and universities were not exempt from this epidemic.[5]

Over the past 30 years, the definition of venereal disease, or STDs, has changed significantly. From the five historically defined STDs—syphilis, gonorrhea, chancroid, lymphogranuloma venereum, and granuloma inguinale—the list has been expanded to include hepatitis A and B, the herpes viruses, human papilloma viruses, HIV, chlamydial infections, and many more. Currently, the United States has the highest rates of STDs in the industrialized world,[6] with 15 million new cases of STDs reported each year.[7] In 1996, approximately 400,000 cases of genital *Chlamydia trachomatis* infections were reported to CDC, making this disease the most commonly reported disease in the United States.[6] At the same time, gonorrhea incidence in the U.S. was 124 per 100,000 (a rate 26 times greater than that of Germany and 50 times greater than that of Sweden) and by

1998, it had increased to 133 per 100,000. Syphilis incidence was approximately 20 cases per 100,000 (13 times higher than Germany and 33 times higher than Sweden). Fortunately, following a national plan to eliminate syphilis in the United States, the rates gradually dropped to 2.5 cases per 100,000 by 1999.[8] Superimposed on this overall prevalence of STDs are higher rates for certain subgroups, including the college population, thus supporting the need for continued intervention by college and university health services.[8,9]

Despite the variations in STD incidence and prevalence and despite the different names given to STDs caused by different organisms, the principles of treating these diseases, both individually and from the viewpoint of public health, remain little different than those outlined by Sir William Osler in 1905:

> Irregular intercourse has existed from the beginning of recorded history, and unless man's nature wholly changes—and of this we can have no hope—will continue. Resisting all attempts at solution, the social evil remains a great blot upon our civilization, and inextricably blended with it is the question of the prevention of syphilis [and one could add here other STDs as well]. Two measures are available—the one personal, the other administrative.

> Personal purity is the prophylaxis which we as physicians are especially bound to advocate. Continence may be a hard condition (to some harder than to others), but it can be borne and it is our duty to urge this lesson upon young and old who seek our advice in matters sexual. Certainly it is better as Saint Paul says, to marry than to burn, but if the former is not feasible, there are other altars than those of Venus upon which a young man may light fires...by which...carnal concupiscence may be cooled and quelled—hard work of body and hard work of mind...

> ...to carry out successfully any administrative measures seems hopeless at any rate in our Anglo Saxon civilization. The state accepts the responsibility of guarding citizens against smallpox or cholera, but in dealing with syphilis, the problem has been too complex and has hitherto baffled solution. Inspection, segregation, and regulation are difficult, if not impossible, to carry out and public sentiment is bitterly opposed to this plan. The compulsory registration of every case of gonorrhea and syphilis with greatly increased facilities for thorough treatment, offers a more acceptable alternative.[10]

These "administrative" measures, for which Osler recognized the need, were not taken seriously (other than during periods of war) until the 1970s, as previously described. Thus, using Osler's approach, the remainder of this chapter is divided into two sections. The first deals with Osler's "administrative measures" (or perhaps now better called "public health" and/or "epidemiological measures") to control STDs, while the second portion discusses certain common STDs and their currently recommended treatments.

ADMINISTRATIVE ASPECTS OF STD CONTROL —PREVENTION AND PUBLIC HEALTH

The prevention of STDs is based on five major concepts:[11]

- Education to reduce the risk of spreading or contracting a disease
- Detection of infected persons—those without symptoms and those who are not likely to seek treatment even with symptoms
- Appropriate diagnosis and treatment of infected persons
- Evaluation, counseling, and treatment if necessary of sexual partners of infected individuals
- Preexposure vaccination for vaccine-preventable STDs[11]

Of these measures, perhaps the most important for primary prevention of STDs is changing behavior through education. By the time young adults begin attendance at a college or university they have almost certainly had some type of instruction regarding sexually transmitted diseases. Unfortunately, in the authors' experience, most of that instruction is limited and revolves primarily around gonorrhea, syphilis, and HIV. While it is undeniable that these are serious problems—particularly the latter—most students seem to have little clear understanding of the full range of diseases which can be spread by sexual activity. As a result, again in the authors' experience, it is not unusual for a student to arrive at a college health clinic requesting an "STD test." Thus, the first step in prevention truly is education about those diseases which actually can be sexually transmitted (and for which treatment may or may not be available or effective) and about potential complications beyond the initial infection.

The second area for primary prevention (or perhaps, secondary prevention depending upon one's perspective) important for college students involves changing high-risk sexual behavior. A study at the mid-part of the last decade by Reinisch et al., involving a random sample of heterosexual undergraduates, documented that 80 percent of males and 73 percent of females had experienced vaginal or anal intercourse, with the average age of first vaginal intercourse at 17.2 years for both men and women.[12] Males reported an average of 8.0 lifetime vaginal intercourse partners while females reported 6.1. Seventeen percent of sexually experienced males and 18 percent of sexually experienced females had participated in heterosexual anal intercourse even though only four years (on the average) had elapsed since the survey participants' first vaginal intercourse.

A similar study by Joffe et al., which involved a cross-sectional survey among single, white, senior college women, measured the association between behavioral risk factors and the acquisition of self-reported STDs during their college years. During the three and one-half college years preceding the survey, the combined prevalence of chlamydia, gonorrhea, genital herpes, HPV, syphilis, and trichomoniasis was nearly 12 percent, and importantly, there was a strong association between the number of sexual partners and the likelihood of having had an STD. For example, women with five or more sexual partners were eight times more likely to report such an infection than those with only one partner.[13]

Two other studies also confirm the relationship of sexual behavior with multiple sexual partners to the frequency of STDs. DeBuono et al., reporting on a series of questionnaires administered to college women in 1975, 1986, and 1989 regarding sexual practices, observed "...despite the existence of major new infectious diseases, sexual practices among...college women did not change markedly in 14 years with respect to the number of sexual partners or specific sexual acts. Although the use of condoms in-creased, the majority of sexually active women surveyed did not report their regular use."[14,p.824] And an update, in 1997, of that same study reported that despite the awareness of new diseases spread by sexual activity, sexual behavior in college women, as mea-sured by frequency of specific sexual practices and numbers of sexual partners, had not changed from 1974 to 1995.[15]

If abstinence—which is the only sure way to prevent contracting or transmitting an STD—is not or cannot (as suggested by Osler) be practiced, lessening the likelihood of sexual transmission of STDs requires certain behaviors. The following recommenda-tions are important for college health providers to relate to students:[11]

- Before initiating sexual intercourse both partners should be tested for STDs, including HIV.
- If sexual activity occurs and the partner's infection status is unknown or if the partner is known to be infected with an STD, at the least, a new condom should be used for each act of intercourse.
- Avoidance or special care should be used in any sexual contact with an injecting drug user; conversely, an injecting drug user should be tested for STDs or avoid intercourse or use the best protective methods available for "safer sex."

Obviously, any discussion about STD transmission must include preventive methods or devices. While currently applicable only to a limited number of STDs, pre-exposure vaccination is extremely important for those diseases for which a vaccination currently exists or may exist in the future. Hepatitis A and B vaccines are currently available. Vaccine trials for other STDs are currently being conducted and may become available over the next several years.

Male condoms, when properly and consistently used (with each act of intercourse), are effective in minimizing the spread of many STDs, including HIV. However, because condoms do not cover all exposed areas, they are more effective in preventing spread by infections transmitted from one mucosal surface to another, rather than those transmit-ted by skin-to-skin contact.

Female condoms have recently become available and although theoretically may represent an effective mechanical barrier to viruses, including HIV, few clinical studies are yet available to evaluate their "in vivo" use. However, it appears that used consis-tently and correctly, the female condom should substantially reduce the risk for trans-mission of certain STDs.

Any discussion of high-risk sexual behavior in college students must include the use and abuse of alcohol and its impact on sexually transmitted disease. Adolescents and young adults are at higher risk for acquiring STDs than are older adults.[16] Further, it is clear from multiple health-risk surveys among colleges and universities (including the authors' institution) that college students who use alcohol are more likely than those who do not use alcohol to participate in high-risk sexual activity, particularly having unpro-tected sex or sex with multiple partners. Thus, any education for prevention must include increasing students' awareness of the association between the use of alcohol and high-risk sexual behavior. And the control of alcohol abuse on college campuses must also become part and parcel of any program to primarily prevent sexually transmitted diseases.

There can be little question that changes in alcohol policy/use/abuse, not only on campus but more generally in society, can impact such issues as STD rates.[17] One important study examined the association between gonorrhea incidence and "alcohol policy indicators," specifically, alcohol taxation and legal drinking age. This study, involving all 50 states and the District of Columbia, covered the period from 1981 to 1995.[18] The analysis compared changes in gonorrhea rates in states *with* a beer tax increase (in a sense, the experimental states) with changes in gonorrhea rates in states *without* a beer tax increase (the "control" states). In general, most increases in beer tax were followed by a relative decrease in gonorrhea rates among young adults. Further, gonorrhea rates were calculated for the year before and the year after changes were made in state alcohol policies, i.e., raising the minimum legal drinking age. Again, most legal-drinking-age increases were followed by a decrease in the gonorrhea rate. The study concluded that higher beer taxes were associated with lower gonorrhea rates in young adults ages 15 to 19 *and* 20 to 24, and that minimum legal-drinking-age increases were associated with lower gonorrhea rates among 15 to 19 year olds.

Finally, disease detection, appropriate treatment, counseling, and, if necessary, treatment of the sex partner deserve some brief comment here, although these issues will be discussed in more detail as related to individual STDs in the next section of this chapter. Any public health intervention strategy for STDs focuses around early detection of disease or "case finding." This approach to control in the United States has been used in some form since World War I, with an increased emphasis in World War II, and has in many respects been the hallmark of public health control, particularly of syphilis and gonorrhea and, more recently, HIV. Obviously, the situation is more complicated now than in the past, with many more diseases documented as potentially spread by sexual contact. Nonetheless, a mechanism to reach the sexual contacts or partners of an individual known to be infected with an STD remains an essential part of control. In a college health service this may require counseling an infected student to notify his or her partner(s), or may require intervention and case finding by the local city or county health department. In the latter case, it is particularly important that state and local laws requiring notification of public health authorities of the occurrence of an STD be adhered to closely.

One unusual difficulty facing many college health services is the problem of the partner of the student infected with an STD not being a student and therefore not eligible for care at the health service. Some health services have seen fit to prescribe medication for a student's partner without ever seeing him/her. That, however, raises medical, legal, and ethical questions. One innovative approach to this issue has recently been tried in a San Francisco health plan[19] by an arrangement allowing physicians to write prescriptions paid for by the plan for anonymous partners of patients diagnosed with chlamydia infections. It is pointed out that treatment is simple and inexpensive, and many of contact patients may be cured with a single course of antibiotic therapy. Chlamydia infection is so prevalent that contact tracing by public health departments, as has been the keystone for other STDs, may not be logistically and financially possible. Nonetheless, Dr. Michael Rian notes that "the upsides probably outweigh the downsides, but the downsides have to be remembered…if you're not interviewing the partner, then you're not doing the contact tracing that…may lead you into a whole network of infection."[19,p.2]

Keeping in mind, then, all these issues related to control of STDs—particularly as these controls apply to college students—the following section deals with individual diseases which may be transmitted sexually. (HIV disease is discussed separately in chapter 9.) It is not the intent to discuss the 25 or more pathogens which may be spread by sexual contact. We have elected to focus our discussion on those STDs which are most common and therefore frequently of most concern in the college age group. Further, we have not included a discussion of diseases such as the hepatitides which may be spread by sexual contact but which are not generally considered to be (primarily) STDs. Once an STD has been diagnosed, correct and timely treatment for the specific disease is absolutely essential. If that cannot be administered within the college health service, referral to a qualified person or an appropriate facility should be done with due diligence. And it is essential to remember that the treatment guidelines discussed in the following section are those *currently* recommended. The reader is advised to confirm a treatment plan using the most current available information from CDC or another reliable source.

RISK ASSESSMENT AND MANAGEMENT OF SEXUALLY TRANSMITTED DISEASES

Over 12 million Americans are infected with sexually transmitted diseases (STDs) annually. The majority of those affected with STDs are in their teens or early twenties, which includes the age of the typical college student. Management of STDs is often difficult because of the need to deal with more than one patient (the index patient and partner). The clinician who neglects the partner misses an opportunity to prevent further transmission of disease and increases the risk that the index patient will be reexposed or reinfected.[20] As part of effective management, the CDC recommends treatment that includes directly observed therapy (in a single session) when possible. [11]

Risk assessment includes a complete sexual history and clinical evaluation. The sexual history should include questions regarding sexual contact with men, women, or both. Ascertaining the mode of sexual practices (oral, anal, vaginal) is particularly important in college students; one recent study reported that 64 percent of college students surveyed had vaginal, 69 percent, oral, and 11 percent, anal sex.[21]

Most STD experts recommend obtaining a history of serologic testing for syphilis and HIV, as well as hepatitis B vaccination. Knowledge of previous antibiotic use is important because antibiotics may mask symptoms of certain STDs or affect sensitivities of the infecting organism. Frequent travel by college students makes travel history and demographic information important in suspecting the possibility of certain STDs.

Clinical evaluation should include a review of systems and a focused physical examination. The information obtained through risk assessment and clinical evaluation directs appropriate confirmatory diagnostic testing or screening. Rapid tests such as wet mounts of vaginal discharge or a urethral Gram stain may aid in starting presumptive therapy.[20] Screening of partners and asymptomatic patients is an important component of STD management.

The following recommendations by the Advisory Committee for HIV and STD Prevention (ACHSP) are particularly pertinent to the typical college population.[23]

- All sexually active women under the age of 25 years who visit a health care provider for any reason should be screened for chlamydia and gonorrhea at least once per year.
- Routine screening of sexually active young men for chlamydia and gonorrhea should be implemented in settings (or for subpopulations) in which the prevalence is >2 percent.
- Older individuals in "high-risk" groups of either gender should be screened yearly for chlamydia and gonorrhea. High-risk groups include substance abusers, persons with a history of STDs, those with more than one sex partner per year, those in correctional facilities, and persons from communities with high rates of STDs.
- Serologic screening for syphilis should be conducted in high-risk persons (those who have multiple sex partners, exchange sex for money or drugs, are incarcerated, or use illicit drugs).
- Persons already infected with HIV should be screened routinely for other STDs.

DISEASES CHARACTERIZED BY GENITAL ULCERS

In the United States, most sexually active patients who have genital ulcers have either genital herpes or syphilis.[11] A diagnosis based only on the patient's history and physical examination is often inaccurate. Evaluation of all patients who have genital ulcers should include a serologic test for syphilis and a diagnostic evaluation for herpes. Newer testing includes the multiplex polymerase chain reaction (PCR) for the diagnosis of *H. ducreyi*, herpes simplex, and *T. pallidum*.[24] Additionally, HIV testing should be performed in the management of patients who have genital ulcers caused by *T. pallidum* or *H. ducreyi* and should be considered if the patient has ulcers caused by herpes simplex virus (HSV).

Chancroid

While uncommon in the U.S., chancroid is endemic in many developing countries. The classic triad of chancroid is an undermined, painful, purulent ulcer with ragged edges. A definitive diagnosis requires identification of *H. ducreyi* on special culture media. A probable diagnosis can be made if the patient has one or more painful genital ulcers, has no evidence of *T. pallidum* infection (by darkfield or serologic testing at least seven days after onset of ulcers), and if the clinical presentation is typical for chancroid, and testing for HSV is negative.[11]

Effective treatment for chancroid cures the infection, resolves the clinical symptoms and prevents transmission to others. The current recommended regimens by the Centers for Disease Control and Prevention (CDC) are outlined below.[11] (Note: Ciprofloxacin is contraindicated for pregnant and lactating women and for persons under age 18.)

- Azithromycin 1 g orally in a single dose
- Ceftriazone 250 mg intramuscularly (IM) in a single dose
- Ciprofloxacin 500 mg orally twice a day for 3 days*
- Erythromycin base 500 mg orally four times a day for 7 days

Syphilis

In 1999, 6,657 cases of primary and secondary syphilis were reported in the United States, with the South continuing to have the highest rate in the country. Nine of the 11 states having rates above the National Health Objective for 2000 are southern states where limited access to health care providers is likely a major factor. Further, the 1999 reported rate of primary and secondary syphilis in blacks was 30 times the rate reported in whites.[8]

The syphilis chancre begins as a papule nine to ninety days after exposure. It then develops into a painless, 2cm to 3cm, ulcer with a hard edge and a clean base. The chancre generally resolves without treatment, disappearing within two to six weeks. Primary, secondary, and early latent syphilis (persons with no clinical syndrome and positive serological tests) of less than one year in duration should be treated with penicillin G benzathine (2.4 million units). Every effort should be made to document a history of penicillin allergy before choosing an alternative regimen.

Parenteral penicillin G is the only therapy with documented efficacy for neurosyphilis or for syphilis during pregnancy. Therefore, when these patients report a penicillin allergy, they should be desensitized and treated with penicillin if possible. Skin testing for penicillin allergy may be useful in some settings.

All patients with a positive nontreponemal test (Venereal Disease Research Laboratory [VDRL] or rapid plasma reagin [RPR]) test should have a confirmatory treponemal test which includes either the microhemagglutinin assay (*Treponema pallidum* [MHA-TP]), fluorescent treponemal antibody absorption test (FTA-ABS), or the newer particle test (Serodia *T. pallidum* particle agglutination [TP-PA]). Using only one test is insufficient for the diagnosis, because false-positive nontreponemal test results occasionally occur secondary to various medical conditions.

HIV-negative patients with early (or congenital) syphilis should have a quantitative VDRL at 6 and 12 months after treatment. Serologic follow-up for HIV-positive patients is recommended at 3, 6, 12 and 24 months.[11] Sequential serologic tests should be performed using the same testing method (e.g., VDRL or RPR) and, preferably, the same laboratory. The VDRL and the RPR are equally valid, but quantitative results from the two tests cannot be directly compared, because RPR titers are often slightly higher than VDRL titers.

When patients are properly treated, the VDRL should decrease by two dilutions at six months, three dilutions at 12 months, and four dilutions at 24 months. Patients should be reevaluated if signs or symptoms persist or if the initial titer fails to decrease fourfold within six months. In these cases, patients may have failed therapy, may have been reinfected, or may be coinfected with HIV.[11, 23]

Herpes Simplex Virus

Genital herpes is the most common cause of genital ulcerative disease (GUD) in the general population and certainly in college students. The herpes simplex virus-1 (HSV-1) and herpes simplex virus-2 (HSV-2) can cause both genital and oral infections. Definitive diagnosis depends on culturing HSV from an open vesicle. Routine viral culture with typing is recommended, as it can be used in counseling patients regarding the risk of recurrence. Ninety percent of people with primary HSV-2 and 60 percent of patients with primary HSV-1 will have a recurrence in the first year of infection.[25] Serological testing for HSV-1 or HSV-2 is not recommended at this time as the high rate of positive results reflecting the 45 million people who have been previously infected with HSV-1 or HSV-2.[25]

The current treatment regimens for primary herpes infection, recurrent herpes infection and suppressive therapy are outlined below.[11,20]

Table 1. Treatment of herpes simplex viral infection

Indication	Drug	Dose	Duration	Comments
First episode of genital herpes	Acyclovir Acyclovir Valacyclovir Famciclovir	200 mg p.o. 5 x/day 400 mg p.o. 3 x/d 1000 mg p.o. 2 x/d 250 mg p.o. 3 x/d	10–14 days	If not healed after 2 weeks of therapy, treat for an additional 7 days.
Recurrent genital herpes	Acyclovir Acyclovir Valacyclovir Famciclovir	400 mg p.o. 3 x/day 200 mg p.o. 5 x/d 500 mg p.o. 2 x/d 125 mg p.o. 2 x/d	5 days	Therapy shortens episode by 1-2 days.
Suppressive therapy	Acyclovir Valacyclovir Valacyclovir Valacyclovir Famciclovir	400 mg p.o. 2 x/day 250 mg p.o. 2 x/d 500 mg p.o. 1 x/d 1000 mg p.o. 1 x/d 250 mg p.o. 2 x/d		A 500 mg dose of valacyclovir may be less effective in patients who have frequent recurrences (>10 episodes per year).

Many patients diagnosed with genital herpes report feelings of depression and isolation and a fear of rejection. Patient counseling should include information about the natural history of herpes infection and reassurance that sexual relationships can continue provided patients take measures to prevent infecting their partners. Advice about prevention and protection primarily involves the correct and consistent use of latex condoms. Condoms do not provide complete protection, because a condom might not properly cover herpetic lesions during periods of viral shedding. It is best to abstain from sex when symptoms are present and use latex condoms consistently between outbreaks.[23]

DISEASES CHARACTERIZED BY URETHRITIS AND CERVICITIS

Chlamydia trachomatis and *Neisseria gonorrhoeae* cause most cases of urethritis and cervicitis. The etiology of most nongonococcal, nonchlamydial urethritis is unknown. Agents that may cause urethritis include *Trichomonas vaginalis*, herpes simplex virus, *Ureaplasma urealyticum* and, possibly, *Mycoplasma genitalium.*[20]

Chlamydia

Infection with *Chlamydia trachomatis* remains the most frequently reported STD in the United States today.[11] Recently the National Committee on Quality Assurance (NCQA) adopted annual screening of young women as a health care quality measure. As a result, annual chlamydia screening of sexually active females 15–25 years of age will be included in the Health Plan Employer Data and Information Set (HEDIS), a set of performance measures to assess the quality of care delivered by managed care plans, and is recommended by the third U.S. Preventive Services Task Force (USPSTF).

Because 50 to 75 percent of patients with chlamydia are asymptomatic, laboratory screening is essential for diagnosis and treatment.[23] Complications of untreated chlamydial infections include pelvic inflammatory disease, infertility, and other serious health problems, including an increased risk of HIV infection. Most chlamydia screening programs use nucleic acid probe (GenProbe®), antigen detection (DFA or EIA), or nucleic acid (NA) amplification techniques (PCR, LCR, or TMA). Antigen or nucleic acid probe tests are performed on cervical specimens, while the chlamydia NA tests can be run on urine or cervical specimens.[24]

Adequate treatment for uncomplicated chlamydia cervicitis or urethritis may be accomplished using doxycycline or azithromycin. Unless symptoms persist or reinfection is suspected, retesting of non-pregnant patients with chlamydia is not recommended.[11] To minimize the risk of reinfection patients should abstain from sexual intercourse until all of their sexual partners are treated. The current CDC treatment guidelines for uncomplicated cervical chlamydia infections are outlined below.[11]

Table 2. Treatment for Uncomplicated Cervical Chlamydial Infection

Recommended Regimens
Azithromycin 1 g orally in a single dose
or
Doxycycline 100 mg orally twice a day for 7 days
Alternative Regimens
Erythromycin base 500 mg orally four times a day for 7 days
or

Erythromycin ethylsuccinate 800 mg orally four times a day for 7 days
or
Ofloxacin 300 mg orally twice a day for 7 days

Doxycycline and ofloxacin are contraindicated for pregnant women. The safety and efficacy of azithromycin use in pregnant and lactating women have not been established. The current CDC treatment regimens for uncomplicated chlamydia cervicitis in pregnant women are outlined below. Repeat testing three weeks after treatment with this regimen is recommended.[11]

Table 3 outlines the current CDC recommendations for uncomplicated chlamydial cervicitis in pregnant women.

(Note: Erythromycin estolate is contraindicated during pregnancy because of drug-related hepatotoxicity. Preliminary data indicate that azithromycin may be safe and effective in pregnancy.)

Table 3. Treatment for Uncomplicated Cervical Chlamydial Infection in Pregnant Women

---

Recommended Regimens
Erythromycin base 500 mg orally four times a day for 7 days
or
Amoxicillin 500 mg orally three times a day for 7 days
Alternative Regimens
Erythromycin base 250 mg orally four times a day for 14 days
or
Erythromycin ethylsuccinate 800 mg orally four times a day for 7 days
or
Erythromycin ethylsuccinate 400 mg orally four times a day for 14 days
or
Azithromycin 1 g orally in a single dose

Gonorrhea

Gonorrhea continues to play a major role in STD prevalence today. Following a 72 percent decline in reported rate from 1975 to 1997, in 1999 the rate increased for the second year in a row.[26] However, it is possible this increase may be due to increased screening and greater sensitivity of newer diagnostic tests. Infection with *Neisseria gonorrhoeae* may cause urethritis, cervicitis, proctitis, prostatitis, pharyngitis, conjunctivitis, and arthritis. Ejaculate and vaginal fluid are considered potentially infectious material and are capable of transmitting gonorrhea.

N. gonorrhoeae conjunctivitis is particularly problematic because of the difficulty in diagnosing infection with routine bacterial swabs. To properly diagnose gonococcal conjunctivitis, the eye should be swabbed and the material immediately streaked on a Thayer-

Martin agar plate with a tight-fitting media bottle lid. Alternatively, an ophthalmic swab specifically designed for gonorrhea is available (GenProbe, blue package).

The current recommended treatment of gonococcal conjunctivitis is 1 gram of ceftriaxone IM, followed by a normal saline lavage of the eye. Follow-up referral to an ophthalmologist is recommended. Patients diagnosed with gonorrhea should also be treated for possible concomitant chlamydial infection.

Antimicrobial resistance of gonorrhea remains an important consideration. Overall, 28.1 percent of isolates collected by the Gonococcal Isolate Surveillance Project (GISP) were resistant to penicillin, tetracycline, or both.[9] Cases of *N. gonorrhoeae* resistant to fluoroquinolones have also been reported by the GISP. Culture and sensitivity testing should be performed on patients who appear to have treatment failure after recommended therapy has been completed. Table 4 outlines the current CDC treatment regimens for uncomplicated gonococcal infections of the cervix, urethra, and rectum.[11] The current CDC treatment regimens for uncomplicated gonococcal infection of the pharynx are outlined in Table 5.[11]

Table 4. Recommended Regimens for Uncomplicated Gonococcal Infections of the Cervix, Urethra, and Rectum

Cefixime 400 mg orally in a single dose
or
Ceftriaxone 125 mg IM in a single dose
or
Ciprofloxacin 500 mg orally in a single dose
or
Ofloxacin 400 mg orally in a single dose,
plus
Azithromycin 1 g orally in a single dose
or
Doxycycline 100 mg orally twice a day for 7 days

Table 5. Recommended Regimens for Uncomplicated Gonococcal Infection of the Pharynx

Ceftriaxone 125 mg IM in a single dose
or
Ciprofloxacin 500 mg orally in a single dose
or
Ofloxacin 400 mg orally in a single dose
plus
Azithromycin 1 g orally in a single dose
or
Doxycycline 100 mg orally twice a day for 7 days

Pregnant women should not be treated with quinolones or tetracyclines. Those infected with *N. gonorrhoeae* should be treated with a recommended cephalosporin regimen plus either erythromycin or amoxicillin for the presumptive or diagnosed *C. trachomatis* infection.

Patients should be instructed to refer their sex partners for evaluation and treatment. Patients should be instructed to avoid sexual intercourse for seven days until both they and their sexual partners are no longer symptomatic.

DISEASES CHARACTERIZED BY VAGINAL DISCHARGE

Vaginitis and vaginal discharge are common complaints prompting college women to visit their student health service. Vaginitis is poorly defined and often ignored. The differential diagnosis for vaginitis is extensive and should include physiologic discharge, chemical or irritant vaginitis, atrophic vaginitis, and vaginitis due to infectious agents. Identifying the cause of vaginitis is paramount. Many over-the-counter products, such as topical antifungals, are widely available and allow women to self-treat, which can make the diagnosis difficult when patients present with partially treated disease.

Bacterial Vaginosis

Bacterial vaginosis (BV) is the most common cause of vaginal discharge among U.S. college women. Signs and symptoms of BV include a foul-smelling, homogeneous, white, adherent vaginal discharge. Vulvovaginal pruritus, burning, and dyspareunia may be associated with BV. While it remains debatable whether BV meets the criteria for an STD, it has been shown that BV occurs more frequently in patients with multiple sex partners.[11] There are concerns that BV may be a cofactor for the acquisition of HIV with the absence of lactobacilli associated with an increased risk of acquiring HIV and gonorrhea.[27] BV appears to be an imbalance of the normal flora of (*Lactobacilllus*) with a mixed flora of *Gardnerella vaginalis, Mycoplasma hominis,* and anaerobes.[28] Diagnosis is usually based on clinical criteria which include any three of the following: (a) homogeneous, uniformly adherent discharge with little evidence of inflammation on examination; (b) vaginal fluid pH >4.5; (c) an amine ("fishy") odor after addition of 10 percent potassium hydroxide (KOH) solution to vaginal fluid; (d) presence of "clue cells" (epithelial cells with coarse granulation and bacterial studding along cell membrane).[11]

Current treatment options for BV are outlined in Table 6.[11] However, standard BV treatment can be followed by a 30 percent relapse rate within one month. Unfortunately, there are no current studies that specifically address management of recurrent BV.[29]

Bacterial vaginosis has been associated with adverse pregnancy outcomes, such as premature rupture of the membranes, pre-term labor, and pre-term birth.[28] Therefore, the CDC recommends that high-risk pregnant women (i.e., those with a history of pre-term labor) be screened and treated for BV in the early weeks of their second trimester. Additionally, low-risk pregnant women with symptomatic BV should be treated (in the second and third trimesters) to relieve symptoms.[11]

It is important to note that clindamycin vaginal cream is *not* recommended for BV treatment during pregnancy, because studies have shown an increased risk of pre-term deliveries among pregnant women treated with this drug.[28]

Tabnle 6. Recommended Treatment for Bacterial Vaginosis

Non-pregnant Women
Metronidazole 500 mg orally twice a day for 7 days
or
Clindamycin cream 2 percent, one full applicator intravaginally at bedtime for 7 days
or
Metronidazole gel 0.75 percent, one full applicator intravaginally twice a day for 5 days
Pregnant Women
Metronidazole 250 mg orally three times a day for 7 days
Alternative regimens (non-pregnant and pregnant women)
Metronidazole 2 g orally in a single dose
or
Clindamycin 300 mg orally twice a day for 7 days

Trichomoniasis

Trichomoniasis is a protozoan infection of the genital tract that in women typically causes a malodorous, yellow-green vaginal discharge and vulvar irritation. In men, it is often asymptomatic. The flagellated organism (*Trichomonas vaginalis*) can be seen on wet mount with normal saline, but this test is only 60 percent sensitive in women and 50–90 percent in men.[30] Newer diagnostic techniques include PCR, which is superior to other conventional methods (culture and wet mount).[24]

The current recommended treatment of trichomoniasis is metronidazole, 2 grams orally in a single dose, or 500 mg twice a day for 7 days. Sexual partners should also be treated. While metronidazole gel is approved for the treatment of BV, it seldom achieves therapeutic levels in the urethra and perivaginal glands and is less efficacious than oral metronidazole for the treatment of trichomoniasis. Therefore, the CDC does not recommend metronidazole gel for the treatment of *Trichomonas vaginalis*.[11]

Studies have associated trichomoniasis during pregnancy with adverse birth outcomes such as pre-term delivery and low birth weight.[30] Cases of resistant trichomoniasis have been reported. The mechanisms of resistance are not known but in some cases can be overcome with larger doses and a longer duration of metronidazole therapy.[30]

PELVIC INFLAMMATORY DISEASE

Pelvic inflammatory disease (PID) comprises a spectrum of inflammatory diseases of the upper female genital tract, including endometritis, salpingitis, tubo-ovarian abscess, and pelvic peritonitis.[11] It is the most common gynecologic disorder in the United States necessitating hospitalization for young women.[31]

The infections can be caused by a variety of organisms, including *N. gonorrhoeae,*

C. trachomatis, gastrointestinal anaerobes, *Gardnerella vaginalis, Haemophilus influenzae, Mycoplasma hominis, Ureaplasma urealyticum, Streptococcus agalactiae,* and enteric Gram-negative rods. The CDC notes that while the precise organism responsible for PID is often difficult to establish, any appreciable delay in treatment can have severe consequences. Therefore, the CDC recommends empiric treatment if the following minimum criteria are present and no other cause for the illness can be identified: lower abdominal tenderness, adnexal tenderness, and cervical motion tenderness. Additional criteria supporting a diagnosis of PID include an oral temperature higher than 101° F (38.5° C), abnormal cervical or vaginal discharge, elevated erythrocyte sedimentation rate, elevated C-reactive protein, and laboratory documentation of cervical infection with either *N. gonorrhoeae* or *C. trachomatis.*[11]

Definitive criteria for a PID diagnosis includes histopathologic evidence of endometritis on endometrial biopsy; transvaginal sonography or other imaging techniques showing thickened fluid-filled tubes, with or without free pelvic fluid; and laparoscopic abnormalities consistent with PID.

The current recommended regimen for outpatient empiric treatment of PID is ofloxacin 400 mg orally twice a day for 14 days, plus metronidazole 500 mg orally twice a day for 14 days; or ceftriaxone 250 mg intramuscularly for 1 day, or another third-generation cephalosporin plus doxycycline 100 mg orally twice a day for 14 days.[11]

Patients who meet any of the following criteria should be hospitalized for treatment of PID.

- Severe illness, nausea, and vomiting, or fever of 102°F or greater
- Pregnancy
- Signs of peritonitis
- Unable to tolerate oral nourishment
- Unlikely to comply with outpatient therapy
- Signs of a pelvic abscess
- Failure to respond to outpatient treatment after 72 hours
- The diagnosis is uncertain

Current inpatient treatment regimens for PID are outlined below.[11] Given the serious reproductive consequences of PID, prevention must be a priority.

Recommended Parenteral Treatment for PID

Regimen A
Cefotetan 2 g intravenous (IV) every 12 hours
or
Cefoxitin 2 g IV every 6 hours
plus
Doxycycline 100 mg IV or orally every 12 hours
Regimen B
Clindamycin 900 mg IV every 8 hours
plus
Gentamycin loading dose (2 mg/kg) IV or IM, followed by a maintenance dose (1.5 mg/kg) every 8 hours

HUMAN PAPILLOMA VIRUS INFECTION

Human papilloma virus (HPV) infections have two important clinical manifestations: external genital warts and cervical squamous intraepithelial lesions. (Refer to chapter 6 for further discussion of the latter topic.) An estimated 24 million Americans are infected with HPV; some experts estimate the incidence of HPV infections to be close to 5 million per year.[32] The 70 HPV genotypes are divided into low-risk types and high-risk types based on their association with anogenital cancers. Because of the resistant nature of HPV, treatment of genital warts is largely confined to the simple removal of visible warts. This approach results in wart-free periods in most patients but does not cure the disease. There is no evidence that current forms of treatment completely eradicate HPV or decrease the likelihood of development of cervical cancer in women infected with HPV high-risk subtypes. Treatment regimens for genital warts include a wide range of provider-administered therapies—cryotherapy, podophyllum resin, trichloroacetic acid, bichloroacetic acid, interferon, and surgery—as well as the patient-applied therapies of podofilox and imiquimod. Success rates vary greatly depending on the size and number of warts, the anatomic site, wart morphology, and patient reliability. Other factors that may be involved in the selection of treatment modality include cost, convenience, adverse effects, and the ability of the patient to apply therapies to the affected areas.[23]

SEXUALLY TRANSMITTED ECTOPARASITIC INFECTIONS

Ectoparasitic infestations are common worldwide. In the United States, both *Pediculosis pubis* (crab lice) and scabies are often sexually transmitted. Both infestations present with severe pruritis. Because of potential central nervous system toxicity associated with lindane (used for both scabies and crab lice), it should be prescribed cautiously. The CDC recommends that lindane not be used immediately after bathing, as this increases its absorption. Lindane is not recommended for persons with extensive dermatitis, children <2 years of age, and pregnant or lactating women.[11,20]

Pediculosis pubis

Crab lice may infest the pubic and perianal areas and can extend to the beard, axilla and eyelashes. Therefore, treatment should be applied to all hairy areas of the body. The CDC currently recommends 1 percent permethrin cream, 1 percent lindane shampoo or pyrethrins with piperonyl butoxide.[11] Cure rates of 60 percent and 57 percent respectively have been reported with 1 percent lindane and 1 percent permethrin. A second treatment one week later may increase the cure rate to 86 percent and 72 percent respectively.[22,33]

Scabies

The CDC currently recommends 5 percent permethrin cream (washed off 8–14 hours later) for the treatment of scabies. One percent lindane (8-hour application) or 6 percent sulfur (apply nightly for three nights) are alternative treatments.[20]

FINAL COMMENTS

It would be naïve to expect a time when STDs are no longer a problem on college and university campuses. That being the case, it is clear that any program to counter this epidemic, which appeared first as syphilis, then as gonorrhea, later as HIV, then as HPV, must be multifaceted. It must involve primary prevention and consideration of "peripheral" issues such as alcohol use; it must include prompt and effective treatment; it must include contact case findings at treatment, whether as individual or a community; and, finally, it must include continued recognition by the community (in this instance, the college or university) of the existence of the problem and the subsequent willingness to commit resources adequate to deal with the problem. In a sense, except for more precise diagnosis and more effective treatment of certain STDs, the issues remain much the same as Osler identified in 1905.

REFERENCES

1. Storey TA. A Summary of the work of the United States Interdepartmental Social Hygiene Board. 1919–1920. *Soc Hygiene.* 1921;7:59–76.

2. Storey TA. The Status of Hygiene Programs in Institutions of Higher Education in the United States: A Report for the President's Committee of Fifty on College Hygiene. Palo Atto: Stanford University Press; 1927.

3. Ferree JW. Education for family living (social hygiene). In: *A Health Program for Colleges.* Report of the Third National Conference on Health in Colleges, May 7–10, 1947. Published by National Tuberculosis Association.

4. Report of the National Commission on Venereal Diseases. U.S. Department of Health, Education, and Welfare. Publication No. (HSM) 72-8125. 1972.

5. Waugh MA. History of clinical development in sexually transmitted diseases. In: Holmes KK, Mardh P, Sparling PF, Wiesner PJ, eds. *Sexually Transmitted Diseases,* 2nd Edition. New York: McGraw Hill;1990.

6. CDC. *MMWR,* Jul 31, 1998, Recommendations and Reports, Vol. 47/No. RR-12.

7. *Healthy People 2010.* Office of Disease Prevention and Health Promotion. U.S. Department of Health & Human Services; 2000.

8. CDC Primary and Secondary Syphilis—United States, 1999. CDC. *MMWR,* Feb 23, 2001;50(07);113–7.

9. Gonorrhea—United States, 1998. CDC. *MMWR,* June 23, 2000; 49(24).

10. Osler W. *The Principles and Practice of Medicine,* 6th Edition. New York: D. Appleton and Company;1905:278–279.

11. CDC. 1998 Guidelines for Treatment of Sexually Transmitted Diseases. *MMWR* Jan. 23, 1997;47(RR-1–116).

12. Reinisch JM, Hill CA, Sanders SA, Ziemba-Davis M. High-risk sexual behavior at a midwestern university: A confirmatory survey. *Fam Plan Perspect.* 1995 Mar-Apr;27(2):79–82.

13. Jaffe GP, Foxman B, Schmidt AJ, Farris KB, Carter RJ, Neumann S, Tolo KA, Walters AM. Multiple partners and partner choice as risk factors for sexually transmitted disease among female college students. *Sex Transm Dis* 1992 Sept-Oct;19(5):272–278.

14. DeBuono BA, Zinner SH, Daamen M, McCormack WM. Sexual behavior of college women in 1975, 1986 and 1989. *NEJM* 322(12):821–825.

15. Zinner SH, McCormack WM. Three decades of research on sexual behavior and sexually transmitted pathogens in college students. *Medicine and Health/Rhode Island.* Oct 1997;80(10).

16. CDC. Sexually Transmitted Disease Surveillance, 1998. Atlanta, GA. U.S. Dept. of Health & Human Services, CDC, Sept, 1999.

17. CDC. Alcohol policy and sexually transmitted disease rates—United States, 1981–1995. *MMWR* Apr 28, 2000;49(16).

18. Chessor H, Harrison P, Kassler WJ. Sex under the influence: The effect of alcohol policy on sexually transmitted disease rates in the U.S. *J Law & Econ* 2000, Apr;XLIII(1):215.

19. Extra meds for sex partner, one approach in public health struggle to curb chlamydia. *American Medical News.* Apr 9, 2001; 44(14):1–2.

20. Thornton A, Adkins D, Arno J. Sexually transmitted diseases. In: Mainous AG III, Pomeroy C, eds. *Management of Antimicrobials in Infectious Diseases.* Totowa, N.J.: Humana Press Inc; 2000.

21. Siegel DM, Klein DI, Roghmann KJ. Sexual behavior, contraception, and risk among college students. *Adolesc Health.* 1999;25:336–343.

22. CDC. HIV prevention through early detection and treatment of other sexually transmitted diseases—US recommendations of the advisory committee for HIV and STD prevention. *MMWR* 1998: 47:1–24.

23. Jennings P, Ridings H, Thornton A. STD update: new CDC guidelines. *Advance for PA's* Aug 1999;7(8).

24. Black CM, Morse SA. The use of molecular techniques for the diagnosis and epidemiologic study of sexually transmitted infections. *Curr Infect Dis Rep.* 2000;2:31–43.

25. Wald A. New therapies and prevention strategies for genital herpes. *Clin Infect Dis.* 1999;28(suppl 1):S4–S13.

26. http://www.sa.psu.edu/UHS/gonorr.htm (Penn State University, June 2001).

27. Martin HL, Richardson BA, Nyange PM, et al. Vaginal lactobacilli, microbial flora, and risk of human immunodeficiency virus type 1 and sexually transmitted disease acquisition. J Inf Dis 1999;180:1863–1864.

28. Joesoef MR, Schmid GP, Hillier SL. Bacterial vaginosis: Review of clinical treatment options and potential clinical indications for therapy. *Clin Infect Dis* 1999;28(suppl 1) S57–65.

29. Hay P. Recurrent bacterial vaginosis, Current Infections Disease Report 2:506–512.

30. Krieger JN, Alderet JF. Trichomonas vaginalis and trichomoniasis. In: Holmes KK, Mardh P-A, Sparling PF, et al. (eds). *Sexually Transmitted Diseases.* New York: McGraw-Hill; 1999:587–604.

31. Walker C, Workowski K, Washington A, Soper D, Sweet R. Anaerobes in pelvic inflammatory disease: Implications for the Centers for Disease Control and Prevention's Guidelines for Treatment of Sexually Transmitted Diseases. *Clin Infect Dis* 1999;28(suppl 1):S29–S36.

32. Cates WJ. The American Social Health Association Panel. Estimates of the incidence and prevalence of sexually transmitted diseases in the U.S. *Sex Transm Di*;1999;26:S2–7.

33. Meinking TL. Infestations. *Curr Probl Dermato.* 1999;11:73–120.

CHAPTER 9

HIV/AIDS in College Health and Higher Education

Richard P. Keeling, MD

The human immunodeficiency virus (HIV) is a recently discovered human T-lymphocytotropic infectious agent that causes a chronic, progressive acquired immunodeficiency state (HIV infection). HIV infection almost invariably becomes symptomatic because of the development of a variety of opportunistic infections and neoplasms typical of T-lymphocyte deficiency states (HIV disease). The most severe phase of HIV disease, characterized by striking reductions in helper T-lymphocyte counts (below 200/mm^3), major, life-threatening opportunistic infections, and/or certain unusual cancers, is called the acquired immunodeficiency syndrome (AIDS). College health, and higher education more generally, have recognized and responded to the significant challenges HIV/AIDS creates for students (and for institutions) with the development of specific policy documents, a variety of prevention programs, specific HIV antibody counseling and testing services, HIV-related personal counseling, sexual health and risk assessment activities, and in some cases, direct clinical care.

HUMAN IMMUNODEFICIENCY VIRUS INFECTION AND DISEASE

Since the first reports in 1981 of confirmed cases of this new acquired adult immunodeficiency disorder, extensive epidemiological, virological, and pathological research has explained the major features of HIV infection. In particular, its pathogenesis is now reasonably well understood. After exposure, HIV establishes both productive (virus-producing) and latent infection in certain populations of immunologically competent cells, especially T_4 (helper) lymphocytes. The rapid reproduction of HIV produces very high blood levels of HIV RNA within days to weeks of infection. A dynamic and proliferative immune response to HIV occurs quickly, with the production of several kinds of specific antibodies directed at various elements of the HIV viral particle. These antibodies have become the usual markers for the presence of HIV infection; they are detected through routine salivary or serum tests (classically, though inappropriately, called "HIV tests"). Prior to the appearance of detectable levels of antibody (approximately four to six weeks after infection, in most cases), it is still possible to document the presence of HIV in the blood through assays for the level of HIV RNA (viral load tests) or by detecting one of HIV's antigens (usually, p24).

Typically, the viral load rises to a peak approximately three to five weeks after infection; helper lymphocyte counts generally plummet during this time (from their usual normal levels of 800–1200 cells/mm^3 to nadirs below 500 cells/mm^3). As antibodies are produced and the full force of a comprehensive immune response is brought to bear, HIV RNA levels fall and helper lymphocyte counts rebound. Within a month or two, blood levels of HIV RNA and the helper lymphocyte count both stabilize (the "set point"); the higher the helper cell number and the lower the viral load at this time, the better the prognosis. The set point appears to represent the emergence of a kind of balance of power between HIV and the immune response.

At least 50 percent of people who acquire HIV infection will experience an illness, called primary HIV infection, in association with their seroconversion to "HIV positive" (the colloquial term used to describe the condition of having a positive test for antibodies to HIV). The proportion of students who develop this illness related to initial infection and seroconversion has not been specifically investigated. Primary HIV infection is generally protean in its manifestations and nonspecific in character; the usual symptoms include fatigue, low-grade fever, anorexia, and, often, a maculopapular rash (suggesting a viral exanthem). In many ways, primary HIV infection mimics the seronegative (heterophile antibody negative or slide test negative), mononucleosis-like illnesses that are exceedingly common among college and university students. Relatively few students (and few health care providers) will regard it as especially significant, unless they recognize the possibility that the symptoms could denote recent HIV infection. In most cases, primary HIV infection resolves spontaneously without being diagnosed. Very rarely, the clinical course is significant enough to require medical evaluation or even hospitalization—especially when the disease is complicated by encephalitis, features suggesting viral hepatitis, or severe rash. It is likely that some students with primary HIV infection have been evaluated for their complaints in college health services, where the protean nature of the symptoms, their resemblance to common minor illnesses in college health, and the nearly universal pattern of at-risk sexual behavior among students can make recognizing the syndrome (and differentiating it from much less consequential, and infinitely more common, mono-like conditions) very difficult. Routine HIV antibody tests are not yet positive during the course of the illness, but tests for p24 antigen or HIV RNA may allow confirmation of the diagnosis before actual seroconversion occurs a few weeks later.

Primary HIV infection ordinarily passes without incident, to be replaced by a long asymptomatic phase (chronic asymptomatic HIV disease). During this time, people who have HIV infection are unaware of any related illness and usually report no symptoms. Students who have been tested for HIV antibodies and are aware of their condition often experience anxiety and may report a variety of minor complaints, such as evanescent adenopathy. It is probable that the great majority of students who have HIV infection are in this chronic asymptomatic period during most, if not all, of the time of their matriculation; many are certainly unaware of their infection while in college.

Even without treatment, chronic asymptomatic HIV disease may last for many years (as many as 12 to15 in some unusual instances), but the absence of clinical activity only masks a dynamic, continuous struggle between HIV and the immune system. A slow, but nonlinear, decline in helper lymphocyte counts (and a panel of other measures of the integrity of cellular immune function) occurs. Conversely, blood levels of HIV RNA rise and fall but tend upward over years. The set point may influence the time to symptomatic disease and time to death, but it also appears that many other factors, including reinfection/coinfection with other strains of HIV, the presence of other immunocompromising illnesses, the use of immunosuppressive medications, and certain health risk behaviors, such as cigarette smoking or injection-drug use, may also contribute.

Eventually, the deterioration of cellular immune functions is enough to permit the development of first minor, and then major, opportunistic infections. It is unusual for anyone with more than 500 helper cells per mm^3 of blood to experience these infections, but as helper cell counts fall, infectious events become increasingly likely. Initially, infections are more annoying than serious: more frequent recurrences of herpes simplex virus infection (both HSV I and HSV II), a chronic eosinophilic folliculitis, crops of aphthous ulcers, or Epstein-Barr virus (EBV)-related hairy leukoplakia of the tongue. If college students present with symptomatic HIV disease, they will probably have one or more of these relatively less intense problems. Later, as helper cell counts decrease below $200/m^3$ (and especially $100/m^3$), far more significant, and often life-threatening, opportunistic infections become common. Thrush, an infection of the mucous membranes of the mouth and throat caused by *Candida albicans,* is an early marker for this transition. Pneumonia, classically caused by the ubiquitous protozoan *Pneumocystis carinii,* can cause extensive morbidity and mortality for people with HIV. Fungal and protozoal meningitis (especially caused by *Cryptococcus neoformans* or *Toxoplasma capsulatum*), systemic and retinal infection with cytomegalovirus, and bacteremia or bowel infection with agents such as *Mycobacterium avium intracellulare* (*Mycobacterium avium* complex), *Cryptosporidium,* or *Isospora belli* are frequent and can be difficult to eradicate permanently. The Centers for Disease Control and Prevention (CDC) has defined a list of 26 opportunistic infections such as these that qualify a person with HIV disease for the diagnosis of AIDS.[1]

People with AIDS may also develop unusual malignancies. Kaposi's sarcoma, a progressive, multicentric epithelial tumor, causes purplish lesions on the skin and mucous membranes; its pathogenesis requires a newly discovered viral agent, human herpesvirus type 8 (HHV-8).[2] Atypical lymphomas, mostly aggressive non-Hodgkins types with anaplastic histology, may develop in unusual primary sites (notably, the central nervous system) and are difficult to treat successfully because of both tumor resistance and the immunocompromising effects of combination chemotherapy regimens. Both cervical and anal carcinomas are also more common in people with AIDS; their development may demonstrate the stimulant effect of HIV-related immunosuppression on the course of human papillomavirus (HPV) disease.[3] In fact, all of the cancers associated with AIDS seem also somehow associated with viruses known or suspected to have oncogenic potential. Only a very few college or university students have developed these cancers while in school.

Although they are seldom seen in people who have received antiretroviral treatment, there are also other late manifestations of AIDS—notably, a profound wasting syndrome and HIV-related neurological disease, including both a progressive multifocal leukoencephalopathy and dementia. Death is usually a result of some overwhelming opportunistic infection; by the time of the terminal illness, most people with AIDS have helper lymphocyte counts well under $100/mm^3$ (and usually under $50/mm^3$) and viral loads of several hundred thousand copies/mm^3. On average, and without treatment, people with HIV will survive 7 to 12 years after infection.

It is distinctly unusual for campus health services to encounter students with any of these advanced manifestations of HIV disease. Most students who have sought care or services related to HIV/AIDS from college health centers have simply requested HIV antibody counseling and testing. The number of new infections documented in college antibody testing programs has been small. Few students have sought comprehensive case management for their HIV infection from college health services, and few college health professionals are currently qualified and experienced in providing expert care for HIV-related problems. When campus clinicians are directly involved in the medical care of students with HIV infection or disease, they are almost always collaborators with other physicians (primarily, specialists in infectious disease) who make most major treatment decisions. Nonetheless, the ability of the college health center staff to offer supportive and cooperative care has made it possible for some students with HIV disease to continue their education and graduate.

PROGRESS IN THERAPY FOR HIV INFECTION AND DISEASE

Both improved anti-infective pharmacotherapy and better antiretroviral treatments have markedly changed the outlook for people with HIV infection. Most of the major opportunistic infections can now be treated successfully (at least on their first occurrence), and many of them can be prevented or modified through the diligent and conscientious application of prophylactic antimicrobials.[4] In many people with HIV, currently available antiretroviral therapies (most of them multidrug regimens) can postpone the development of symptomatic disease for several years and restore to productive life those who have already experienced serious complications related to their immunodeficiency state. People with HIV disease are hospitalized far less frequently now than a decade ago, and on average, they lose less time from work, are less likely to be disabled, and are more likely to be able to continue in school.

At the same time, it is clear that (1) these antiretroviral regimens are not effective for everybody with HIV, (2) the toxicity of many of them produces unacceptable complications for many users, and (3) any number of realities in life can prevent sustained adherence to the complex, demanding dosing requirements of most modern combination therapies. Even if efficacy and side effects were not major concerns, antiretroviral treatment would still not be helpful to everyone with HIV because of inequities in access to care or the detrimental influence of larger life issues and social problems (such as drug addiction and poverty). And it is painfully clear that no currently available antiretroviral regimen will cure HIV infection. Levels of HIV in the blood rise quickly again whenever treatment is paused or discontinued; careful assays have shown that HIV remains latent during antiretroviral therapy even when viral levels in the blood are rendered undetectable. However, it is important to acknowledge both the extraordinary progress that has been made in the treatment of HIV infection and disease since 1990 and the pressing need for better, more durable, less toxic therapies.

It is possible that the earlier consideration, recognition, and diagnosis of primary HIV infection would improve the management of people with HIV infection by permitting the immediate institution of antiretroviral therapy for the purpose of reducing the set point, but such an aggressive approach to recent infection remains controversial and unproven.[5] It is not clear that early intensive antiretroviral therapy produces benefits in terms of eventual morbidity or survival.[6] There may also be unanticipated toxicities from the prolonged use of the pharmaceuticals required. There are, however, many reasons to advocate the earliest possible detection of new HIV infections. From a public health perspective, earlier diagnosis helps facilitate the prevention of further transmission, and from a clinical point of view, it permits health care providers and people with HIV to begin monitoring the clinical course of infection, intervening to prevent complications, and applying health promotion strategies to strengthen immune function.

There is substantial reason for optimism about the future prospects for progressively better treatments; therefore, preserving the immunological capacities of people with HIV as long as possible is an especially important and hopeful strategy—today's treatments may make it possible for people with HIV to survive until better, more definitive therapies are available. Easily accessible, barrier-free HIV antibody counseling and testing services are key elements of such an approach. Providing or guaranteeing easy referral to such testing services is an essential and core responsibility of college health programs.

TRANSMISSION OF HIV

The transmission of HIV has been well understood since early in the epidemic (1983–1984). HIV is passed from one person to another exclusively in certain body fluids—blood, semen, vaginal secretions, and breast milk. HIV is infectious (able to be transmitted from person to person) but not contagious (casually transmitted from someone who has it to incidental contacts, as through respiratory droplets or fomites). After almost two decades of surveillance, it is clear that HIV is not transmitted by any ordinary non-intimate interpersonal contact. Virtually all cases can be explained by intimate sexual contact with an infected person, by exposure to infected blood (usually through sharing needles used to inject illegal drugs, exceedingly rarely now, through the transfusion of infected blood or blood products, and very uncommonly as a result of accidents in health care or emergency services) by perinatal transmission from mother to her child during pregnancy or, through breastfeeding, after birth.

HIV is thus both a blood-borne pathogen and a sexually transmitted infectious agent. Clearly, certain sexual practices are most commonly associated with HIV infection (vaginal or anal intercourse, with the receptive partner at greater risk). However, it is becoming increasingly clear that some other instances of HIV transmission occur through oral intercourse. Fellatio may uncommonly result in the transmission of HIV to the performing partner through either semen or pre-ejaculatory fluid.[7] Many other intimate and sexual acts (kissing, mutual masturbation, and touching, as examples) do not entertain any risk of acquiring HIV. Latex condoms, properly and timely used, significantly reduce the risk of transmitting HIV when used for vaginal or anal intercourse.

The effect of antiretroviral therapy on the transmissibility of HIV is not completely clear and, in individual cases, is not predictable. While combination regimens can reduce the viral load to undetectable levels and sustain them there for months, there is no evidence that an undetectable viral load correlates with any specific reduction in the transmissibility of HIV in blood, semen, or vaginal secretions. Common sense suggests that a lower viral load may reduce transmissibility, but the degree of protection provided is not known. People with HIV who are being treated with antiretroviral drugs still need to take all appropriate precautions to prevent transmitting HIV to others.

EPIDEMIOLOGY AND RISK OF HIV INFECTION

The epidemiology of HIV infection first suggested, and later confirmed, the mechanisms of transmission of the virus. Persons who become infected with HIV are most often the sexual or needle-sharing partners of people who already have HIV; far less frequently, they are the babies of women with HIV, recipients of HIV-infected blood or blood products, or workers who are exposed to HIV in the course of their professions (usually, health care or emergency service workers).

In the United States (in 1999), CDC estimated that 70 percent of all new HIV infections were among men, with men who have sex with men accounting for the majority (60 percent) of these infections. Heterosexual exposure accounted for 15 percent and injection drug use, 25 percent of infections among men. Women accounted for 30 percent of new infections, with the majority of women (75 percent) infected sexually. Overall, 25 percent of new infections were associated with injection-drug use.

Further, people of color in the U.S. were reported at disproportionate risk. Approximately 63 percent of all women and 42 percent of all men reported with AIDS in 1999 were African American. And Hispanics (who represent some 13 percent of the U.S. population) account for 19 percent of new AIDS cases.[8]

In many other countries, though (especially in Central and South America, the Caribbean, Africa, and Southeast Asia), most of the transmission of HIV has always occurred through heterosexual contact. And, after more than a decade of progress in reducing the incidence of new HIV infections among gay and bisexual men, a resurgence of HIV transmission has occurred, especially among younger men.

The sexual transmission of HIV requires three things: (1) the performance of an act of intercourse that can sustain the transmission of the virus through the exchange of certain body fluids, (2) the absence of a functional, effective latex barrier to prevent exposure to those fluids, and (3) a partner who is infected with HIV. Accordingly, assessing the risk of HIV infection for a given person equally requires assessments of (1) sexual behavior and practices, (2) the reliability, frequency, and predictability of risk reduction measures, and (3) the prevalence of HIV infection in the sexual partnership networks in which that person participates. Even a pattern of multi-partner unprotected intercourse creates no risk of HIV infection if none of the partners involved is infected. Thus, the commonly quoted prevention message, "It's not who you are, it's what you do,"is fundamentally flawed. AIDS is certainly not a gay disease—not in college, not anywhere—but HIV infection is definitely associated with certain sexual networks. So, in fact, it *is* who you are (in the sense that who you are governs who you have sex with), as well as what you do, that determines the risk of HIV infection.

PREVENTING THE TRANSMISSION OF HIV

"Safer sex" consists of the regular use of condoms for intercourse (every time) or the substitution of other sexual behaviors for intercourse.[9] It is not, however, possible to assure anyone that condoms render the chance of HIV infection zero. The degree of protection provided by other supposedly protective devices, such as dental dams and latex squares, is not known. The presence of other conditions that affect the integrity of the genital mucous membranes or skin (genital ulcer diseases, including genital herpes) increases the probability of the transmission of HIV in any given sexual act.

The only certain way to avoid infection with HIV through sexual contact is to avoid all sexual intercourse (oral, vaginal, and anal) or to have intercourse only with a partner, or partners, who assuredly do not have HIV infection. Since abstinence from intercourse, though expedient, is not universally desired, and since it is rarely possible to guarantee with absolute certainty that any given partner is not infected with HIV (or that a theoretically exclusive sexual partner actually behaves in an exclusive manner), HIV prevention is more realistically directed at risk reduction than complete risk elimination. An approach to prevention called "harm reduction," now popular in college health, emphasizes incremental helpful changes that ameliorate risk (sometimes in a stepwise, progressive manner, and sometimes in an episodic, ad hoc way), rather than absolute prohibitions, restrictions, or requirements that may not be always and everywhere applicable, appropriate, or possible. Having unprotected intercourse with fewer partners, using condoms in a higher proportion of sexual encounters, and terminating fellatio before ejaculation are all examples of harm reduction strategies.

Similarly, harm reduction approaches are more valuable than "just say no"strategies in preventing the spread of HIV through needle sharing associated with injecting drug use.[8] Making clean needles available, instituting needle exchange programs, and helping drug users learn how to use bleach to clean their "works"are typical examples. Few college health centers will have reason to employ any of these activities unless the proportion of students who inject drugs and share needles changes in some dramatic and unexpected way.

It is clear from 15 years of research in college health that knowledge alone is not sufficient to prevent the sexual transmission of HIV, and that HIV prevention strategies must work in a practical way within the specific context of life and relationships for each individual. Students, like everyone else, make health-related choices within complex internal and social environments. Their decisions about HIV-related sexual behaviors are likely determined and reinforced by a wealth of factors, from the intensity of desire to the influence of advertising. It is likely, in fact, that each person?s prevention needs are different, even unique—and, therefore, that effective HIV prevention approaches will require extensive customization. At the same time, it also seems clear that the support of others matters, whether that support is felt in specific intimate relationships or through a greater sense of community. The experience of the American urban gay community from 1982 through 1990 would strongly suggest that knowledge, contextually appropriate skills, and accessible social support can materially reduce HIV risks on a population-wide basis.

UNIQUE PATTERNS OF HIV EPIDEMIOLOGY ON CAMPUS

Among college and university students in the United States, the prevalence of HIV infection appears to be very low, despite the presence among students of patterns of sexual behavior that could be (and sometimes are) associated with a significant risk of the acquisition of sexually transmitted infections. Many research studies have confirmed that most students are already well educated about HIV and AIDS prior to their matriculation in college; that college-level HIV education programs add marginal, incremental knowledge to preexisting information; that more than 80 percent of college undergraduates have had sexual intercourse; that a history of intercourse with several partners is common among both female and male students; and that students' use of condoms, though more predictable than a decade ago, remains inconsistent. At the same time, the frequency of HIV infection among students does not suggest that they are in any way at elevated risk; students are certainly not a "high-risk group,"to use the (unfortunate) terminology of the 1980s.

The only reliable nationwide study of the seroprevalence of HIV infection among students was conducted in 1988-89 by the American College Health Association (ACHA) on behalf of the federal Centers for Disease Control and Prevention.[10] Seventeen moderate-and large-sized state universities participated, submitting blood samples from students who had visited their campus health centers (for any reason) for HIV antibody testing. The results of that study were simple: about 0.2 percent, or 1 in 500, of the students tested showed HIV antibodies in their blood. Men were 22 times more likely to have HIV infection than women, and among men, HIV seropositivity was additionally associated with older age and enrollment on a large campus (more than 25,000 students). Interestingly, race, which is a significant factor in the probability of seropositivity in other U.S. populations, did not influence results among students. These seroprevalence data strongly suggest that the great majority of HIV infections occurring among college and university students have resulted from male-to-male sexual contact. For most sexually transmitted infections, the female-to-male ratio tilts toward women; this is also true for sexually transmitted diseases on campus. In the case of HIV, though, that ratio overwhelmingly emphasizes men. The only explanation for these observations—given that there is a negligible rate of injection drug use and needle sharing among students—is homosexual contact. This conclusion is strongly supported by the actual experience of most college health centers, which is that almost all students who test positive for HIV antibodies are men who have had unprotected sexual contact with other men. Similarly, almost all students who seek care from campus clinicians because of HIV infection are gay or bisexual men.

Despite patterns of sexual behavior associated with risk and the absence of consistent precautions against the transmission of HIV, it is highly unlikely that most college students who are not injecting drug users, whose relationships are primarily with other students, and who have exclusively heterosexual patterns of behavior will be infected with HIV. Despite the democratization of higher education, class and socioeconomic status still influence the probability of admission and enrollment. Since HIV infection among heterosexual adults is strongly associated with poverty and/or injecting drug use, most college students are not in sexual networks that will include a significant proportion of heterosexual partners who have HIV.

The same is not true for men on campus who have sex with other men. Unfortunately, the prevalence of HIV among gay and bisexual men in the U.S. is high enough, and the probability of sexual contact with partners who are not college students is significant enough, that unprotected intercourse with another man may well expose male students to HIV. All taken together, these elements of risk assessment and prediction are perfectly consistent with both the available seroepidemiological data and the known experience of college and university health centers. Few health centers have any substantial direct experience in providing medical care to students with HIV, and when they do have, that experience is almost exclusively with students who are men who have sex with other men or students now arriving in college who have been infected with HIV years before as a result of their treatment for hemophilia.

At the same time, it is clear that the diversity among college students means that overall, population-based studies may miss important nuances that affect the risk of HIV infection for certain subpopulations. For example: students in some urban environments attend predominantly nonresidential colleges; their relationship communities may extend far beyond other students, and their risk of HIV infection is accordingly not determined by their student status, but by the prevalence of HIV infection in their primary communities. Similarly, it is important to remember that a decade has passed since the original nationwide campus HIV seroprevalence studies were completed; the snapshot they provided may have changed in the interim. On the other hand, there is no evidence whatever, either from surrogate indicators such as the rate of other sexually transmitted diseases or the frequency of pregnancies or from actual clinical experience, to suggest that there has been any change.

HIV PREVENTION IN COLLEGE HEALTH

Despite the clear and strong associations between HIV/AIDS and the lives of gay and bisexual male students, U.S. colleges and universities have addressed HIV largely by developing task forces and programs, thinking of HIV as a universal problem, rather than by creating programs for the special needs of men who have sex with other men. Educational programs have depended on an equitable, but epidemiologically unsound, paradigm: Anybody can be infected with HIV. Although early informal prevention activities (1983–85) often specifically attended to the needs of gay and bisexual men, most regularized campus HIV prevention work thereafter emphasized the chance that any-body—any student—was at risk.

Many campus-based HIV risk-reduction programs therefore targeted the wrong students with the wrong message. The risk of HIV infection is in fact not universally equal, and an occasional lapse in sexual behavior does not produce the same concern in all circumstances. Teaching low- or zero- risk women that a single unprotected sexual encounter could leave them infected with HIV, while true in a technical sense, is not necessarily relevant for college students in an epidemiological sense. So it is that campus-based HIV-antibody testing programs are unnecessarily and wastefully flooded with (often repeated) testing of very low-risk individuals. Similarly, informing HIV risk-reduction programs with standard prevention rhetoric (such as "It's not who you are," etc.) misinforms students and contradicts their own life experience (which is that it very much *is* who you are, as well as what you do).

On the other hand, the diversion of message, money, and emphasis in college HIV prevention activities toward the comprehensive reduction of some imagined, and universal, high-risk pattern of sexual networking, has left poorly attended and neglected critical and pressing prevention needs of gay and bisexual male students. Although the climate for GLBT students improved remarkably on many campuses during the 1990s, homophobia persists and continues to create substantial pressure toward silence. Nonetheless, especially in the past five years, some college health services have instituted HIV-prevention projects that truly do address the unique needs, social contexts, and community structures of gay and bisexual men. Often, these programs are framed within larger "gay health" initiatives.

CURRENT TRENDS AND FUTURE PROSPECTS

During the 1980s and early 1990s, HIV/AIDS was a very visible issue on most campuses. Many institutions appointed task forces, developed policy statements (most of them opposing discrimination against students with HIV), experimented with various prevention activities (most notably, peer education programs), and implemented HIV risk assessment services (sometimes including HIV antibody testing) in their health or counseling centers. Special presentations about HIV/AIDS were common; students' interest in learning about HIV was high. Students were, in fact, generally concerned enough that health educators would use HIV as a vehicle for other, somewhat related health concerns such as pregnancy prevention or "responsible drinking" (because it was widely felt that alcohol impaired judgment in sexual partner selection, reduced the probability of successful sexual communication, and undermined students' commitments to use condoms for intercourse).

As the 1990s wore on, however, HIV/AIDS became less important on campus, just as it became less critical to most Americans. The anticipated "breakout" of HIV into the so-called general population never occurred (for all the sound epidemiological reasons discussed earlier), and the development of better antiretroviral therapies (many of which, like the protease inhibitor "cocktails," got extensive press coverage) seemed to reduce the perceived danger of infection. The sense of HIV/AIDS as a "crisis" dissipated as the startling increases in the incidence of new HIV infections or AIDS diagnoses common in the 1980s slowed and were replaced with annual declines. HIV prevention education had become de rigeur in high schools and, even though the quality of the work varied a great deal, and the tone of it was often constrained by political realities—such as the emphasis on abstinence only—most students arrived in college with high levels of knowledge about how HIV was transmitted, and how to prevent that from happening. By the mid- to late 1990s, few students would choose to attend "AIDS talks,"most campus task forces had stopped meeting, and the HIV/AIDS-specific educational programs, including "AIDS peer educators," had largely disappeared.

However, at the beginning of the 2000s, HIV/AIDS remains important in higher education. There are fundamental, critical reasons for colleges, universities, and communities to work very hard in responding to the issues, concerns, and needs created by HIV/AIDS, no matter what the level of public concern might be or what the specifics of its epidemiology. Regardless of the question of personal risk, HIV/AIDS is an important social, cultural, and global problem that demands the attention of every student, school, community, and society. Responding to problems that primarily affect other people is basic to citizenship and community. And education about HIV/AIDS is education for life. Our graduates will work, manage, and lead in a complex society; they will have to handle concerns about HIV/AIDS in a variety of settings and roles, and they should be prepared to think and decide in a careful and informed manner. Learning about HIV/AIDS will prepare them to deal with a great many other complex human issues. Our students will graduate into a "shrinking world"with fluid international boundaries, global markets, and shared health problems.

HIV/AIDS also forces us to confront very difficult questions of difference, diversity, prejudice, and inequity—not only within American society but across nations. And HIV/AIDS demands a clear focus on issues of inclusion that bear not only on social and health problems, but also on critical thinking. Postmodern epistemology, feminist thought, and challenges to the "Western canon" are not just academic issues; they will be infused in the way graduates work, think, and learn in the future. HIV is also emblematic of the problem of new emerging global infectious diseases, most of them viral (e.g., Ebola virus, hantavirus). Understanding their patterns and coping with their impact will be essential for 21st-century citizens.

The patterns of HIV/AIDS among most U.S. students are not illustrative of the whole epidemic. There are multiple "subepidemics" within the larger one, and in some populations and communities, and indeed, entire countries, HIV continues to be devastating. Some students, particularly if they are nontraditional, urban, returning adults, or international students, live and work in those deeply affected communities. To ignore HIV/AIDS is to neglect critical realities of those students' lives.

SUGGESTED READINGS

Burns, William David (editor). Learning for Our Common Health: How an Academic Focus on HIV/AIDS Will Improve Education and Health. Washington, D.C.: Association of American Colleges & Universities, 1999.

Keeling, Richard P. (editor). Effective AIDS Education on Campus. New directions in student services series, number 57. San Francisco: Jossey-Bass Publishers, 1992.

Keeling, Richard P. HIV and Higher Education: From Isolation to Engagement. Liberal Education 82(4): 36–43, 1996.

Rotello, Gabriel. Sexual Ecology: AIDS and the Destiny of Gay Men. New York: Dutton/Penguin Books, 1997.

REFERENCES

1. Centers for Disease Control. Surveillance for AIDS-Defining Opportunistic Infections, 1992–1997. *MMWR-CDC Surveillance Summaries,* Vol. 48/No. SS-2. April 16, 1999.

2. Bevis P, Waldvogel. Hematologic Alterations in Infectious Disease Patients. In *Clinical and Infectious* Diseases, RK Root, Editor-in-Chief. New York: Oxford University Press. 1999.

3. Stranford SA, Levy JA. AIDS Immunology.

4. Centers for Disease Control. 1999 USPHS/FDSA. Guidelines for the Prevention of Opportunistic Infections in Persons Infected with Human Immunodeficiency Virus. *MMWR*, Vol. 48, No. RR-10, August 20, 1999.

5. Centers for Disease Control. Report of the NIH Panel to Define Principles of Therapy of HIV Infection and Guidelines for the Use of Antiretroviral Agents in HIV-Infected Adults and Adolescents. *MMWR*, Vol. 47, No. RR-5. April 24, 1998.

6. Centers for Disease Control. PHS Report Summarizes Current Scientific Knowledge in the Use of Post-exposure Antiretroviral Therapy for Non-occupational Exposures, Fact Sheet, CDC website, March 23, 2001.

7. Centers for Disease Control. Primary HIV Infection Associated with Oral Transmission, Division of HIV/AIDS Prevention. Fact Sheet, CDC website, March 23, 2001.

8. Centers for Disease Control. HIV Prevention Strategic Plan Through 2005. January 2001.

9. Centers for Disease Control. HIV and Its Transmission. Fact Sheet, CDC website, March 23, 2001.

10. Keeling R., ed. *AIDS on the College Campus: A Special Report*, 2nd ed. Rockville Md.-American College Health Association. 1999.

CHAPTER 10

MENTAL HEALTH ISSUES IN COLLEGE HEALTH

Leighton C. Whitaker, PhD, ABPP

A BRIEF HISTORY

Campus mental health and counseling programs began in the early to mid-twentieth century. The need for these programs was fostered by student personnel programming and was related to the emergence of the mental hygiene movement, the advent of psychiatry as a full-fledged medical specialty, and the growth of psychology as a profession.[1] Robert Arnstein, psychiatrist and longtime leader of Yale University's student mental health program, has given an excellent account of the historical diversity of early developments in the field.[2]

Typically, "mental health" services are part of university health services, while "counseling" or "psychological" services are free-standing units in student affairs or are affiliated with psychology departments. Some universities have merged mental health and counseling services. For example, in 1972 Stanford University created an interdisciplinary center with a broad mandate for both direct and indirect clinical and consultative services.[3] In 1976 Harvard University consolidated its psychology and psychiatry services into one mental health service.[4] During the past quarter century, many other universities have merged services.

Several early conceptualizers laid the foundation for campus mental health services. In 1899 University of Chicago president William Rainey Harper delivered an address, "The Scientific Study of the Student," suggesting "a general diagnosis of each student" in terms of character, intellectual and special capacities, and social nature.[1] In 1910, Stewart Paton, neuro-anatomist and psychiatrist at Princeton University, formulated the first specific conceptualization of the need to study personality and its development in United States colleges and universities, and he began clinical work with students.[1,2]

Subsequently, Paton had many conversations with James Rowland Angell, a psychologist and personality theorist, who became president of Yale University in 1921.[1,2] As Clifford Reifler, psychiatrist, epidemiologist, and distinguished longtime leader in college health, noted in his 1989 address at Yale, "Angell emphasized a psychological approach to education on the broadest front—from selection of students through the development of psychological incentives and the provision of psychological services."[5, p. 6] In 1925 Yale and Harvard each made their first appointment of a psychiatrist to serve students at their universities. Similar services had been started in 1914 by Smiley Blanton at the University of Wisconsin, and in 1920 by Karl Menninger at Topeka's Washburn College and Harry Kearns at the United States Military Academy. Dartmouth instituted services in 1921; Vassar in 1923.[2]

Eighteen psychiatrists from institutions of higher learning attended the 1927 Commonwealth Fund's "mental hygiene" meeting, giving evidence that the movement had gained a foothold. By 1953, eighty-seven colleges and universities had a mental health program under psychiatric direction, and about 51 percent of all U.S. institutions of higher learning had some kind of program to deal with the emotional problems of students.[1]

Like most developments that broadly affect society, campus mental health services were both supported and resisted. Yale University had such solid leadership support that in 1933 President Angell said Yale had "the most extensive organized staff for dealing with (student mental hygiene) problems to be found in any American institution."[5 p. 8]

But not every institution of higher learning was ready to acknowledge that its students might be psychologically troubled or need help in coping with the considerable emotional and developmental challenges of college or university. The stigma associated with admitting mental health problems, together with tight budgets and the wish to focus only on academics, has often constrained, or even set back, the development of services. One major university's mental health program, highly rated by a national panel,[6] was halved in size when a new university administrator declared that students would not have need for it if they played sports. (Although those who played sports in college can attest to the benefits, many research studies have shown no dearth of mental health problems among athletes. For example, a recent study of over 50,000 students at 125 institutions showed "that the use of alcohol and consequences related to substance abuse were generally greater as the degree of involvement in sport increased.") [7, p. 187]

NEEDS AND UTILIZATION IN RECENT DECADES

In contrast to the myth of universal normality in the student population, college mental health practitioners know that virtually all mental disorders, including the most severe that are found in the general population, are also found on campuses. But denial and stigma, though lessened in recent decades, continue as cultural resistances. As a result, student mental health problems are still often hidden. Furthermore, the task of documenting need has been complicated by institutions' worries about their images, and questions about whether the central mission of academic learning is served by helping students with mental health and emotional challenges.

Need is not adequately measured by utilization rates of mental health services for the student population overall, or even for particular subpopulations. Lower utilization rates may not acknowledge hard-to-reach groups on campus that have serious problems such as substance abuse, "closet" eating disorders, or depressive withdrawal.

Male students generally use mental health services at about half the rate of female students, not due to their lower need, but due to greater male reluctance to reach out for help. The "paradox of masculinity," as Capraro has termed it,[8] links alcohol and masculinity in ways that make men more likely to become problem drinkers and, more broadly, the macho orientation in men is linked to higher rates of morbidity overall, including far greater male rates of suicide and homicide.[9] From a community mental health standpoint, the inverse relationship between male student need and utilization is a major, largely unanswered, challenge.

"Estimates of prevalence of psychiatric disorders which are obtained by doing a survey of a population have routinely given figures which were higher than those obtained from facility usage."[5, p. 11] It is no surprise that this finding applies to college campuses as well. Furthermore, the degree to which an institution and its students are motivated and sophisticated enough to make good use of a mental health program must be taken into account. Dana Farnsworth, psychiatrist and longtime leader of Harvard University's student mental health program, wisely observed in 1974: "The widely accepted estimate that 10 to 12 percent of all college students have emotional conflicts of sufficient severity to warrant professional help may be too conservative for institutions whose populations are relatively sophisticated about the nature of emotional conflict" [10, p. 774] Bearing out this observation, utilization rates among institutions vary greatly. Small, highly selective institutions show annual student mental health service utilization rates of 20 percent or higher while some large public universities have rates as low as 5 percent. Further, graduate students use services more than undergraduates, attributable to their generally greater life experience and sophistication, which results in increased readiness and perceived need for professional help.[11]

In addition to size, selectivity, gender distribution, the sophistication of its students, and how well it funds its mental health program, an institution's utilization rate is affected by two other important factors: the distance students are from home and the availability of off-campus mental health resources. Depending on the interplay of these factors, as many as a third or as few as a tenth of students will use their campus mental health facilities sometime during their undergraduate careers.

Major societal changes in recent decades have further added to the complexity of the relationship between need and utilization:

- The practice of in loco parentis, common through the 1950s, began fading in the 1960s and the decline continues to the present. (Even so, some colleges and universities began in the 1990's to rethink their orientation, particularly in terms of restrictions on alcohol use.)
- The passage of Section 504 of the 1973 National Rehabilitation Act, prohibiting discrimination against the handicapped, allows mentally, as well as physically, handicapped persons easier enrollment and more protection from dismissal.[12]
- The acceleration in the 1970's of the mental hospital deinstitutionalization movement encouraging many previously isolated mentally disturbed persons to attempt higher education.
- The increase in several forms of mental disturbance since the 1950's (e.g., eating disorders, alcohol and illegal drug use and abuse, suicide and violence).

- The "women's movement," facilitating recognition of womens' rights and their mental health and career needs.
- The increased acceptance of homosexuality with gay students asserting their needs for services.
- Affirmative action programs and (hopefully) less bigotry in society, encouraging minority persons to seek more education.
- Foreign students coming to the U.S. in increasing numbers for higher education.
- Older, returning students greatly increasing in numbers.
- Managed care's rapid growth influencing virtually all mental health practices, including those on campuses.
- Prescribed psychiatric drug use in society and on campuses rapidly increasing.

Every college and university needs to be attuned to these enormous societal changes; their mental health programs must reflect the changes in terms of staffing, sensitivity, and services. As the stigma against using mental health services has lessened, students have become more outspoken in their demands for services that will help them with both mental disturbances and developmental challenges.

PROGRAM CONCEPTUALIZATION AND SERVICES

Campus mental health programs antedated the community mental health movement that began in the 1960s. They are probably the first examples of the mental health movement's goals of comprehensiveness, continuity of care, and community relatedness. As an integrated facet of a university health service, a campus mental health service can help meet the needs and preferences of its particular student population in tailor-made fashion

However, the threats impeding the health and well-being of people in society at large also threaten programs for students. Murray DeArmond,[13] psychiatrist and longtime director of the University of Arizona Health Service, warned against "an overwhelming focus on symptoms, on pieces"; "the authority dimension in medicine"; and "quantitative science" p. 290 which "by medicalizing our lives ... run the risk of treating ourselves as parts in need of repairs, medicine as engineering." p. 291 In contrast, he also saw a great opportunity in student health to offer " ... a commitment to the whole person ... being ever mindful that we relate to students in the dynamic context of young adult development ..." p. 291

Thus, the following discussion of types of services should be viewed in the context of the overriding importance of the larger mission—not just facilitating academic learning and treating disorders. Ideally, campus communities all work toward helping students maintain and/or develop their health and well-being to actualize their constructive potentials.

Psychotherapy and Counseling

As Robert Arnstein suggested, a campus mental health service's primary offering should be therapy, including emergency care.[14] Since psychotherapy is bound by strict confidentiality restrictions and since its methods and values are not easily observable, college psychotherapists may have to convince their institutions of the need for it.[15, 16] Still, even when people are given good information about psychotherapy, it often remains a mysterious process except to those who have experienced it directly.

The term *psychotherapy,* which connotes helping to alleviate mental disturbance, typically overlaps with the broader term *counseling,* which connotes various approaches to helping, including eliciting and building on students' mental assets. Most college student psychotherapy is short-term, dictated by the nature of the student calendar, students' needs and preferences, and financial limitations. Frequent breaks in the school year, including entire summers where the student is off-campus, mitigate against longer-term, continuous therapy. Furthermore, even relatively sophisticated undergraduate students tend to desire or tolerate only a short series of sessions as they try to become more independent of adults by periodically seeking help and taking breaks of their own. As Richard Webb and Jane Widseth stated, "Undergraduate college students in a liberal arts college both will seek psychotherapy which helps them explore their inner worlds and then seek respite from this exploration." [17, p.5] Fortunately, brief therapy has been shown to be largely successful for the majority of students, though it is certainly not the treatment of choice for all students.[18]

Many schools commonly limit to 12 or 15 the number of psychotherapy sessions allowed per student per year. Fortunately, even small, well endowed, highly selective, private colleges with a limitation on number of visits to the mental health clinic find that the modal number of sessions is one, the next highest frequency is two, and so on. Psychotherapy utilization rates tend to be higher at small, highly selective, non-urban colleges, some of which have rates of 20 percent per year or more, while many large universities may see as few as 5 percent of the student population. Most college and university mental health programs recognize the need to provide latitude for some relatively longer-term therapy, albeit often not continuous.

Group psychotherapy can be highly useful, either by itself or in conjunction with individual therapy. But students at small colleges, with enrollments of 1500 or less, typically think that confidentiality is more difficult to ensure, so they may shy away from group therapy and strongly prefer individual sessions.

Many colleges and universities have peer counseling programs, which might seem to represent potentially powerful helpful influences. Such programs, however, do not always live up to that potential. (*Peer Counseling: Skills, Ethics and Perspectives* [2nd ed.] is an excellent state of the art book covering the many considerations that should be addressed in any serious effort to develop or improve student peer counseling resources.)[19]

Evaluation and Referral

Because a significant portion of students need and want more therapy than is available on campus, they may be evaluated and referred to outside therapists. But several problems may interfere with successful referral. Quality services may not be readily accessible without private transportation, students may not be able to afford the costs of such referrals, or they may be reluctant—often for privacy reasons—to try to use their family's health insurance. Furthermore, in an era of increasing domination by managed care, students may find themselves not covered for long-term therapy or not covered at all for away-from-home mental health services. In contrast, campus services provide easy geographic and financial accessibility, obviate students having to inform parents, and provide the opportunity to talk with a therapist highly familiar with the challenges of the college environment.

Consequently, the campus therapist trying to "refer students out" must take into account these problems while explaining to the students why they cannot be seen on campus. Not surprisingly, the rate of successful referrals tends to be quite low, unless the campus therapist understands how to make an "artful" referral.[20]

Emergency and Hospitalization Services

Every campus community experiences situations calling for immediate, intensive responses by deans and/or mental health staff. Some colleges, and virtually all universities, maintain an emergency on-call system with at least one mental health staff person readily available after regular service hours. Large universities, especially those with medical schools, usually provide psychiatric emergency and inpatient services for students at nearby hospitals or on campus. Smaller institutions typically have a close working arrangement with a nearby hospital.

Some have questioned why an institution of higher learning should have to respond with emergency or hospitalization services when, presumably, students themselves could contact off-campus mental health facilities if they had an urgent need. Student resourcefulness can be limited in such circumstances due to many factors. Most notably, students from far away, though residing on campus, may be unfamiliar with local facilities, and their health coverage may be limited to their home areas, particularly now that so much health care is under the aegis of managed care. Students with out-of-area coverage may not be able or willing to involve their parents by giving evidence of their family insurance policy. Furthermore, the common lack of parity between mental health and physical health coverage can mean lack of readily available adequate off-campus coverage for mental health emergencies even when students have some mental health insurance coverage.

Consultation and Education

The goal of community and, indeed, individual well-being as the centerpiece of both community mental health and public health models means being available to, and reaching out to, the entire campus community. Achieving this goal requires, at the very least, making sure everyone on campus is given information about available services and mental health staff available to consult not only with students but with faculty, staff, and dormitory resident assistants (RAs). Deans and RAs are of prime importance because they often see problems first and may need to apprise and involve others. Further, not only will these individuals want to present problems, but they will need information and assistance in dealing with particular situations.

Confidentiality, the cornerstone of successful mental health services, demands that mental health staff limit their answers and advice to acceptance of referrals and to other measures that respect student privacy. Even so, the consultant can be quite valuable in several ways. First, just listening empathically can be helpful, as it is in psychotherapy. Second, in the process of discussion, consultees can clarify their concerns with the consultant being a sounding board and suggesting what might be good options "in such situations." Third, regular consultation may lead to the development of policies and practices to address not only the current problematic situation but other similar situations which might arise in the future.

Gerald Amada has shown how mental health consultants can be highly effective in helping deans and faculty with disciplinary matters in his text *Coping with Misconduct in the College Classroom*,[21] in which he advises on how to deal with ten common disruptive classroom behaviors. A meeting with faculty advisors and university deans can serve to make them much more familiar with campus mental health services, to hear what they consider their most common and pressing problems, and to formulate with them ways of talking with students to facilitate referrals or to prevent misunderstandings about student behavior.

A further type of consultation can be of a public health nature; for example, agreement that certain "celebrations" characterized by binge drinking and serious damage to people and property should be limited or eliminated. Every college or university desires to do more to prevent alcohol-related deaths, accidents, and disruptions of campus life. The use of mental health expertise in formulating alcohol policies which help limit consumption and counter the widespread assumption that "drinking is what college is all about" can be important to the public health. Timely and proper consultation/education can serve to prevent much of what otherwise might become crises or, at the least, more serious problems.

Mental health education efforts must be geared to gain student attention in such a manner as to be taken seriously. Simply handing out fliers, for example, seldom influences those students who are resistant to the information but may need it the most. Educational sessions may disproportionately attract the already converted. Mental health practitioners may not feel qualified to reach out to (and influence groups of) students, but getting students involved in the planning and operation of campus educational programs is more likely to make programs successful.

Effective teachers, as well as psychotherapists, cultivate understanding in ways that strongly appeal to students by providing knowledge and wisdom that fascinate and lead them to further, creative exploration. Direct relationships with students afford the advantage of making such learning tailor made. But even more generic forms of mental health education can be remarkably appealing and helpful if the providers know the important questions being asked by students and have the wisdom and skill to answer them. (*Beating the College Blues*,[22] by Paul Grayson and Philip Meilman, addresses the most frequent student concerns with wise answers that take into account differences among students and their situations. The authors give basic information, make suggestions for resolving concerns, and apprise students of resources, thereby maximizing the helpfulness of the generic approach but also noting its limitations and students' needs for direct services. *Helping Students Adapt to Graduate School*[11] by the College Student Group for the Advancement of Psychiatry [GAP] exemplifies how mental health education can be helpful to both students and to university administrators. It shows how universities can anticipate the most important needs of students, ranging from the decision to attend through life in graduate school and into the transition from graduate school to their lives beyond.)

Psychotropic Drug Treatment

Nicholi (1983) addressed problematic issues with psychotropic drug treatment among the college age group, citing misuse of sedatives and tranquilizers.[23] And in 1989 psychiatrist Victor Schwartz spoke to the "'Somatization' of Psychiatric Disorders."[24] But, until the 1990s, psychotropic drugs were not commonly prescribed on college and university campuses. Thus, texts on college mental health, including that by the Group for the Advancement of Psychiatry (GAP, 1990)[25] gave the topic only passing mention. However, by 2000, GAP observed: "As the number and variety of drugs increases, psychopharmacology becomes ever more complex. Psychiatrists must learn about drug interactions and the effects of drugs on different individuals and in different age groups, and so prescribing appropriate medications is no longer a simple procedure."[11 p. 80]

Since 1990, prescribing of psychotropic drugs in the United States has grown so rapidly that it is now common even among preschoolers. The use of these drugs is encouraged by the drug companies with apparently little regard for traditional physician prescribing responsibilities. Television and magazine ads extol the virtues of their particular antidepressant or antianxiety drug and advise viewers to seek out "anyone" who will prescribe that drug. Further, these drug commercials now urge consumers to seek drug treatment for innumerable conditions, even including what were formerly considered rather ordinary childhood and adolescent developmental challenges, such as "social anxiety."

In 1991 psychiatric drug prescribing by psychiatrists accounted for only 17.3 percent of the 135,896,000 such prescriptions. Both internists (22.3 percent) and family practitioners (23.0 percemt) prescribed more than psychiatrists,[26] typically on the basis of a patient's symptom reporting in a single office visit of fifteen minutes or less. Meanwhile, the numbers of non-physician prescribers (physician assistants and nurse practitioners) continue to grow and it appears possible that psychologists may soon acquire prescribing privileges as well. What was already a $3.1 billion industry in 1991 in the United States mushroomed in the 1990s with huge increases in the numbers and kinds of prescribing for all age groups.

As more and more students arrive at college having already been prescribed psychotropic medications, they often pressure the college or university health service to assume prescribing, monitoring, and treatment outcome responsibilities. The central issue for campus mental health centers has become *not* whether judiciously prescribed psychiatric drugs can be helpful to students but *how* centers can deal with the pressures and complexities involved. In 1997, Grayson, Schwartz, and Commerford highlighted the broader implications of what they called the "drug boom":[27] "Drug treatment entails far more than taking a pill. Along with related trends like managed care and the influx of deeply disturbed students to campus, it is transforming the character of college student mental health. Drug therapy is not on the periphery anymore. More and more, what happens in the campus clinic is tied to events taking place in the laboratories and marketing departments of the major pharmaceutical companies." [p. 32]

Campus psychiatrists, who in the past were the final arbiters of whether psychotropics should be prescribed for students, are pressured to prescribe "on demand" as the national campaigns, mounted by the pharmaceutical industry, are specifically targeted at college students. Consequently, campus psychiatrists may find themselves relegated to merely providing quick "medication evaluations" or being bypassed in favor of non-psychiatrist prescribers. Either way, campus mental health centers are increasingly subject to financial, ethical and legal dilemmas which are largely not of their own making. If they do not acquiesce to the pressure, they may be seen as old fashioned, too cautious or derelict in their duty to "correct" presumably biological deficits such as "biochemical imbalances." If they do prescribe, however, they may find themselves liable for adverse reactions, drug overdoses, unfortunate admixtures of drugs (polypharmacy), patient non-compliance problems, including "rebound effects" from stopping medications on their own, or failure to warn of the adverse effects of taking, or ceasing to take, what is prescribed.

Many students, prior to college, have had *only* drug treatment available to them. In college, psychotherapy becomes available to them, often at no expense. Accordingly, an important issue facing campus mental health practitioners is sorting through various expectations and assumptions students bring with them, including wanting simply to be continued on their medications without any real focus on the benefits of the psychotherapeutic process.

Ideally, prescribing both on-campus and off-campus will occur only when, after careful evaluation, it appears that prescription drugs would be helpful in conjunction with psychotherapy or, at least, with careful, continued monitoring. Avoidance of what one campus psychiatrist called "promiscuous prescribing" may help to avoid legal liability as well.

Confidentiality and Relationships with Medical Care

Integrating mental health and physical health care can provide great benefit to the student if issues of confidentiality and style of communication can be resolved. The especially strict confidentiality standards in mental health care, required ethically and legally, limit what mental health practitioners can communicate even to their in-house medical colleagues. Information must be shared, however, about topics vitally related to students' health and safety.

First, students' drug use history, both legal and illegal, needs to be elicited and shared between mental health and medical services, at least through chart notes about types, doses, and usage regimens. Otherwise, the health center may unwittingly contribute to hazardous drug interactions or prescribe drugs that will be used in non-therapeutic ways[23] or simply fail to take into account drugs that students bring with them to campus. Second, information about threat-to-life situations must be shared with persons in a position to minimize the threat. Potential suicides, homicides, and psychotic breakdowns all require some sharing of information on a "need to know" basis, for legal as well as clinical care reasons.

Sharing information with other health service clinicians about clinical concerns can also be very helpful to students, provided that the students themselves give permission. As every mental health or medical practitioner knows, many disorders are caused by combinations of biological and psychological factors that should be addressed collaboratively for optimal care. Typically, medical practitioners neither need to know, nor are they interested in knowing, detailed information about students' psychotherapy. Rather, they are particularly concerned to know how they and the mental health practitioner can be of practical help, for which even very brief consultations may be sufficient. Although the confidentiality/care dilemma is never fully resolved by simply agreeing on procedures, it can be further eased by an atmosphere of good will among caregivers who can be trusted to practice respect and to make carefully considered judgments of the "need to know" in any given case.

ETHICAL, LEGAL, AND ADMINISTRATIVE ISSUES

The growing complexity of challenges in student mental health in recent decades requires an increasing sophistication about ethical, legal, and administrative issues. Of these closely interrelated areas of concern, ethical guidelines have remained the most solid foundation of policy and practice. Thus, Arnstein's 1986 discussion of "Ethical and Value Issues in Psychotherapy with College Students"[28] continues to provide a basic orientation to this area in terms of cultural values and definitions of mental health; undisclosed goals maintained by the therapist that may differ from the patient's, as well as recommendations for types of treatment; and the psychotherapeutic method with its emphasis on the therapeutic relationship and its encouragement of openness of patient communication and, accordingly its guarantee—albeit qualified—of confidentiality.

The 1976 Tarasoff Decision and Beyond

Just as mental health professionals must routinely practice more stringent confidentiality standards than other health professionals, there are also more legal limitations in their privileges to disclose in exceptional circumstances, including in a court of law. But the traditional guarantee of confidentiality or patient privacy was greatly qualified by the 1976 landmark case of *Tarasoff vs. Regents of the University of California*,[29] which established a definite exception to confidentiality. *Tarasoff* has established a legal precedent requiring a "duty-to-warn" by a psychiatrist or psychologist in certain cases. Thus, the confidentiality requirement comes into conflict with a duty to warn others of the threat of harm by the patient. The court in *Tarasoff* stated:

> We realize that the open and confidential character of psychotherapeutic dialogue encourages patients to express threats of violence, few of which are ever executed. Certainly a therapist should not be encouraged routinely to reveal such threats; such disclosures could

seriously disrupt the patient's relationship with the therapist and the person threatened. To the contrary, the therapist's obligations to his patient requires that he not disclose a confidence unless such disclosure is necessary to avert danger to others, and even then that he do so discreetly, and in a fashion that would preserve the privacy of his patient to the fullest extent compatible with the prevention of the threatened danger.[29]

The therapist was left to judge the degree of danger and its imminence; how best to warn the threatened party; and how to preserve, if possible, the confidence of the patient in the therapist. Accordingly, the therapist is well advised to consult with colleagues and, perhaps, legal counsel to plan strategy in such cases.

The *Tarasoff* precedent may be interpreted somewhat differently depending upon legal jurisdiction, but recent decisions elsewhere suggest essentially the same formulation, for example, *Emerich vs. Philadelphia Center for Human Development*.[30] "Thus, drawing on the wisdom of prior analysis, and common sense, we believe that a duty to warn arises only where a specific and immediate threat of serious bodily injury has been conveyed by the patient to the professional regarding a specifically identified or readily identifiable victim."[30]

Suicide threats and attempts pose similar ethical and legal dilemmas. The treating professional has an obligation to protect the patient from imminent self harm, possibly by involving others who are in a position to prevent the harm, but he/she also may have to deal with the suicidal student's objection to notifying others, especially if hospitalization is being considered.

Education to Minimize Threats to Life and Lawsuits

Campus mental health centers should prepare for and prevent threat-to-life crises as much as possible by knowing how to assess suicide, homicide and psychosis risks among students; the psychodynamic, epidemiologic, and situational causal factors; various prevention and intervention strategies; and methods of working collaboratively with other staff.[31, 32, 33, 34] Failure to carefully assess risks may result in lawsuits such as happened when a court found that an intake history was inadequate to ferret out patients with suicidal tendencies, and when a university was sued after a student committed suicide following a brief walk-in clinic evaluation.[35]

Contrary to the time pressures exerted by some managed care organizations and the spread of their influence onto campuses, initial evaluations should be at least forty-five minutes to meet the usual standards of practice and to demonstrate to students that their concerns are being taken seriously. Students should be clearly apprised of the mental health center's confidentiality policy, emphasizing both its strictness *and* the exception if the student poses an imminent threat to life and therefore a need to notify others who may be in a position to lessen the threat.

As noted earlier, the rapid acceleration of prescribed psychotropic drug use has added to ethical and legal responsibilities and hazards in campus mental health, especially given the greater numbers of seriously disturbed students who may already be taking or requesting such medications. Paranoid, schizophrenic, and borderline patients, in addition to presenting major therapeutic challenges, may present difficult medication management and monitoring problems both because of "side effects" and non-compliance with medication regimens common among these patients. For example, patients who suddenly stop use of "antipsychotic drugs" often have rebound reactions resulting in considerable worsening of their psychosis and possibly a greater tendency to become destructive.

Expanded responsibilities for students' mental health have involved practitioners in areas beyond therapy and medication management. Campus practitioners have increasingly been invited, persuaded, or told they must help in deciding on matters of student discipline, mandatory psychotherapy, "psychiatric leaves," or even dismissal from the institution. These matters often involve practitioners in knotty ethical, legal, and administrative issues. On the one hand, practitioners take on responsibilities that may instill a sense of making a greater contribution to the institution and help justify their positions, while on the other, they must negotiate the complex intersections of mental health, institutional policy, and the legal system. When one considers the complexity of the interactions, it is not surprising that practitioners disagree among themselves about policy and practice.

Some student behaviors clearly threaten the safety and well-being not only of individuals but also portions, or even all, of the campus community. Student suicides and homicides, for example, invariably traumatize the entire community. Because campus mental health staff have a definite obligation for the well-being of the community as a whole and not just to certain individuals, they must take some responsibility in such matters. Inevitably, deans, faculty, staff, students and parents have strong concerns about what should be done in terms of policy and practice.

Most student affairs staff probably cannot imagine carrying out their own disciplinary and dismissal functions without calling on mental health professionals for at least referral and consultation, particularly if there is any question of an emotional/mental component to the behavior requiring action. This area of concern becomes especially problematic if the campus mental health center is expected, essentially on its own, to solve questions of discipline or dismissal. Deans may not relish their disciplinary role for fear of loss of popularity or of lawsuits, especially since their authority has weakened with the demise of *in loco parentis*, while at the same time society's litigiousness has grown. (One relatively small university, historically rather unaccustomed to legal difficulties, reportedly found itself, by the early 1990s, the object of over two hundred lawsuits and felt the need to gird itself with five full-time lawyers.)

Defining the Limits of Responsibility

College and university administrators have been increasingly tempted to assign more responsibility to the mental health center, via an expanded definition of "mental health related" disciplinary and dismissal cases. A partial answer to this expectation is to develop a clear understanding in writing, approved at the highest administrative level of the college or university, that while the mental health staff may assist in disciplinary matters, the final decision and responsibility must belong to the dean or another non-mental health institutional official.

Campus mental health practitioners disagree about whether they should accept referrals for "mandatory treatment," usually meaning counseling or psychotherapy, but possibly also involving drug treatment. Some therapists cite ethical, legal, clinical, disciplinary and administrative contraindications to mandatory psychotherapy of students[36] and give specific arguments against it,[37] noting that most such referrals involve students who are not a threat to themselves or others. But some therapists hold that they should at least try to help students who may perpetrate verbal and/or physical aggression to learn nonaggressive ways of dealing with anger and frustration;[38] these therapists criticize arguments for eliminating involuntary treatment as simplistic and short-sighted.[39]

Similarly, practitioners disagree about the need for *psychiatric leave policies*, some arguing that "time away" requirements and "screening interviews" for readmission are not predictive of successful reintegration into the society of the institution and that continued academic enrollment may facilitate treatment and recovery for many students.[40] Others feel that not permitting re-enrollment for a semester after psychiatric withdrawal is a wise idea, that the "screening" interview for re-admission can be useful,[41] and that students often make good use of their time out of college.[42] Still others think that it is not ethical, for any reason, to deny a student's return to school following a withdrawal.[43] Further, some schools have no system of psychiatric or mental health leave,[44] presumably feeling no need for it.

Obviously, practitioners who assume responsibility for cases in which several major hazardous avenues of practice intersect are quite vulnerable to dire outcomes even if they are expert clinicians and administrators. As a result, an increasingly common reaction is to practice as defensively as possible, to the extreme of doing no appreciable good (rather like the maximally defensive driver who seldom leaves the garage).

An example of such a dire outcome was given by Dr. Myron Liptzin,[45] in the annual David Dorosin Memorial Lecture at the American College Health Association for the year 2000. Liptzin, a psychiatrist and longtime director of the University of North Carolina Mental Health Service, focused on the hazards of assuming care for a complex situation involving a difficult second-year law student. The student, who killed two people eight months after his last session with Liptzin, was found not guilty by reason of insanity. In an action filed by the ex-patient against the psychiatrist, the jury decided unanimously against the psychiatrist/plaintiff and in favor of his ex-patient, to whom they awarded a substantial settlement. Although the verdict was later reversed on appeal, the case still illustrates well the unique potential pitfalls of college mental health practice. A year and a half prior to seeing Liptzin, the student had been hospitalized but had refused treatment and was deemed not dangerous to himself or others. Then, while in law school, he had been disruptive in class, where he wanted to prove he was telepathic. A beleaguered law school dean asked the mental health service for advice. Liptzin saw the student six times, was able to gain some rapport with him, and treated him, apparently successfully, including prescribing an antipsychotic medication. But after completion of his second year of law school (and while living away from campus), the student failed to follow Liptzin's advice regarding follow-up with an outside clinic or physician. Furthermore, as was learned retrospectively, he had stopped taking the prescribed medication on his own, ten days after leaving campus.

The many hazards in this case included the student's initial resistance to treatment, a period when he drank heavily and used marijuana, his failure to follow his psychiatrist's recommendation for follow-up while living away from the university, and stopping medication on his own. The student's apparently favorable response to the medication and to sessions with his campus psychiatrist was thus severely compromised by the student himself. Nevertheless, the jury decided that the psychiatrist-defendant was negligent and that the student was not responsible for contributory negligence. While such cases lend themselves to endless discussion and public debate, and their handling in the legal justice system may seem to compound, rather than correct, an injustice, there can be little question that they create extreme difficulties for the practice of the college mental health specialist.

Preparing for Hazardous Duty

What is to be learned from such disagreement and qualification about the interface of mental health with ethical, legal, and administrative considerations?

- The issues are complex and not always readily resolved, even by astute practitioners
- Practitioners should apprise themselves of the complexities with a view to the benefits and hazards that might accrue in their particular institutions
- Since legal jurisdictions matter, practitioners, together with their college and university administrations, should become familiar with the ethical and legal principles of their particular state. (In Pennsylvania, for example, applicable principles, case examples and precedents are reviewed in workshops and in book form)[46]
- The hazards are multiplied when especially difficult areas of practice are combined (for example, treating psychotic or borderline students under duress and/or with psychotropic drugs and being held responsible for their behavior outside of sessions, even during breaks in the college calendar or after the student has left school and may no longer even be eligible for care at the student mental health service)
- Policy-making may be aided by obtaining outside consultation to maximize prevention of harm in these difficult situations

Clearly, administration of college and university mental health programs is increasingly a challenge. In addition to becoming familiar with the many issues involved, the mental health director should be sure to cultivate as much understanding and good will as possible among all constituents of the institution. New, uninformed, and untested college presidents and deans may add to difficulties, rather than protect the mental health center from hazardous and even unjust actions. Similarly, students, who by definition, are newly exposed to much of the knowledge and sophistication they will need in life, need to be apprised of and involved in discussion of mental health issues. Thus, regular meetings with presidents and/or deans and with students is of critical importance. Student advisory boards can help the center to learn about student concerns and impact the center's thinking about policy and practices.

STAFFING AND TRAINING

The changing pattern of staffing and training gives some insight into the future of campus mental health programs. Increasingly, medical degrees and doctorates in psychology are being conferred on women and minorities, and clinical social work programs continue to produce principally women graduates. The "feminization of clinical and counseling psychology" has been so dramatic in the past two decades that, ironically, considering the previous preponderance of males in these professions, universities have begun struggling to increase male enrollment in these areas of study. However, while the number of minority psychologists has more than tripled, the numbers of minority practitioners in campus mental health programs are still not representative of the overall minority population.[47]

Such major changes in staffing, together with the myriad societal changes previously noted, mean that staff need far better understanding of the complex issues confronting them. Campus mental health training programs for psychiatric residents and psychology and social work interns help keep staff "on their toes" and provide well-prepared staff for the future.

If history is any predictor, campus mental health practitioners will continue to find their work with college and university students, while challenging, extremely meaningful and rewarding.

REFERENCES

1. Reinhold, JE. The origins and early development of mental health services in American colleges and universities. *J Coll Student Psychotherapy.* 1991; 6(1): 3-13.

2. Arnstein, RL. Psychiatry and the college student. Chapter 19, pp. 393-407 in S. Arieti (ed.) Volume V, *American handbook of psychiatry,* 2nd ed., 1974.

3. D'Andrea, VJ. A history of counseling and psychological services at Stanford University. *J Coll Student Psychotherapy.* 1992; 7(1): 3-13.

4. Dinklage, KT, Gould, NB, Blaine, GB Jr. Evolution of the mental health service of Harvard University's health services. *J Coll Student Psychotherapy.* 1992; 7(2); 5-33.

5. Reifler, CB. Clements Fry, if you could see us now —The Robert L. Arnstein retirement lecture. *J Coll Student Psychotherapy.* 1990; 5(1): 3-18.

6. Glasscote, R, Fishman, ME. *Mental health on the campus: A field study.* Washington, DC: Amer Psychiatic Assoc & Natl Assoc for Mental Hlth; 1973.

7. Meilman, PW, Leichliter, MA, Presley, CA. Greeks and athletes: Who drinks more? *J Am Coll Health.* 1999; 47:187-190

8. Capraro, RL. Why college men drink: Alcohol, adventure, and the paradox of masculinity. *J Amer Coll Health,* 2000, 48(6), 307-315.

9. Whitaker, LC. Macho and morbidity: The emotional need vs. fear dilemma in men. *J Coll Stdt Psychotherapy,* 1987, 1(4), 33-47.

10. Farnsworth, DL, Mental health programs in colleges. Chapter 52, pp. 773-799. in Volume II of S. Arieti (ed.) *American handbook of psychiatry,* 2nd ed., 1974.

11. College Student Group for the Advancement of Psychiatry (GAP). *Helping students adapt to graduate school: Making the grade.* New York: Haworth Press, 1999. Co-published simultaneously as *J Coll Student Psychotherapy,* 14(2).

12. Pavela, G. *The dismissal of students with mental disorders: Legal issues; policy considerations; and alternative responses.* Asheville, NC: College Administration Publications, Inc., 1985.

13. DeArmond, MM. A response. *J Amer Coll Health.* 1999; 47: 290-291.

14. Arnstein, RL. A student mental health service as a place to work: What is its role in the university, and how does that affect the therapeutic effort? *J Coll Stdt Psychotherapy.* 1990; 5(1): 19-33.

15. Whitaker, LC. Communicating the value of psychotherapy with college students. *J Amer Coll Health.* 1985; 33: 159-161.

16. May, R. Basic requirements and survival strategies for a college psychotherapy service. *J Coll Stdt. Psychotherapy.* 2000; 15(1): 3-13.

17. Webb, R, Widseth, J. Facilitating students' going into and stepping back from their inner worlds: Psychotherapy and the college student. *J Coll Stdt Psychotherapy,* 1988; 3(1): 5-15.

18. Cooper, S, Archer, J. Brief therapy in college counseling and mental health. *J Amer Coll Health.* 1999; 48:21-28.

19. D'Andrea, VJ, Salovey, P (eds.) *Peer counseling: Skills, ethics and perspectives,* 2nd edition. Palo Alto, CA: Science and Behavior Books, 1996.

20. Zuriff, GE. The art of referral in a university health center. *J Coll Student Psychotherapy,* 2000; 15(1) in press.

21. Amada, G. *Coping with misconduct in the college classroom: A practical model.* Asheville, NC: College Administration Publications; 1999.

22. Grayson, PA.& Meilman, PW. *Beating the college blues* (2nd edition). New York: Facts on File, Inc., 1999.

23. Nicholi, AM. The nontherapeutic use of psychoatherapeutic drugs among the college age group: The sedatives and tranquilizers. *J Amer Coll Health.* 1983: 33, 87-90.

24. Schwartz, V. ÒSomatizationÓ of psychiatric disorders. *Am J Psychiatry,* 1989:146, 4, 570.

25. Group for the Advancement of Psychiatry. *Psychotherapy with college students.* New York: Bruner/ Mazel, 1990.

26. Grayson, PA, Schwartz, V. & Commerford, M. Brave new world? Drug therapy and college mental health. *J Coll Student Psychotherapy,* 1997; 11(4): 23-32.

27. DeLeon, PH. Prescription privileges: Continuing progress scope of practice issue. *Register Report, The Newsletter of Psychologist Health Service Providers,* 1992; 18, pp. 3,4,15,16.

28. Arnstein, RL. Ethical and value issues in psychotherapy with college students. *J Coll Student Psychotherapy,* 1986; 1(1), 3-20.

29. Tarasoff vs Regents of the University of California, 551 P. 2nd 334 (Cal., 1976)

30. Emerich v Philadelphia Center for Human Development, 720 A.2nd 1032 (Pa., 1998)

31. Whitaker, LC. Suicide and other crises. Chapter 3, pp. 48-70 in P Grayson & K Causley (eds.) *College psychotherapy.* New York: Guilford Press, 1989.

32. Schwartz, AJ, Whitaker, LC. Suicide among college students: Assessment, treatment, and intervention. Chapter 12, pp. 303-340, in SJ Blumenthal, DJ Kupfer (eds.) *Suicide over the life cycle: Risk factors, assessment, and treatment of suicidal patients.* Washington, DC: American Psychiatric Press, 1990.

33. Whitaker, LC, Slimak, RE (eds.) *College student suicide.* Binghamton, New York: Haworth Press, 1990. Published simultaneously as Journal of Coll Student Psychotherapy, 4 (3/4).

34. Whitaker, LC, Pollard, JW (eds.) *Campus violence: Kinds, causes, and cures.* Binghamton, New York: Haworth Press. Published simultaneously as *J Coll Student Psychotherapy* 8 (1/2), 1993.

35. Thomas Speer, Administrator v. State of Connecticut, 4 Conn. App. 535 (1985).

36. Gilbert, SP, Sheiman, JA. Mandatory counseling of university students: An oxymoron? *J Coll Student Psychotherapy.* 1995, 9 (4), 3-21.

37. Amada, G. Mandatory psychotherapy: A commentary on mandatory counseling of university students: An oxymoron? and Anger and aggression groups: Expanding the scope of college mental health provider services. *J Coll Student Psychotherapy,* 1995, 9(4), 33-44.

38. Castronovo, NR. Anger and Aggression groups: Expanding the scope of college mental health provider services. *J Coll Student Psychotherapy,* 1995, 9(4), 23-32.

39. Pollard, JW. Involuntary treatment: Counseling or consequence? *J Coll Student Psychotherapy,* 1995, 9(4), 45-55.

40. Hoffman, FL, Mastrianni, X. Psychiatric leave policies: Myth and reality. *J Coll Student Psychotherapy,* 1991,6(2), 3-20, 53-57.

41. Arnstein, RL. Psychiatric leave policies: Myth and reality—A commentary thereon. *J Coll Student Psychotherapy,* 1991, 6(2), 21-24.

42. Liptzin, MB. Reflections on policy: Commentary on psychiatric leave policies: Myth and reality. *J Coll Student Psychotherapy*, 1991, 6(2), 25-35.

43. Marsh, KF. A public university view of psychiatric leave policies: Myth and reality. *J Coll Student Psychotherapy*, 1991, 6(2), 37-42.

44. May, R. Discussion of Psychiatric leave policies: Myth and reality. *J Coll Student Psychotherapy*, 1991, 6(2), 43-52.

45. Liptzin, MB. Violence by an ex-patient and how a psychiatrist got blamed. David Dorosin Memorial Lecture at the annnual meeting of the American College Health Association, Toronto, Canada, June 3, 2000.

46. Tepper, AM, Segal, AM. *Ethical and legal principles in the everyday practice of the mental health professional in Pennsylvania*. Altoona, Wisconsin: Medical Educational Services, Inc., 1999.

47. Berg-Cross, L, Mason, K, & Normington, J. The training of minority psychologists—Trends and changes during the last 15 years. *J Coll Student Psychotherapy*, 1997, 12(1), 3-13.

CHAPTER 11

SUBSTANCE ABUSE ISSUES IN COLLEGE HEALTH

Alcohol, Tobacco, and Other Drugs of Abuse

Betty Reppert, PA-C, MPH, and Betty Anne Johnson, MD, PhD

Heroin, cocaine, marijuana, and PCP have received much public attention in our society as drugs of abuse. However, the two substances that have the most potential for increasing morbidity or mortality of college students, in the short or long run, are alcohol and tobacco. This chapter provides an overview of substance abuse on college campuses, with a concentration on those two substances.

ALCOHOL

Alcohol abuse is associated with significant morbidity and mortality throughout the United States. The American college student is no exception. Alcohol abuse puts students at increased risk for motor vehicle accidents, poor academic performance, violence, unwanted pregnancy and sexually transmitted infections. Motor vehicle fatalities are the leading cause of death among American youth and alcohol is involved in nearly half of the cases.[1]

Statistics on College Students and Alcohol

The *National College Health Risk Behavior Survey (NCHRBS)*, conducted in 1995, surveyed 4,838 undergraduate students from 136 two- and four-year colleges and universities in the United States. Survey data revealed 68.2 percent of college students had at least one drink of alcohol during the previous 30 days. More than one-third (34.5 percent) of college students reported having had 5 or more drinks at one sitting on at least one occasion during the past 30 days (defined by the Centers for Disease Control and Prevention (CDC) as "current episodic heavy drinking", sometimes called "binge drinking"). Binge drinking was more common among male students (43.8 percent) than female students (27 percent). White students (34.5 percent) had a higher binge drinking rate than Hispanic (22.6 percent) or black college students (12.5 percent). Students in the 18 to 24 year age range were more frequent binge drinkers than those age 25.[3] Further, 27.4 percent of students surveyed reported having driven a vehicle after drinking alcohol, whereas 35.1 percent had ridden with a driver who had been drinking alcohol.[2]

The Monitoring the Future Study (MTF) is an annual survey conducted by the University of Michigan for the National Institute on Drug Abuse. Drug use data (including alcohol) is collected on middle school, high school and college students and tracked from year to year. In 1998, the binge-drinking rate among college students was slightly higher (38.9 percent) than in the 1995 NCHRBS (defined in this survey as five or more drinks in one sitting in the previous two weeks). Binge-drinking rates in college students declined by 1.7 percent between 1997 and 1998 according to MTF data.[3]

Binge-drinking rates have also been measured in the Harvard School of Public Health College Alcohol Study (CAS) conducted in 1993, 1997, and 1999. The 1999 reported binge-drinking rate was 44 percent (defined in this study as the consumption of at least five drinks in a row for men or four drinks in a row for women during the two weeks prior to the survey). This is the same rate as in 1993. Abstainers increased to 19 percent and frequent binge drinkers (those who binged three or more times in the 2 weeks prior to the survey) increased to 23 percent.[4]

Although media attention surrounding the release of the 1999 CAS data focused on the increase in heavy binge drinking on campus, there were important positive findings:

- Abstinence rates continued to climb nationally.
- *Overall* binge drinking rates were *not* increasing.
- A small percentage of students accounted for most of the serious alcohol problems.
- Most college students drink moderately or not at all.

Many colleges and universities are now collecting data about their own students' drinking habits. College health professionals benefit from knowing the "norms" surrounding drinking on their campus. Reinforcing the positive campus norms with students ("Did you know the majority of your fellow students are either not drinking alcohol, or are drinking in a low-risk manner?") is a way to avoid reinforcing the myth that "all college students binge drink." It has been well documented that students who are binge drinkers are at higher risk for alcohol-related problems such as poor academic performance, being injured, injuring others, not using protection when having sex, or engaging in unplanned sexual activity.[5]

Non-binge drinkers may experience a different set of alcohol-related consequences than "bingers," labeled "second-hand effects" of binge drinking. These effects are perpetrated upon those in the immediate vicinity of the binge drinkers. These second-hand effects have been followed in the CAS.[4] They include property damage, interrupted studying or sleep, unwanted sexual advances, or becoming a victim of sexual assault. Obviously, these second-hand effects are experienced more frequently by students on campuses with higher binge-drinking rates.

There is evidence that low-to-moderate consumption of alcohol may be protective against coronary heart disease (CHD), ischemic stroke, and cholelithiasis.[6] Explanations for the cardioprotective effect of alcohol at low consumption levels include an increase in HDL, an antioxidant effect, or a decrease in platelet aggregation and coagulation. No one type of alcoholic beverage has been singled out as the most cardioprotective. In young populations, however (e.g. traditional college-aged students), risks associated with heavy alcohol consumption are of primary concern, and these risks may more than balance any CHD benefit from low-risk drinking.[7] Therefore, clinicians need to be cautious in counseling students concerning possible health benefits.

Most students who are experiencing ill consequences related to abuse of alcohol will not present to the clinician complaining of a drinking problem. Instead, they are more likely to complain of such problems as gastritis, injuries (secondary to falling, fights or other trauma), headaches, depression, unintended pregnancy, or sexually transmitted infections. They are often in denial that their drinking patterns are related to their problems. Events or symptoms such as headaches, dyspepsia, diarrhea, insomnia, palpitations, blackouts, sexual dysfunction, anxiety, or depression or reports of repeated trauma, relationship violence, academic woes, DWI's, or multiple emergency room visits should alert the clinician to question the student about alcohol abuse.

Objective findings on physical examination in a traditional-aged college student are usually sparse, if present at all. They can include mild elevation in blood pressure, unexplained tachycardia, tremors, or the smell of alcohol on the breath. Abnormal laboratory tests might detect mild liver function abnormalities or an increase in mean corpuscular volume (MCV).[8]

Acutely life-threatening alcohol-related problems often present to the Emergency Department (ED) rather than the student health service. These include alcohol-related motor vehicle accidents and acute alcohol poisoning. Information is sparse concerning alcohol-related ED visits by college students. Some universities have fairly accurate tracking mechanisms for ED admissions, especially if there is only one ED nearby which the students primarily use and if the student body is primarily residential. (One such university did track alcohol-related emergencies that presented to their university-affiliated ED. Of the 616 undergraduate students who were seen in the ED during the academic year, 101 [16 percent] presented with an alcohol-related problem.)[9] In contrast, many large, urban universities are unable to track these visits due to such factors as multiple ED sites, a high percentage of commuter students who may present to out-of-town emergency rooms, and confidentiality issues hampering accurate data collection.

Screening Tools

Many screening tools have been developed to detect problem drinking and alcoholism. The sensitivity and specificity of the Michigan Alcohol Screening Test (MAST), CAGE, Alcohol Use Disorders Identification Test (AUDIT), and TWEAK questionnaires have been reviewed.[10] No one screening tool has been shown to be consistently more reliable in either general or specific populations. However, one of the most widely accepted tools is the CAGE Questionnaire.

The CAGE Questionnaire is a brief, four-question assessment has been tested in many different primary care settings. Questions have been raised about the reliability of the CAGE tool in the college population, especially with college women.[11, 12] The dichotomous format, the use of an "eye opener," and the fact that the questions may be more pertinent with lifetime use rather than more recent problems have all been cited as drawbacks. One study combined the use of the CAGE Questionnaire, the Perceived Benefit of Drinking Scale (PBDS), information about use of tobacco, and the best friend's drinking patterns to screen students for current and future problem drinking.[13] Other campuses have developed their own screening tools such as the College Alcohol Problem Scale (CAPS) to screen students cited for a first offense of university drinking policies.[14]

CAGE Questionnaire

1. Have you ever felt you ought to <u>C</u>ut down on your drinking?
2. Have people <u>A</u>nnoyed you by criticizing your drinking?
3. Have you ever felt bad or <u>G</u>uilty about your drinking?
4. Have you ever had a drink first thing in the morning (<u>E</u>ye-opener) to steady your nerves or get rid of a hangover?

One or more "yes" responses indicate a positive screening test.

A brief screening questionnaire such as CAGE can be a catalyst for discussion with a student regarding alcohol use and perceived risks, but the CAGE questionnaire is more reliable if used in the context of a face-to-face interview rather than when self-administered. It is important to remember that no screening test, including CAGE, is diagnostic. Any such test should be incorporated into the entire clinical picture. Many institutions have found it useful to include a few questions inquiring about the frequency and quantity of alcohol consumption in a health history form to be completed by each student presenting to the health service. In such cases, special attention should be given to students at high risk, particularly those who are in recovery from substance abuse of any kind or those with a significant family history of alcohol abuse.

Substance Abuse Terminology

Clarification of diagnostic criteria is appropriate before discussing the clinical diagnosis of alcohol-related problems. The following widely accepted definitions are frequently used to discuss substance abuse.

Experimental use Trying a drug once or a few times to learn about the experience (often in adolescents)

Recreational use Moderate use of a drug to experience pleasurable effects (often known as "social use" or "social drinking")

Binge drinking Consuming five or more drinks on one occasion

Compulsive use Continued consumption of a drug despite adverse consequences

Drug abuse Any use of drugs that causes physical, psychological, economic, legal, or social harm to the user or others

Drug addiction Chronic disorder characterized by compulsive use of a substance resulting in progressive harm to user or others

Psychological dependence Emotional state of craving a drug either for its positive effect or to avoid negative effects associated with its absence

Physical dependence A physiological state of adaptation to a drug, usually characterized by the development of tolerance to effects and emergence of withdrawal syndrome during abstinence

One drink (alcohol) 12 g of pure alcohol which is equal to one 12 oz. can of beer, one 5 oz. glass of wine, 1 oz. of 100-proof distilled spirits

Some controversy surrounds the CDC National College Health Risk Behavior Survey's definition of binge drinking. Some prefer to use the terms "high-risk drinking," "heavy drinking," or "heavy episodic drinking." Some also amend the definition to be gender-specific and reduce the threshold to "four or more" drinks for women.

The National Institute on Alcohol Abuse and Alcoholism (NIAAA) categorizes heavy drinkers into three groups:[15]

At risk drinkers
- Men who have more than 14 drinks per week or more than 4 drinks per occasion
- Women who have more than 11 drinks per week or more than 3 per occasion
- No current medical, social, or psychological consequences of drinking
- A positive CAGE score or a personal or family history of alcohol-related problems

Problem drinkers
- Patients with current alcohol-related problems (physical, psychological, family, social, employment, academic, or legal)
- usually score 1 or 2 on CAGE questionnaire
- usually drink at or above the level of at risk drinkers

Alcohol-dependent drinkers
- Compulsion to drink, increased tolerance, withdrawal symptoms may be present
- CAGE score of 3 or 4

The DSM-IV criteria for alcohol abuse and alcohol dependence are also useful in differentiating between different degrees of alcohol-related problems.[16]

Primary Care Intervention

College health clinicians may either feel inadequate to address "problem" or "at-risk" drinking patterns in students, or may feel too pressed for time to follow through on a "red flag" from the student's history, thus ignoring the problem or deciding to address it on the next visit. Worse, the clinician may perceive heavy drinking as a "rite of passage" for college students that will resolve upon graduation. Some clinicians believe there are no effective intervention strategies for the short duration the college student is present. None of these behaviors or beliefs are acceptable. College health professionals must address alcohol abuse as an important clinical/behavioral issue.

And there *are* several intervention strategies that have proven effective in primary care settings.

Combined data from history, risk assessment, screening tools, and physical examination are all important in reaching a clinical decision. If a student is assessed as an "at risk" or "problem" drinker, the end point of therapy should be drinking at low-risk limits. This will be the most common scenario faced by the student health practitioner. Abstinence should be recommended if the student is pregnant or takes medications which may react with alcohol. If the student is assessed as alcohol dependent, the therapeutic end point is abstinence from alcohol, and a judgment should be made about whether this student can best be treated at the health service, or referred to an outpatient or inpatient alcohol treatment program.

Techniques for Enhancing Change

Perhaps the most practical model for intervening at the college level is "motivational interviewing," or "motivational enhancement."[17] This type of interviewing is intended to enhance the patient's motivation to change drinking behavior. The interview is focused on the patient's goals, motivation, and choices. Patient autonomy is of paramount importance to this model, since it is the *patient's* understanding of the problem and choice of solutions to the problem rather than the *health care practitioner's* viewpoint that is most likely to result in behavioral change. This may be difficult for some practitioners who are more comfortable in the role of "expert" (i.e., handing down information to patients in order to "make them better").

Another important goal of motivational interviewing is to aid the patient in understanding his/her ambivalence about changing their drinking behavior. Throughout the interview, the patient is encouraged to clarify the "pros" and "cons" of drinking and of not drinking, personal goals, and ways in which alcohol is interfering with these goals. Discussing these issues may make the patient aware of the discordance of his/her behavior with stated life goals.

Presenting campus norms for low-risk drinking behavior is also appropriate when counseling students concerning their high-risk drinking patterns. Students need to be informed that the majority of their classmates do not engage in binge-drinking behavior.

The *transtheoretical model of change*[18] is a useful tool for determining how receptive a student may be to changing his/her drinking behavior. This model is based on the theory that individuals going through any kind of behavioral change, whether reduction of alcohol intake, tobacco cessation, or dieting, move through various "stages of change." (See Appendix 1 for details of this model.) Many students are in the *precontemplative* stage of changing drinking behavior. With a youthful sense of invulnerability to consequences, they may not sense the connection between their behavior and things going awry in their lives. Even at this stage, however, the clinician can still help the student take a step toward the next stage in the continuum by simply having the student list the pros and cons of drinking and not drinking. Sometimes it is also helpful to have the student keep a diary of alcohol use.

There are times when a brief intervention in the health clinic is not the most appropriate choice. For students who may need more intensive or ongoing intervention, college health professionals must be aware of other resources available in the university and surrounding community. Some of these resources may offer different approaches to patients with alcohol-related problems, including the disease model (12-step models), cognitive-behavioral therapies, or family/couples therapy. Clinicians also need to be familiar with the concepts behind self-help organizations such as Alcoholics Anonymous, if they include such options in their referrals.

Alcohol Withdrawal

The signs of alcohol withdrawal are elevated blood pressure, pulse, and temperature; hyperarousal, agitation, restlessness, cutaneous flushing, tremors, diaphoresis, midriasis, ataxia, clouding of consciousness, and disorientation. Symptoms include anxiety, panic, paranoid delusions, and visual and auditory hallucinations. The duration of these signs and symptoms is usually five to seven days; the peak period is one to three days.

Some college health clinicians feel comfortable prescribing outpatient drug therapy for students withdrawing from alcohol. While thorough coverage of this type of therapy is beyond the scope of this chapter, Swift has written an informative review article.[19]

Prevention

It is essential that college health personnel stay abreast of the latest public health/health promotion approaches to reduction of harmful drinking on college campuses. There is at present a move away from relying solely on educational lectures and brochures concerning alcohol, and a move toward "environmental approaches". These may include changes in alcohol-related policies on campus (stiffer penalties, lessened availability of alcohol), social marketing campaigns designed to re-set the student's perceived norms about drinking on their campus,[20] and work with the surrounding community (bars, restaurants and other area merchants) in order to promote the idea of low risk drinking among students. "Harm reduction" is being emphasized, focusing on reduction of harmful consequences rather than solely focusing on drinking rates. Using this approach, recent research at the University of Washington concluded that screening of high-risk students at the beginning of their university career, and offering these students a brief educational "harm reduction" session, may reduce harmful drinking in that population.[21]

Other approaches include curriculum infusion, and using and peer educators to teach decision-making skills to provide another venue for social norms setting. It is not clear which of these methods is or will be the most effective decreasing alcohol abuse. Most likely a combination of public health efforts, in addition to a caring and knowledgeable health service staff, will provide students with the best chance to reduce harm from alcohol abuse.

TOBACCO

Smoking rates among college students fell in the 1970s, stabilized in the 1980s, and rose again in the 1990s. Many factors have played a part in the resurgence of tobacco use among youth. They include influence from peers, the perceived "coolness" factor among some groups, cigarette advertising with youth oriented messages, the availability of "excess" spending money for use on tobacco products, easy access to tobacco, the apparent long delay between tobacco use and its serious health effects, and the general sense of invulnerability to negative health consequences.

College health professionals can make a difference in this mix of societal factors which encourage tobacco use, by creating an on-campus environment supporting the choice to be a non-smoker. At the same time, the health service setting provides an excellent opportunity to encourage students who are already smokers to quit.

Health Consequences of Tobacco

Tobacco kills more Americans each year than alcohol, cocaine, crack, heroin, homicide, suicide, car crashes, fires, and AIDS combined. About 400,000 deaths a year are attributable to cigarette smoking. The morbidity and mortality are due to an increased risk of premature coronary heart disease, cardiomyopathy, stroke, chronic bronchitis, emphysema, and cancer. About 30 percent of all cancer deaths are due to tobacco. These cancers include lung, mouth, larynx, pharynx, esophagus, stomach, pancreas, cervix, kidney, ureter, and bladder. Alcohol and tobacco work synergistically to contribute to 75–95 percent of all oral, esophageal, and laryngeal cancers.[22] Effects of smoking on pregnancy include increased rates of stillbirths, low birth weight infants, and higher infant mortality during the neonatal period.

The health consequences of smokeless tobacco (chewing tobacco and snuff) include an increase in susceptibility to oral cancer, gingival disease, and oral leukoplakia. In female users, an increase in low birth weight infants and premature delivery has been observed.[23]

Incidence/Prevalence of Tobacco Use in College

Cigarette smoking prevalence rates were measured by the Harvard School of Public Health in 1993 and again in 1997. Over that four-year period the prevalence of current smoking (defined as having smoked at least one day out of the previous 30) rose from 22.3 percent to 28.5 percent.[24] Smoking levels increased among all student subgroups (men, women, all ethnic groups measured, and each year in school). Increasingly, students arrive at colleges and universities as smokers. According to the Monitoring the Future Study,[3] 35 percent of high school seniors smoked at least once in the last 30 days. Nationwide, 5.4 percent of college students have used smokeless tobacco at least once in the last 30 days.[2] Male students are much more likely to use smokeless tobacco (11.7 percent) than female students (0.3 percent); male athletes are the highest risk group.

Clinical Management

A question concerning tobacco use frequency and type should be included on the health history form in the student's medical record to alert the clinician to the problem. *Individual counseling* may be initiated at the request of the student ("I've decided I want to quit smoking. Can you help me?") or by the practitioner ("I see you are on the birth control pill and you are a smoker. Did you know this puts you at a higher risk for health problems on the pill? Have you thought about quitting?"). As with alcohol, the stages of change model can help practitioners assess the readiness of students to quit and assist in selecting the most appropriate approach for each student (Appendix 1).

In addition to the strategies detailed in the stages of change model, the following "Why Do You Smoke?" quiz, adapted from the National Cancer Institute, is a useful tool. This assessment helps smokers recognize the main reasons they smoke. The reasons fall into six categories: stimulation, handling, pleasure, relaxation/tension reduction, craving, and habit.

Once the student recognizes which factors are the most important to them as a smoker, they can tailor their cessation efforts to help their challenge areas. This quiz can be given to the student to score at home with a follow-up appointment to review the plan of action and discuss a definite quit date.

Why Do I Smoke? Quiz

	Always	Frequently	Occasionally	Seldom	Never
A I smoke cigarettes to keep from slowing down.	5	4	3	2	1
B Handling a cigarette is part of the enjoyment of smoking.	5	4	3	2	1
C Smoking cigarettes is pleasant and relaxing.	5	4	3	2	1
D I light up a cigarette when I am upset about something.	5	4	3	2	1
E When I run out of cigarettes, I find it almost unbearable.	5	4	3	2	1
F I smoke automatically without even being aware of it.	5	4	3	2	1
G I smoke to perk myself up.	5	4	3	2	1
H Part of the enjoyment of smoking comes from the steps I take to light up.	5	4	3	2	1
I I find cigarettes pleasurable.	5	4	3	2	1
J When I feel uncomfortable about something, I light up a cigarette.	5	4	3	2	1
K I am very much aware of the fact when I am not smoking.	5	4	3	2	1
L I light up a cigarette without realizing I still have one burning in the ashtray.	5	4	3	2	1
M I smoke to give myself a "lift."	5	4	3	2	1
N Part of the enjoyment of smoking is watching the smoke I inhale.	5	4	3	2	1
O I want a cigarette most when I am comfortable and relaxed.	5	4	3	2	1

Why Do I Smoke? Quiz (continued)

	Always	Frequently	Occasionally	Seldom	Never
P When I feel "blue" or want to take my mind off my cares, I smoke a cigarette.	5	4	3	2	1
Q I get a real craving for a cigarette when I haven't smoked in a while.	5	4	3	2	1
R I've found a cigarette in my mouth and didn't remember having put it there.	5	4	3	2	1

Scoring

1. Enter the circled number for each statement in the space provided, putting the number for statement A on line A and so on.

2. Add the three scores on each line; for example, the sum of your scores on lines A, G, and M gives you a total score for the "stimulation" category.

A ____ G ____ M ____   Stimulation
B ____ H ____ N ____   Handling
C ____ I ____ O ____   Pleasure
D ____ J ____ P ____   Relaxation/Tension Reduction
E ____ K ____ Q ____   Craving
F ____ L ____ R ____   Habit

The higher your score, the more important the reason for your smoking. A score of 11 or more (15 is the highest) in one category indicates an important reason for you. If you have a high score in more than one area, you may find quitting more difficult. Don't worry; when you understand what you derive from smoking, you can look for satisfying substitutes. Remember your high-scoring reasons. Later in the program we'll help you plan strategies for overcoming them.

Some college health professionals have the misperception that smoking cessation counseling is futile in college because college students are too young to want to quit. In fact, two-thirds of adolescent smokers say they want to quit, and 70 percent say they would not have started smoking if they could choose again.[25] More than one-half (58.7 percent) of college students have tried to quit at least once.[2] Quitting smoking is very difficult for most smokers given the addictive nature of nicotine. In addition, the repetitive behaviors that become associated with the act of smoking have been reinforced countless times, even in the relatively young smoker. It is essential that students have available a full slate of smoking cessation services. These services may be offered in different university and community locations, such as a student health clinic, health promotion office or wellness center, counseling center, school of psychology, and off-campus programs such as the American Lung or American Cancer Association. Services offered may include individual or group counseling, self-help materials, support groups or "buddy systems," pharmacological interventions, or computer/Internet support services.

Pharmacological Interventions

Clinicians should consider recommending medication as part of the tobacco cessation strategy for students who are having a difficult time quitting. Students who might particularly benefit from medication include those who:

- smoke within one half hour of waking in the morning
- smoke one half to one pack per day or more
- are bothered by cravings for nicotine
- have tried to quit without medications and have failed

The two types of medications currently available for tobacco cessation are nicotine replacement products and bupropion. Nicotine replacement products are available over the counter in the patch and in gum form. Prescriptions are required for the spray and the inhaler. These products blunt the physical withdrawal symptoms. The inhaler may also provide a substitute activity that mimics the act of smoking a cigarette.

Bupropion has been prescribed for years as an antidepressant. It was observed that many depressed smokers who were put on this medication had a lessened desire to smoke. This oral medication has both dopaminergic and adrenergic actions and decreases both craving and withdrawal symptoms. More recently bupropion has been released under the trade name specific for smoking cessation, Zyban® (Glaxo-Wellcome). Clinicians should screen for seizure or eating disorder history before placing students on Zyban.®

A few studies have compared the success rates of these two types of pharmacological interventions. One compared the twelve-month quit rates of patients in four groups: bupropion alone, nicotine replacement patch alone, a combination of the patch and bupropion, and placebo. It was found that bupropion alone or in combination with the patch resulted in a significantly higher quit rate at twelve months than either the nicotine patch alone or placebo.[26] One review article presented multiple studies measuring six month quit rates of the various forms of nicotine replacement products and bupropion. The conclusion was reached that patient preference was the most important factor in selecting a treatment option.[27]

Smokeless Tobacco

Although the majority of tobacco users on campus are smokers, a small fraction of students use smokeless tobacco in both snuff and chewing tobacco. Students may start chewing one of the sweeter varieties of chewing tobacco (which is usually lower in nicotine) and then graduate to a higher nicotine product once a tolerance develops. The use of nicotine replacement products such as gum and the patch have not met with as much success as in smokers. Research continues using higher doses of nicotine replacement products and bupropion.

Other Important Points to Remember When Counseling Smoking Patients

- Be knowledgeable about what physical withdrawal symptoms students may experience during withdrawal. These may include insomnia, drowsiness, irritability, headaches, constipation, diarrhea, increased appetite, and decreased tolerance to caffeine.
- Heavy smokers should be screened for alcohol or other drug use.
- Many students link smoking with drinking. Since drinking alcohol can lower the resolve to stay a non-smoker, students may need to be advised to avoid alcohol, at least during the early part of smoking cessation efforts.
- Cost tends to be a factor when students are considering medications for smoking cessation. Clinicians should remind students that, unless they are "bumming" the vast majority of their cigarettes, they are probably spending as much on their tobacco products as they would for the prescription.
- Above all, treat smokers with respect and in a positive way. Being non-judgmental and recognizing how difficult it is to quit smoking is important in relating to patients who smoke.

Remembering the "Big Picture"

Student health professionals must stay up-to-date on the environmental change strategies and other tobacco reduction efforts on campus. A recent consensus statement in the *Journal of the American Medical Association* summarizes the U.S. Public Health Service's report "Treating Tobacco Use and Dependence: A Clinical Practice Guideline." This article provides specific recommendations regarding tobacco cessation interventions and system-level changes.[28] System-level changes for college campuses includes the encouragement of smoke-free residence hall environments, cyberspace support for smokers trying to quit (list serves and cyberspace quit "buddies"), and social marketing campaigns to reset norms.

OTHER DRUGS OF ABUSE

Other drugs of abuse on college campuses include marijuana, hallucinogens, stimulants (cocaine, methamphetamine, and Ritalin), sedatives, inhalants, opiates (e.g. heroin), steroids, and a whole host of drugs, recently labeled "club drugs." Also common are narcotics (morphine, meperidine, and methadone), MDMA ("Ecstasy"), Rohypnol®, gamma-hydroxybutyrate (GHB), inhalants, antibiotic steroids, and sedatives (barbiturates, methaqualone). Combinations of prescription drugs such as Xanax®, Valium®, Percocet®, Oxycontin®, with alcohol or other drugs may have potentially lethal results. Unfortunately, students may have a false sense of security when taking a "prescription drug" versus a "street drug," believing that they, at least, have a "pure" form of the drug.

The 1960s heralded a dramatic increase in illicit drug use among American college students. This increase spread rapidly to non-college same-age peers and eventually to middle and high school youth. College students were the "trend setters" in the 1960s and early 1970s in the illicit drug arena. (This trend-setting role now seems to have shifted to youth of middle and high school age.) Although the use of other drugs of abuse is not as widespread as alcohol and tobacco, college health professionals need to be attuned to which drugs are being used on their campuses and to be familiar with prevention, detection, and treatment modalities for each.

The percentage of college students using marijuana and other illicit drugs has been tracked by several large surveys, including the Monitoring the Future (MTF) Study, the Core Alcohol and Drug Survey,[29] and the National College Health Risk Behavior Survey (NCHRBS). Findings consistently reveal that marijuana is the most commonly used illicit drug on campuses across the United States.

Overall trends of illicit drug use among youth in the U.S. have been tracked through the MTF study. In general, illicit drug use peaked in all age groups in the mid-to-late 1970s. It then steadily declined until the early 1990s when secondary school students exhibited a significant increase in use of marijuana, cocaine, hallucinogens, and inhalants. This behavior was believed to be related to the softening of attitudes about drugs (as confirmed by questions on the MTF study about the perceived risks of drug use and the disapproval of use). In 1997, illicit drug use again began to decline in the 8th grade cohort, to be followed by a decline in drug use in the 10th grade, 12th grade, and in college. It remains to be seen whether these trends will continue.

The 1998 data tracking individual illicit drugs indicate that there have been minimal changes in the use of most drugs, albeit a slight increase in use of marijuana, cocaine, and MDMA. Amphetamine use dropped slightly from 1997 to 1998. Inhalant use has decreased since 1996, possibly secondary to an ad campaign launched that year.

The majority of college students who use drugs are "recreational" or "experimental" drug users. It is important to recognize the difference between an occasional user and someone who has a more serious problem.

Marijuana

Marijuana is the illicit drug most widely used by the college population and in the United States. Thirty-two percent of college students reported marijuana use at least once within the last year, and 19 percent reported use within the last 30 days on the 1998 Core Alcohol and Drug Survey.[29] Most students who smoke marijuana in college started smoking in middle or high school. Marijuana is used as a mixture of dried, shredded flowers and leaves of the plant *Cannabis sativa*. Although there have been more than four thousand chemicals isolated from this plant, the main active ingredient is THC (delta-9-tetrahydrocannabinol). It is known that there are specific THC receptors in the human brain. Once THC binds to these receptors, a series of cellular reactions occur which leads to the "high" experience by users. This high usually begins with relaxation and mood elevation. Within thirty minutes, the user becomes sedated. However, conversely, some users can become anxious or fearful after a heavy dose of THC.

The amount of THC absorbed into the body depends on the route of delivery. Marijuana cigarette smoking results in absorption of 10 to 20 percent of the THC, pipe smoking delivers 40 to 50 percent, and water pipe (bong) use results in close to 100 percent absorption of the THC. Marijuana can also be ingested orally resulting in a lower absorption of the drug.

Health Risks of Marijuana Use

Recent generations of college students tend to downplay the potential for any harmful effects from smoking marijuana. However, marijuana does have adverse health effects:[30]

- It interferes with coordination, short-term memory, and the ability to make decisions. Marijuana users are twice as likely to become involved in car crashes. (This effect is placed first on the list since it applies to any student who smokes marijuana, whether he/she smokes one "joint" a year or two per day.)
- Smoking marijuana is associated with an increased rate of lung, esophageal, and bladder cancer. One "joint" contains as much carbon monoxide as 4 to 5 tobacco cigarettes and as much tar as 3 to 5 tobacco cigarettes.
- THC temporarily increases the heart rate and blood pressure by as much as 50 percent, potentially causing problems for those with underlying heart disease, elevated blood pressure, or abnormal heart rhythms.
- An increase in anovulatory menstrual cycles occurs in women who are heavy users.
- An increase in low birth-weight infants has been noted in women who use marijuana during pregnancy. THC is also passed to the infant through breastfeeding, and a decrease in milk production in nursing mothers can occur.
- Regular use in men is associated with decreased levels of testosterone and sperm count. Erectile dysfunction and gynecomastia can occur.
- Amotivational syndrome is a syndrome associated with chronic heavy marijuana use. It is characterized as a state of passive withdrawal from usual work and recreational activities.
- There is potential for drug interactions: marijuana use, in conjunction with alcohol, diazepam, antihistamines, phenothiazines, barbiturates, and narcotics, can potentiate sedation. Use with cocaine and amphetamines potentiates stimulation. THC antagonizes the effects of phenytoin, propranolol, and insulin.[24]

There is still much to be learned about the long-term effects of marijuana use. One study examined cognitive effects on college students who were heavy marijuana users (had smoked a median of 29 out of the previous 30 days). Heavy users were compared to light users (had smoked 1 day in the previous 30) on a battery of written and verbal vocabulary and memory tests. Heavy users were found to have residual neuropsychological effects even after a day of abstinence. However, it was unclear whether this effect was due to a residue of drug in the brain, a withdrawal effect, or a neurotoxic effect of the drug.[31]

Clinical Presentation

The student medical history should explore the frequency and quantity of marijuana use. Complaints about declining academic performance, frequent cough, menstrual irregularities, and erectile dysfunction should prompt the clinician to ask about marijuana use. If marijuana use is identified, special emphasis should be placed on counseling about its negative effects on coordination, which places students at higher risk for motor vehicle accidents and other trauma.

Although users can develop psychological dependence, signs and symptoms of physical withdrawal from marijuana are mild, if present at all. Even with very high doses imposed on humans in studies, physical withdrawal symptoms have not been shown to occur universally.[32] Some heavy users may experience irritability and restlessness during an abrupt withdrawal period.

Hallucinogens

Approximately 7.3 percent of college students used hallucinogens at least once over the previous year, with 2.4 percent using within the previous 30 days.[29] This class of drugs includes LSD, peyote, mescaline, psilocyben, DMT, morning glory seeds, nutmeg, STP, jimsonweed, and PCP. LSD is the most commonly used of this group.

The usual dose of LSD is 25-100 mg. sold as tablets, gelatin squares, or applied to small pieces of paper, decals or stickers. Any dose more than 250 mg. is considered especially dangerous. Most users describe a seemingly mild "trip" with colorful visual images, sound enhancement, and light sensations. There may be a loss of time sense and loss of ego boundaries. LSD can also produce reactive psychoses, flashbacks, and the well-known "bad trip," which can induce panic and a sense of "going crazy." It is critical to remember that there is no "quality control" of illicit drugs. Product sold as LSD may contain no LSD, be laced with other drugs, or contain a higher dose than the user expects.

Stimulants

Cocaine has been used by 4.4 percent of college students within the previous year, and 1.8 percent within the previous 30 days.[29] Other drugs used by college students in this category include amphetamines such as methamphetamine, and Ritalin®. Stimulants may appeal to students due to their ability to increase attention, stimulate alertness, decrease appetite, and eliminate fatigue.

Cocaine

Cocaine is a powerfully addictive drug that is snorted, injected, or smoked (free-base or crack cocaine). All routes of administration can pose a great risk to the user. As with other illicit drugs, what is sold as cocaine on the street may be mixed with cornstarch, sugar, baby laxatives, or other substances. The actual cocaine content may vary from 5–35 percent. Cocaine is a strong central nervous system stimulant, resulting in an almost immediate euphoric effect and a sense of increase in energy. Heart rate, respiratory rate, blood pressure and temperature increase, and the user has an increased sense of mental alertness. Pupils are dilated. There is a decrease in appetite and there may be an alteration in sensory awareness. The user may display constant repetitive physical motions. These symptoms last about 30 minutes and may be followed by a period of depression. Large doses of cocaine can result in violent or bizarre behavior. Death from cocaine use is usually the result of cardiac arrest or seizures followed by respiratory arrest.

Regular cocaine users can become restless, irritable, and anxious. The presenting clinical picture can include weight loss, insomnia, chest pains, and palpitations. If the student smokes crack, a cough ("crack hack") may be evident. If snorting is frequent, nasal findings can include sinusitis, epistaxis, nasal ulcerations, or septal perforation. Lab findings may include an elevated creatine kinase (CK).[33] Supportive rather than specific measures are used for patients undergoing cocaine withdrawal. Observation for depression and suicidal ideation are advised. The use of an antidepressant may be necessary.

Methamphetamine

Methamphetamine is another stimulant which has a very high potential for abuse and dependence. Modes of administration include snorting, smoking, intravenous injection, or oral ingestion. Methamphetamine hydrochloride, clear chunky crystals known as "ice," can be inhaled by smoking. The euphoria and withdrawal symptoms are similar to those experienced by cocaine users.

Methylphenidate (Ritalin)®

The vast majority of methylphenidate users in college are using the drug to treat the symptoms of attention-deficit hyperactivity disorder (ADHD). While Ritalin® has a focusing effect on those with ADHD, it is a CNS stimulant, and therefore has potential for abuse. Abusers most often take the drug in the pill form. A mild high is produced lasting 2 to 4 hours. Users have also crushed the pills and injected the medication or snorted the resultant powder. Although Ritalin® abuse is relatively rare on college campuses, college health professionals need to be aware that this drug has a potential market for students other than those they may be treating for ADHD.

Heroin

Heroin is the most commonly abused opiate on college campuses. According to the 1998 MTF study, 0.6 percent of college students had used heroin at least once within the previous year. Though herion has been traditionally thought of as an IV administered drug, both smoking and snorting heroin have recently gained popularity, along with the misconception that it is safer if used this way. Although inhalation of the drug decreases the chance for transmission of HIV or hepatitis B or C from sharing IV "works," the drug is still extremely physically and psychologically addictive, regardless of the mode of administration.

Heroin acts on the opiate receptors in the brain, causing an intense euphoria almost immediately. This is followed by a dreamlike state that can last up to a few hours. Other symptoms can include decreased pain sensitivity, lower respiratory rate, miosis, and flushed skin. Nausea and vomiting can occur in addition to constipation and difficulty urinating.

Tolerance to heroin develops rapidly, with the user requiring greater quantities to achieve the same euphoria. Dependency can result within a few weeks of use. Heroin overdoses are most common with IV use, but can occur with any dosage form if enough is taken. Overdoses can be lethal, usually from respiratory arrest. Overdoses are not a result of a cumulative effect of the drug, as they can happen on the very first dose.

Withdrawal from heroin is very unpleasant, but not life-threatening. Signs and symptoms include yawning, watery eyes, rhinorrhea, sweating, tremors, vomiting and muscle spasms. Persistent craving can last for years following the acute withdrawal. Medications such as methadone can be administered in treatment programs to decrease craving.

"Club Drugs"

Health service clinicians need to be aware of a class of drugs labeled "club drugs" because they are frequently being taken at all-night dance parties (sometimes called "raves"), dance bars, or clubs. Drugs included in this category are MDMA (Ecstasy), GHB, Rohypnol®, ketamine, methamphetamine, and LSD.

MDMA (3-4 methylenedioxymethamphetamine), known commonly as "Ecstasy," gained the reputation of being a drug that would stimulate empathy and good feelings for others. In fact, it has risks similar to those found with amphetamines and cocaine, including increases in heart rate and blood pressure, involuntary teeth clenching, nausea, sleep disruption, blurred vision, nystagmus, chills or sweating,· and syncope. Psychological difficulties can include confusion, depression, severe anxiety, and paranoia. Psychotic episodes have been reported. Research findings also link frequent MDMA use to memory impairment that persists for at least two weeks after the cessation of the drug.

Flunitrazepam (Rohypnol®) is commonly known as a "date rape" drug. An unsuspecting student may be given the drug (often mixed in a drink containing alcohol), which can incapacitate the victim and prevent resistance to (or even remembrance of) a sexual assault. The predominant clinical manifestations are drowsiness, impaired motor skills, and anterograde amnesia. Rohypnol® is also used by heroin and cocaine abusers to produce an even more profound intoxication, boost the high of heroin, and modulate the effects of cocaine. Rohypnol® can produce physical and psychological dependence and may be lethal when mixed with alcohol or other depressants.

Few statistics exist on how often this drug is involved in rape, partly because the victim is often unable to supply historical clues of the rape. Students who present acutely with a history of sexual assault and who appear intoxicated or have anterograde amnesia should be suspected of having ingested flunitrazepam. Congress recently passed the "Drug-Induced Rape Prevention and Punishment Act of 1996" which increased federal penalties for use of any controlled substance such as Rohypnol® to aid in sexual assault.

GHB

GHB is a CNS depressant that is being used by some college students for its euphoric, sedative, and anabolic effects. Although widely available in health food stores during the 1980s, GHB has not been sold over the counter in the U.S. since 1992. Liquid GHB is used in the club scene to produce effects similar to those of Rohypnol®. As with Rohypnol®, it has been associated with sexual assault cases. Coma, seizure, and death can occur following use of GHB. When combined with methamphetamine, an increased risk for seizure has been noted.

Inhalants

Two percent of college students reported the use of inhalants over the previous year and 0.9 percent within the previous 30 days on the 1998 Core survey.[29] Students may use inhalants chiefly because they are cheap and readily available.

A large range of substances have been inhaled including paint thinners and solvents, degreasers (dry-cleaning fluids), gasoline, glue, correction fluid, felt-tip-marker fluid, electronic cleaners, butane lighter fluid, propane, whipping cream aerosols or dispensers, refrigerant gases, hair spray, deodorant spray, fabric protector sprays, anesthetic gases (e.g. ether, chloroform, halothane, and nitrous oxide), and nitrites (amyl nitrite is available by prescription only; butyl nitrite is now an illegal substance).

Although different in chemical structure, almost all inhalants produce an anesthetic type effect. Intoxication may last a few minutes or several hours, if sniffed repeatedly. Following an initial "head rush," or intoxicating effect, the user experiences lethargy and an increasing loss of control. Death from inhalants usually occurs after inhalation of large doses or by inhaling from a paper or plastic bag placed over the head.

Amyl and butyl nitrites use has a high association with development of Kaposi's Sarcoma (KS), a cancer commonly found in AIDS patients. Research continues to explore the cause of a possible link between nitrite inhalation and KS.

Health risks of using inhalants include hearing loss (toluene and trichloroethylene), peripheral neuropathies (glues, gasoline, nitrous oxide), CNS damage (toluene), bone marrow suppression (benzene), liver and kidney damage (toluene, chlorinated hydrocarbons), and blood oxygen depletion (nitrites, methylene chloride).

Anabolic Steroids

Anabolic steroids are synthetic derivatives of testosterone and are used to enhance sports performance by "bulking up" muscle mass. Steroids are most often taken orally, but can be injected. While athletes often take these drugs in cycles of weeks or months, and may take more than one kind of steroid at a time, only 0.5 percent of college students reported having used anabolic steroids in the last 30 days on the 1998 Core Alcohol and Drug Survey.[29] Young people may be persuaded to use these drugs in order to emulate prominent athletes who have had record-breaking seasons after using anabolic steroids during their periods of success.

Health hazards associated with anabolic steroid use include elevated blood pressure, fluid retention, increases in LDL and decreases in HDL, severe acne, tremor, hepatitis, and hepatic tumors. In men, testicular atrophy, reduced sperm count, baldness, and gynecomastia can occur. In women, hirsutism, irregular menses or amenorrhea, clitoral enlargement, and deepened voice may develop. Adolescents may experience growth halted prematurely through premature skeletal maturation and accelerated puberty changes. There are also reports that anabolic steroid use can result in behavior changes such as extreme mood swings and an increased propensity to violence.

The Injecting Drug User

For students who have a history of IV drug use, it is important to counsel them about the risks of sharing needles and transmission of HIV and Hepatitis B and C. Unique signs are observable on physical examination if IV drug use is suspected. Puncture wounds, track marks, and "tattooing" may be present. (Tattooing is caused by deposition of carbon particles in the user who "sterilizes" the needle by holding it over a flame.) The injecting drug user may also have sclerosis of superficial veins, lymphatic streaking, or ecchymosis in the anterolateral supraclavicular region, caused by attempts to inject a drug directly into the jugular vein (called a "pocket shot").

Treatment for Other Drugs of Abuse

Description of treatment modalities for all of these drugs is beyond the scope of this chapter. The transtheoretical model of change is a model that can be used to determine student readiness to change drug use behavior. The principles of motivational interviewing as outlined in the alcohol section apply to these drugs as well. As with alcohol treatment, it is important for college health professionals to be familiar with the treatment options, both inpatient and outpatient, which are available to students who are abusing drugs. The National Institute on Drug Abuse (NIDA) provides useful resources for those interested in a guide to the treatment of drug addiction.[34]

SUMMARY

Substance abuse remains a persistent problem in the college years. College health professionals can impact substance abuse prevention and treatment. Each university should strive toward a comprehensive approach to substance abuse with concentration on the two substances that cause the most morbidity and mortality in the college-age population—alcohol and tobacco. Primary prevention strategies should be multi-faceted and include such public health strategies as norm-setting social marketing campaigns, campus policies on alcohol and other drugs, smoke-free environments (including residence halls), peer educator programs, and community coalitions designed to reshape the environment both on- and off-campus. High risk groups can be targeted to increase the impact of these programs. Ongoing outcomes-based research will guide public health professionals in selecting the most effective prevention strategies.

Early detection and treatment for individuals at risk of substance abuse in the college setting is imperative. The use of effective screening tools in addition to skilled interviewing techniques provides college health professionals with the background to be effective in this challenging area. The challenge often consists in moving a student from the "precontemplative" stage to a stage where action is being considered for a behavior change. Knowledge of appropriate referral resources both on and off campus is another step in providing the best care possible for students who may need further help.

Appendix 1—Stage of Change[18] Model

Precontemplation

Students in this stage have no intention of changing behavior in the foreseeable future. Some are in denial that a problem exists at all.

What can you do?

Alcohol: Have posters and literature in many locations. Use clinic visits to point out, in a non-judgmental fashion, what appear to be consequences of the student's drinking. Social-norms marketing may work here.

Tobacco: Have eye-catching posters and fliers around. Some universities are trying social-norms marketing campaigns to reach this group of smokers.

Contemplation

Students are aware that a problem exists and are thinking about changing, but have not yet made a commitment to change.

What can you do?

Alcohol: Have the student list pros and cons of drinking and not drinking and keep a diary of alcohol use. Suggest considering a trial of abstinence or reduction in quantity of drinking. Provide quality pamphlets, and offer any educational program you have on campus that addresses assessment of student risk and drinking.

Tobacco: Use motivational interviewing techniques in order to link reasons for change to quitting. Talk to the student briefly about other services available, such as support groups and prescription medication. Encourage exercise.

Preparation

At this stage, students are intending to take action to change behavior within the near future. They may have already begun some preliminary attempts, such as reduction of drinking or smoking.

What can you do?

Alcohol: Help the student set definitive goals for abstinence or low-risk drinking. Discuss available treatment options. Review family and social supports for change.

Tobacco: Provide detailed and specific information about strategies to quit, including medication options. Encourage them to set a specific quit date. Review their personal roadblocks and how they plan to overcome these.

Action

Students will modify their behavior at this stage.

What can you do?

Alcohol: Continue to provide support for this decision. Reinforce reasons for reduction or cessation of drinking and review the student's network of support. Discuss how they will handle specific situations.

Tobacco: Provide counseling and medications if appropriate. Encourage the building of support systems among friends and family. Point out any support groups available (including cyberspace options), and talk to the student about how to best cope with cravings. Signing a contract is effective in some cases.

Maintenance

For most substance abuse-related behavior, relapse is a very real possibility. Each conversation with a student in this stage of change can include positive reinforcement for behavior changes as well as preparation for any relapses.

What can you do?

Alcohol: Continue reinforcing the decision to change drinking behavior.

Tobacco: Support students in their behavior change. Point out the benefits they now have as non-smokers. Review possible relapse triggers.

REFERENCES

1. CDC National Center for Health Statistics. National Vital Statistics Reports, Vol. 47, No. 25, October 5, 1999.

2. Centers for Disease Control and Prevention. Youth risk behavior surveillance: National College Health Risk Behavior Survey. Morbidity and Mortality Weekly Report 1997; 46(SS-6), 1–56.

3. National Institute on Drug Abuse. National survey results on drug use from the monitoring the future study, 1975–1998. Vol 2: College students and young adults. Bethesda, Md. 1999.

4. Wechsler H, Lee JE, Kuo M, Lee H. College binge drinking in the 1990s: a continuing problem. Results of the Harvard School of Public Health 1999 College Alcohol Study. J. Am. Col. Health 2000;48:199–210.

5. Wechsler H, Davenport A, Dowdall G, et al. Health and behavioral consequences of binge drinking in college. JAMA 1994;272:1672–1677.

6. Thaccer KD. An overview of health risks and benefits of alcohol consumption. Alcoholism: Clinical and Experimental Research 1998;22:285S–298S.

7. Rehm J, Ashley MF, Dubois G. Alcohol and health: individual and population perspectives. Addiction 1997;92:S109–15.

8. Burge SK, Schneider FD. Alcohol-related problems: recognition and intervention. Am Fam Phy 1999;59:361–370.

9. Wright SW, Norton VC, Dake AD, Pinkston JR, Slovis CM. Alcohol on campus: alcohol-related emergencies in undergraduate college students. So Med J 1998;91:909–913.

10. Schorling JB, Buchsbaum DG. Screening for alcohol and drug abuse. Medical Clinics of North America 1997;81:845–865.

11. Heck EJ, Williams MD. Using the CAGE to screen for drinking-related problems in college students. J of Studies on Alcohol 1995;56:282–286.

12. O'Hare T, Tran TV. Predicting problem drinking in college students: gender differences and the CAGE questionnaire. Addictive Behav 1996;22:13–21.

13. Werner MJ, Walker JS, Greene JW. Concurrent and prospective screening for problem drinking among college students. J of Adol Health 1996;18:276–285.

14. O'Hare T. Measuring problem drinking in first time offenders. J of Subst Abuse Treat 1997; 14:383–387.

15. National Institute on Alcohol Abuse and Alcoholism: Physicians' guide to helping patients with alcohol problems. Washington, DC, National Institutes of Health Publication No. 95-3769, 1995.

16. American Psychiatric Association. Diagnostic and statistical manual of mental disorders. 4th ed. Washington, DC: American Psychiatric Association, 1994.

17. Barnes HN, Samet JH. Brief interventions with substance-abusing patients. Med Clinics of NA, 1997;81:867–879.

18. Prochaska JO, DiClemente CC, Norcross JC. In search of how people change: applications to addictive behaviors. Am Psychologist. 1992;47:1102–1114.

19. Swift R. Drug therapy for alcohol dependence. NEJM 1999;340:1482–1490.

20. Haines MS, Spear SF. Changing the perception of the norm: a strategy to decrease binge drinking among college students. J of Am Coll Health 1996;45:134–140.

21. Marlatt GA, Baer JS, Kivlahan DR, Dimeff LA, Larimer ME, Quigley LA, Somers JM, Williams E. Screening and brief intervention for high-risk college student drinkers: results from a 2-year follow-up assessment. J of Consulting and Clinical Psychology 1998;66:604–165.

22. Centers for Disease Control and Prevention. The Surgeon General's 1990 Report on the Health Benefits of Smoking Cessation Executive Summary. Morbidity and Mortality Weekly Report 1990;39(RR-12);2–10.

23. Neinstein L. Tobacco. Adolescent Health Care: A Practical Guide, 3rd edition (pp 1018–1031). Baltimore, MD: Williams & Wilkins, 1996.

24. Wechsler H, Rigotti NA, Gledhill-Hoyt J., Lee H. Increased levels of cigarette use among college students. JAMA 1998;280:1673–1678.

25. U.S. Department of Health and Human Services. Preventing tobacco use among young people: a report of the Surgeon General. Office of Smoking and Health. Atlanta, GA: USDHHS, CDC, Publication S/N 017-001-00491-0, 1994.

26. Jorenby DE, et al. A controlled trial of sustained-release bupropion, a nicotine patch, or both for smoking cessation. N Engl J Med 1999;340:685–691.

27. Hughes JR, Goldstein MG, Hurt RD, Shiffman S. Recent advances in the pharmacotherapy of smoking. JAMA 1999;281:72–76.

28. Journal of American Medical Association. A Clinical Practice Guideline for Treating Tobacco Use and Dependence. Vol. 283, No. 24, June 28, 2000.

29. Core Institute. 1998 statistics on alcohol and other drug use on American campuses. Southern Illinois University.

30. Neinstein L. Marijuana. Adolescent Health Care: A Practical Guide, 3rd edition (pp1033–1037) Baltimore, MD: Williams & Wilkins, 1996.

31. Pope HG, Yurgelun-Todd D. The residual cognitive effects of heavy marijuana use in college students. JAMA 1996;275:521–527.

32. Kuhn C, Swartzwelder S, Wilson W. Buzzed. 1998. WW Norton & Co., New York.

33. Meyers MJ. Substance abuse and the family physician: making the diagnosis. Fam Prac Recert 1999;21:53–76.

34. National Institute on Drug Abuse. "Principles of Drug Addiction Treatment—A research-Based Guide." National Institutes of Health Publication No. 99-4180, 1999.

CHAPTER 12

UNIQUE HEALTH CARE NEEDS IN HEALTH SCIENCE STUDENTS

Wylie Hembree, MD

Health science students make up a unique, definable constituency of student health services. Their education and/or training occurs exclusively, or in part, in the health care setting. Even before the writings of Hippocrates, it was recognized that students in medicine were at risk of contracting the illnesses they were trying to cure. In addition, they were noted to be responsible for communicating disease to their patients.* Thus student health services have the dual responsibility of protecting both student and patient—a charge uniquely occasioned by the nature of the academic curriculum of health science students.

Assuming the responsibility of certifying that students are physically and mentally capable of minimizing risks to their own health, as well as that of patients, presents liability concerns for the health service and the institution. Therefore, student health services must be authorized to have easy access to the students (required enrollment or attendance at the student health service for certain programs) as well as to services that protect both student and patient. Occupational exposures represent only one of several concerns that illustrate difficulties brought about by the assumption of responsibility for the physical and mental health of health science students. Occupational Safety and Health Administration (OSHA) regulations provide the guidelines for services required, although in many states "students" are not considered "health care workers," resulting, thereby, in limited access to testing, counseling, and medications.[2] Thus related services and costs may fall to the student health service.

---

*Perhaps the most dramatic and well-documented story of the danger students brought to the health care setting was the situation recognized and remedied by Semmelweiss. Women who delivered babies on a ward tended by students, who were also active in postmortum dissections, had more than twice the incidence of puerperal fever as did the women in the ward attended by midwives. As we know, the simple expediency of cleanliness reduced the incidence nine-fold on the student ward.[1]

For geographic, political and practical reasons, it may be difficult to define the extent to which health care needs for health science students require different and/or additional services from the remainder of the students. A program of services specifically designed for health science students is not necessarily more difficult, complicated, important or interesting than that for other students. It is, however, different and experience suggests that it is more costly.[3]

Because health services often have no direct access to, and almost universally no authority in, the curriculum arena where risks occur, close collaboration between the academic administration and the health professionals in the clinical setting is essential for effective risk reduction and prevention. In addition, health services are uniquely qualified to minimize the impact of the "morbidity of risk perception" upon the educational goals of the students. Thus, health services given the responsibility for providing services for health science students must precisely define the extent of their role, insure they have the authority to carry out this role and make certain that the financial and administrative structure of the health service (including the insurance base) is adequate to perform these functions.

As a format for addressing these special concerns, the discussion herein focuses upon both the unique health care needs of health science students as well as those services that, while not unique, may need to be structured differently from other students'. These concerns include pre-matriculation requirements, immunizations, health risk surveillance and compliance, occupational exposures, psychiatric care, impairment, reproductive health issues, medication use, travel, the balance between primary care and specialty referrals, and preventive services. Further, and of particular importance to a student health service, the requirement for and nature of health education for the health science student is radically altered by the nature of the health science curriculum. Nonetheless, it is essential that health services recognize the educational role they play as students learn to care for others, in part, by learning how to care for themselves.[4]

During these learning processes, it is evident that health science students are burdened by a "double vulnerability" that shapes their responses to illness and health risks. The first dimension of this vulnerability is that experienced by all patients whose illness and its outcome appear to be out of their control. The second dimension is that which results from exposure to a large body of medical knowledge, only a small fraction of which has been integrated into a realistic perspective. This second dimension is often represented by the stereotype of the neurotic second-year medical student who gets every disease he studies—a figure in whom we often find humor. Failure to recognize the importance of this dimension, however, may result in unproductive health behavior exhibited by health professionals.[5] Since this dimension may alter the outcome of recommended health interventions (compliance, access, follow-up), it must be addressed by the student health service.

It is also likely that adverse outcomes for students, as they become professionals, will shape their responses to similar needs of patients. The extent to which students learn to care for their own health, through successful interaction with the health care system, may predict their effectiveness as providers of health care. This dimension of the health care provided for health science students should be viewed as part of the curriculum for which the student health service is the responsible educator, as well as provider, and should be one of our highest priorities.

DEMOGRAPHICS

Health science students, as defined above, are, of course, found in schools of medicine, osteopathy, dentistry, nursing, occupational and physical therapy, speech therapy, music therapy, osteopathy, pharmacy, graduate science, allied health, public health and others. While the number of programs, students and their characteristics can be approximated from data provided by national education organizations, actual published data are limited in scope. In 1993, there were more than 350,000 health science students,[6] increasing by 1999 by approximately 20 percent, primarily in nursing, allied health science, paramedics, graduate students and nursing. The number and percentage of women in health science have risen, although precise numbers in some programs are not known. Women medical students have increased from 36 percent to 42 percent, and women dental students from 26 percent to 35 percent.[7,8] The fraction of male students in nursing and occupational therapy has remained at approximately 10 percent.[9] Within most health profession schools, colleges of medicine represent the largest enrollment, although, overall, there are almost four times as many nursing schools and three times as many students.[10] The number of allied health professional students is nearly that of medical students.

Access to health care is determined both by the proximity of the professional school to clinical resources and by the location where students spend most of their time. For example, there are 125 medical schools;[7] however, only 48 of 54 dental schools are located on a campus with a medical school.[8] In contrast, although 82 of the medical campuses have nursing schools, only 26 percent of the nursing schools are located within academic medical centers.[9] This isolation is more pronounced for occupational and physical therapy programs, most of which have less than 120 students and are located on campuses where there are no other health science students.[9,11] There are 178 programs in physical therapy (PT) and 138 programs in occupational therapy (OT), with only 34 percent and 35 percent, respectively, located within academic medical centers. Although 66 of the 125 medical schools have programs in OT or PT, one third of these programs are located geographically away from the medical center. The majority of health profession schools are located on campuses where their students make up less than 10 percent of the student body.[6]

Only dental[8] and medical[7] schools have precise information regarding ethnic and racial background. In 1999, African American, Hispanic, Native American, and Asian students accounted for 3.5 percent, 4.8 percent, 0.4 percent, and 24 percent of first-year dental students. In the same year, for first-year medical students, the percent of African Americans was higher (7.9 percent), although Hispanic (6.5 percent), Native American (0.9 percent), and Asian (19.1 percent) students were similar. The number of students born and/or raised outside the United States has not been documented, but identifying them is important for tuberculosis screening and immunization programs.

The American Association of Dental Schools (AADS) has published age data for its students.[8] Incoming Dental students for the year 1999-2000 ranged in age from 19 to 46 with an average age of 23.6 years and 6 percent over the age of 30.[7] The average age is 26.8 years, the median age is 30 years, 26 percent are 30 to 39 years old, 8 percent are 40 to 49 years old, and 1 percent are over 50 years old. The percent over 30 years old ranges between 11 percent (medical) to 43 percent (nursing). This range of ages clearly demonstrates that services offered for health science students must extend well beyond those required for the "typical" college or university student.

PRE-MATRICULATION REQUIREMENTS

The pre-matriculation requirements which should be considered for health science students include a complete medical history, physical examination, mandatory insurance, required and recommended immunizations, and baseline tuberculin testing. Many student health services require completion of a medical form which documents medical and family history, immunizations, physical exam, medication use, allergies, and health risk data. The Association of American Medical Colleges (AAMC) has recommended that medical students have a pre-matriculation physical examination.[12] Although complete medical screening of this young, healthy population may not be cost effective, it is important for addressing individual health problems and to assess health risks of the population. Review of health data by health service medical and psychiatric staff makes it possible to request complete medical records, maintain continuity of care, and institute prevention efforts for those with health risks.

Mandatory health insurance and required enrollment in the student health service allows the student easy access to primary, specialty and emergency care, ancillary services and medications. It also insures the health maintenance and surveillance important to participating in a curriculum in a health care setting. Graduate and professional student health care may be more expensive than that of undergraduates, and the unique services necessary for participating in health care may not be covered by many student health insurance plans.[3,13] Health science student health services, in collaboration with their health professional schools, can provide services not covered by insurance yet necessary to certify the safety and health of both students and their patients.

All states have immunization requirements for primary and secondary schools; many have requirements for college-level students. Only recently, a few states have begun requiring hepatitis B immunization for secondary school enrollment.[14] Thus, it is likely that at the time of matriculation most health science students, particularly those born in the United States, will have had a wide array of immunizations. However, compliance and documentation of compliance by elementary schools, secondary schools and post secondary schools have never been 100 percent. Further, as mentioned, certain immunizations, considered necessary by most academic medical centers for their health science students, are not typically a prematriculation immunization requirement (PIR) in a general college or university. (The pre-matriculation immunizations recommended by ACHA are limited to MMR, hepatitis B, polio, varicella, and a tetanus booster.)[15]

Specific documentation of immunity deserves comment. Proof required may vary from only certification of disease immunization by a health care provider, to recent serologic proof of immunity. One reason for these differences is the outcome sought by the agency requiring immunizations. States, health departments and universities are charged with preventing epidemics of airborne and contact illnesses that are more likely to occur in closed populations. Their focus upon hepatitis B is also one of public health. However, amongst health science students the goal is to also protect both student and patient, requiring a higher level of herd immunity (hopefully 100 percent) than for the student population at large.

As a result, two policy issues must be addressed in monitoring compliance with immunizations and documenting immunity status. First, the level of immunity desired for the student population must be determined. The benchmark should be 100 percent. Second, the specific type of documentation must be designated. In this respect, health services must integrate their efforts with the requirements for documentation used in affiliated clinical training sites for students. Many may require serologic proof of immunity for MMR, hepatitis B and varicella, even though > 90 percent serologic immunity is observed in those providing proof of immunization or clinical disease.[16,17,18] When serologic proof of immunity is required, a small percentage of students with absence of a serologic response to immunization will be detected. As a result, the potential underlying health problems suggested by this lack of immune response should be addressed.

The Centers for Disease Control and Prevention (CDC) recently published a Core Curriculum on Tuberculosis,[19] recommending that health care workers at risk for exposure to tuberculosis should be part of a skin-testing program which includes an initial test, repeat tests at intervals determined by the nature of their risk of exposure and a prevention/education program. Baseline tuberculin screening should be performed before a student is allowed into any clinical setting. For health science students coming from high-risk settings (foreign-born, medically underserved populations, high-risk populations, persons at personal high risk), testing will detect latent tuberculosis infection (LBTI) and permit early treatment. Documentation of a history of a positive tuberculin skin test in a student should include full details of the test, a review of the chest x-ray and written records of treatment. Otherwise, re-evaluation and treatment are appropriate for consideration.

Traditionally, annual tuberculin skin testing of negative health care workers (HCW) and annual chest x-rays of tuberculin-positive HCWs have been required by states and hospitals. "Routine" x-rays are no longer recommended and many hospitals retest only if annual health assessments indicate high risk for exposure or symptoms of disease.[19] (Many states, however, still have a requirement for annual tuberculin testing in hospital employees.) Health science students should be tested, at a minimum, upon entry, prior to the major clinical curriculum and at least three months prior to graduation. It is important to detect and initiate treatment of latent tuberculosis infection which has occurred during health profession education prior to post-graduate training or employment.

IMMUNIZATIONS

CDC published recommendations for immunization of health care workers in December 1997,[20] all of which are also included in the CDC recommendations for vaccination of adolescents[21] and, with the exception of hepatitis A, in the Recommendations for Institutional Prematriculation Immunizations (RIPI) published by the American College Health Association.[15] CDC recommendations fall into three categories:

- Immunizations to prevent special risks of health care workers (hepatitis B, influenza, measles, mumps, rubella and varicella)
- Immunizations indicated in special circumstances (tuberculosis, hepatitis A, meningococcal disease, typhoid fever, vaccinia, perhaps pertussis)
- Immunizations recommended for all adults (tetanus, diphtheria, pneumococcal disease)

In 1998, the American Medical Association (AMA) accepted the recommendations of its Council on Scientific Affairs, "calling for universal immunization, including medical students, for hepatitis B and health insurance coverage for hepatitis B immunization."[22] The OSHA federal standard requirement that employees be provided hepatitis B vaccine at no cost,[2] has been emphasized by CDC.[23] Although required by only 10 percent of student health services, 90 percent of medical schools require hepatitis B vaccination and 22 percent pay for the vaccination and serologies; students pay in 68 percent, and less than 15 percent restrict clinical contact without proof of immunity.[24] It has been estimated that 30 percent of health care workers are not immune to hepatitis B and that compliance rates of medical students' immunization range between 40 and 80 percent.[25] Compliance rates are higher when immunization is paid for by insurance, the school or the student health service.[26,27]

Procedures vary for attempting to achieve universal immunization to hepatitis B. Pre-immunization serologies are not indicated unless found to be cost effective for the population to be immunized. One study has demonstrated pre-immunization immunity in 6 percent and carrier status in 0.3 percent of medical students.[25] Positive serologic tests that screen for immunity should be followed, when indicated, by medical history and antibody testing specific for surface and core antigens.

Influenza vaccine is recommended for all health care workers, especially those caring for high-risk patients. Because health science students are exposed to a diverse group of patients in the clinical setting, they should have annual vaccines.[28]

Proof of measles, mumps and rubella immunity, as noted above, is required for school enrollment in most states for any student born after 1957. One of the following is generally considered acceptable for documentation:[16]

- Written physician documentation of two MMR vaccine injections after one year of age
- Written physician documentation of rubeola and mumps disease
- Laboratory report of positive rubella, rubeola and mumps titers

Neither documentation of rubella disease nor birth before 1957 is conclusive evidence for rubella immunity in women of childbearing age who can become pregnant[16] and "documented" physician-diagnosed rubella alone is not sufficient for health care workers, international travelers or post-high school educational institutions.[16] Unvaccinated students born before 1957, without a documented history of rubeola and without laboratory documentation of rubella immunity, should have MMR immunization.

Health science students should be required to demonstrate immunity to varicella. Serologic immunity to varicella is observed in 97 to 99 percent of adults with a positive history of the disease and in 71 to 93 percent with a negative or uncertain history.[18] Prematriculation requirements should include physician documentation of two vaccine injections or laboratory proof of immunity. However, it should be noted that seroconversion after vaccination does not guarantee full protection after exposure to varicella.[18] Thus, it is recommended that vaccinated students with known exposures to varicella be tested and, if negative, have no patient contact for an appropriate period while monitoring for disease onset. There is a minimal risk that students vaccinated for varicella may transmit vaccine virus to contacts. After the first injection, 5.5 percent of adults develop rash, as do 0.9 percent after the second injection, with up to 15 percent of contacts of vaccinated children developing the disease.[18] Therefore, there must be surveillance procedures in place for students receiving the vaccine.

Although routine immunization of health care workers or health science students is not recommended for several illnesses that can be prevented by immunoprophylaxis, special circumstances may arise during their education in which immunization should be considered. Many students elect clinical rotations where infection control procedures are poor and/or where drug-resistant tuberculosis is common. Policies regarding health and safety of students should be developed by health professional schools before allowing students to rotate "outside" clinical sites. These policies should include criteria for acceptable levels of infection control and for access to health care, especially for occupational exposures. Within these guidelines, if approval of a clinical rotation site is given at which tuberculosis transmission is a high risk, students should be counseled regarding the value of BCG vaccination.[29]

Routine hepatitis A vaccination is not recommend for healthy health science students, although it is valuable for students with certain health risks.[30] For health science students who elect clinical rotations where hepatitis A is endemic, passive immunization with intramuscular immunoglobulin (when available) and active immunization with hepatitis A vaccine are equally effective in preventing disease. Immunoglobulin is immediately protective whereas vaccination may not confer protection for 30 days. The prolonged protection available from the vaccine makes it cost effective for the student.

Control, prevalence and vaccine prevention of meningococcal disease have received much attention in the recent past. This information is summarized in CDC recommendations.[30,31] Where the apparent higher risk of meningococcal disease to college freshmen living in dormitories is applicable to health science students, access to a vaccine program should be provided. Students traveling to countries where the disease is hyperendemic or epidemic should be vaccinated.

Students who work in laboratories where exposure to *Salmonella typhi* is possible should update typhoid immunity every two to five years (depending upon the vaccine used).

Immunization surveillance for health science students should include medical documentation of completion of DTaP immunization (diphtheria, tetanus, pertussis) in child-hood.[20,21,22] Non-immunized individuals should receive the complete course, unless medi-cally contraindicated. Documentation of a tetanus booster every ten years should be part of the pre-matriculation requirement, and updated if needed. The rarity of diphtheria and the high level of immunization compliance with DTaP immunization in childhood obvi-ate concerns about diphtheria.

It is of interest that polio vaccination is not mentioned in the CDC recommendations for health care workers,[20] although it is addressed in a recent CDC Report.[32] Populations of students born in the United States exhibit nearly 100 percent immunity attributable to immunization programs which began in the early 1950s. The annual number of cases of paralytic disease is eight or nine and, of the 152 cases reported since 1980, 144 were associated with oral polio vaccine administration. The current recommendation is for unvaccinated students to have three doses of the inactivated virus vaccination (IPV) and vaccinated students who are at risk (travel to endemic or epidemic areas, laboratory contact, high-risk patient contact) to have a single booster of IPV.

Other immunizations, such as those required for curriculum-related travel, pneumo-coccal vaccine for those with health risks and special needs for immunocompromised or HIV-infected students, are critical for health maintenance and disease prevention in se-lected health science students.[20]

Occupational Exposures

In 1987, "universal precautions" were published and adoption recommended in all health care settings, especially outpatient settings and provider offices.[33] In 1990, the CDC recommended AZT prophylaxis post-exposure in high-risk cases for HIV exposure[34] and, in 1991, OSHA promulgated rules and procedures for institutional management of exposures of health care workers.[2] However, students were not specifically named as health care workers and their status as such was, and has remained, ambiguous and undefined. Further, initially, neither insurance nor clinical rotation settings supported the cost of the services required when students were exposed. Today, most hospital infection control plans require incident reports, counseling and provision of one to three days of antiviral prophylaxis ("starter doses") for all employees exposed in a health care setting. Although in 1998, students were included in the CDC guidelines for management of exposures, many are still not covered in hospital control plans.[23]

The estimated rate of infection after percutaneous exposure to blood and body fluids is 26 percent, 6 percent, and 0.3 percent for hepatitis B, hepatitis C, and HIV.[35,36] The rate, reporting rate, and consequences of occupational exposures have been documented in multiple studies.[37,38,39,40] The actual risk for occupational exposures for medical and dental students has been estimated,[41] and the number of students likely to experience an exposure can be calculated.

Important required features of the management of occupational exposures, particu-larly to bloodborne pathogen exposures, include the following:

- training for prevention

- pre-exposure immunizations and surveillance
- post-exposure risk counseling
- post-exposure testing of source patient and exposed patient (student)
- access to post-exposure prophylaxis (PEP) with monitoring
- follow-up care and testing

In most colleges and universities, either the hospital, the health service and/or the academic program provides the facilities, equipment and training to minimize and prevent exposures. Immunizations are typically required as previously mentioned for matriculation with the health service responsible for compliance. Counseling, treatment, and follow-up for students are best handled in the same manner as for any university employees, preferably by one person/department who is trained in post-exposure counseling, recognizing the broad spectrum of risk that extends beyond HIV and hepatitis B.[42,43] This will ensure that appropriate testing is done and, if necessary, PEP provided, with follow-up care. Frequently, occupational exposures occur in a health care setting outside students' institutions. Because program quality may vary, all students should be expected to report and follow up all exposures with their home institution.

Because of the expenses associated with a post-exposure prophylaxis program, it is important to address this issue. In 1996, 59 percent of health services in which health science students were enrolled had protocols for occupational exposures, although only 15 percent provided post-exposure prophylaxis at no cost.[44] In 1998, 71 percent of medical schools relied upon occupational health services at the clinical site to provide testing and medication for health science students.[45] In early 2000, less than 50 percent of 26 major health plans covered post-exposure prophylaxis; this percentage is increasing as the awareness of the problem becomes more widespread.[46] Further, it is increasingly common for many institutions, particularly medical schools, to cover the cost of testing of the source patient and/or the student if they are not otherwise covered by student health or its insurance program. In many cases, occupational exposure programs at health care settings provide a portion of the PEP, typically the first three days, at no cost.

Self-reporting of bloodborne pathogen exposures by health care workers and health science students remains a serious problem. Reporting frequency ranges from 15–75 percent and has increased during the past decade.[47,48] Importantly, a "user-friendly" reporting procedure is essential. It must be characterized by designated access, efficiency, competence, confidentiality, low cost, and it must address broader aspects of risk, consequences, and follow up. Otherwise, the medical and psychological impact of exposures cannot be assessed. Despite a decade of surveillance by the CDC, only 56 persons are known to have seroconverted to HIV+ after an occupational exposure.[49] None of these were students. Therefore, CDC no longer maintains its surveillance program.[50]

It is not known how many medical students have had percutaneous exposures to HIV. Osborn et al. reported 84 such exposures in medical students over seven years in a setting wherein the maximum HIV infection was 23 percent.[51] Thus, approximately twenty students may have had HIV exposures; none were known to have been infected. Turner et al. reported 298 incidents in one year, only three (1 percent) of which were HIV exposures.[41] Eight percent of these incidents occurred to health science students. Further, Turner et al. calculated the "attack rate" for health care workers and health science students at their institution. Using either Osborn's or Turner's data, it is estimated that it would take approximately 140 years for a single seroconversion to occur in a health science student and, with antiviral PEP, one seroconversion should occur only every 700 years.

Exposures reported are predominantly percutaneous, presumably because of the known higher risk and the need for access to PEP. Cutaneous and mucocutaneous exposures are reported by post-exposure surveys of populations at risk, but seroconversion is rarely reported.[52] Nonetheless, these low-risk data do not preclude HIV infections of students occurring at any time. In addition, although the risk of hepatitis B infection following an occupational exposure is nearly 100 percent preventable by pre-exposure immunization, recent studies suggest that health care workers in general and, specifically, some health science students are less than 100 percent compliant.[25] Thus, effective prevention programs and efficient post-exposure services for all types of exposures must be maintained. Student health services whose responsibilities include occupational health for the employees and/or faculty of the medical center have a distinct advantage in providing the services needed to health science students.[41]

Another dimension of a program for students at risk for chronic infection with HIV or hepatitis virus, B or C, is the management and counseling of the infected health science student. Carrier status of hepatitis B or C can be treated, reducing morbidity and mortality from chronic infection, as well as reducing infectivity of such students.[35] Since 1991, when the CDC published recommendations for preventing patient infections by infected health care workers, careful surveillance has demonstrated that the risk to patients is extremely low.[53] Yet, procedural, ethical, and institutional priorities are often unclear and in conflict when faced with the issue of the health science student who contracts a bloodborne pathogen infection. Until recently there were no clear policy guidelines in the United States for institutions to follow for students (nor are there yet clear guidelines for fully trained health care workers). A conference at the University of Kentucky Medical Center in November 2000 addressed the medical, legal, and ethical aspects of this problem and reached a consensus from which specific, clear recommendations for the student who is infected with a bloodborne pathogen were developed.[54]

PEP for HIV exposure through sexual and IV drug use has been proposed.[55] New York State provides a protocol of PEP for cases of sexual assault. However, attempts to balance cost and toxicity against the frequent uncertainty of the health status of the source and the risk assessment of the exposure make the decision to treat difficult. Few have adopted protocols and policies regarding students eligible for such treatment, except perhaps in cases of involuntary exposures by known HIV-positive persons (assault, rape and injury) or of cases of inadvertent exposure during sexual contact. Most troubling is the lack of efficacy data, despite obvious rationale, and, therefore, the high risk/benefit and cost/benefit ratios.[56]

ACCESS TO PRIMARY AND EMERGENCY CARE

While there are not major differences between health science students and other students in relation to their general health care needs or needs for emergency care, a few comments are important. Certain barriers to obtaining health care exist for health science students, particularly medical students, which do not apply to others. These may include time constraints, geography (i.e., remote clinical assignments), denial of health concerns, lack of available insurance, costs, privacy concerns and, particularly unique to this setting, alternative sources of health care ("hallway medicine"). Thus, a health service that deals with the unique needs of health science students must consider each of these when establishing policies and procedures that relate to health science student care.

The perception of lack of privacy and confidentiality remains an issue of great concern among health science students. The major areas of concern focus upon, first, the relationship of the health service personnel to the academic faculty and administrative staff of schools/programs and, second, the protection of psychiatric data. Adoption, publication and strict adherence to policies regarding the separation of a student's *personal* health care from the academic arena are essential.

Health science students require and demand a disproportionately greater number of services than do other students. Although no systematic studies have been published, the author has presented data at American College Health Association and Association of American Medical Colleges meetings characterizing health science students' patterns of utilization of health services .[57,58,59,60,61,62] High utilization rates are a constant, varying little from year to year despite a 30 percent annual turnover of students. Significantly different patterns of use between men and women are also consistently observed. Women visit the health service more frequently and require a greater number of laboratory studies and medications. Even when diagnostic codes referable to female reproductive issues/organs are excluded from the analysis, these differences persist. For example, in 1998 at the author's institution, women constituted 59 percent of the enrollment but accounted for 68 percent of the labs, 73 percent of the medications and 64 percent of the referrals. Although these data may not be representative, they do point out that patterns of health care use by health science students must be considered when programs are designed.

Finally, one very important issue in delivering health care to health science students requires mention. The student with an infectious disease poses a public health concern to individuals whose health may already be compromised, particularly those immunosuppressed. Therefore, any treatment and recommended course of action must include counseling, education and, at times, furlough for students from clinical contact.

MENTAL HEALTH CARE

Traditionally, it has been assumed that the curriculum for health science students is their major stressor while in school. There is no question that the curriculum does influence the students' response to their own illnesses. The reality is, however, that difficulties in school represent only a small fraction of the reasons why health science students seek psychiatric care. The incidence of suicide has been well documented amongst certain health professionals to be higher than the norm and prevention thereof has traditionally been one of the major goals of mental health services for health science students. However, some published reports have not documented a higher than expected rate for medical students.[63] Only anecdotal information is available for students in dental, nursing, and other health professions.

Few published articles about the impact of stress management interventions upon medical personnel have used rigorous methodology despite promising results reported in a number of limited studies.[64] A longitudinal study from Manchester University, England, measured "psychological distress" in a single medical class over five years.[65] Repeatedly high scores were found in a small group (18/172), suggesting that those who exhibit distress throughout school may be at high risk for emotional disturbances in later training. There were no gender differences in this study. However, a large Canadian study[66] comparing medical students, residents, and graduate science students demonstrated higher stress scores in women for all three groups, but, interestingly, a beneficial effect of stress was self-reported in each category and, overall, the level of stress was low. A Hong Kong study of academic performance documented a correlation between higher stress levels and poor performance.[67] In addition, the data led the authors to propose that coping with stress correlated with improved performance. Taken together, these and other studies suggest that stress may play both positive and negative roles, with both high stress levels and adequate stress management being important predictors for, respectively, negative or positive performance.

Depression in medical students has also been studied and found to increase above the expected incidence during progression through school, with women exhibiting significantly greater increases.[68] The amount of both stress and depression was lower in medical students than in law or graduate science students, but both increased after transition to clinical training.[69] However, stress did not correlate with depression in medical students.[70]

The single most serious threat to students in the usual age group of health science students is posed by psychological illness, specifically distortions of development and personality and the relevant spectrum of psychiatric syndromes. The data reported in epidemiological studies of the prevalence of illness, type of illnesses, gender distribution and barriers to care[71,72] are reflected in the experiences at the author's own institution. Further, at the same university, student health service psychiatric utilization rate is 14 percent, having increased gradually from 10 percent in 1990. More specifically, the utilization rate of medical students has been stable at about 19 percent, for nursing students at 23 percent and at 4 percent for dental students. Twenty-five percent of the students who consult the psychiatric service have had a previous mental health consultation, usually in their mid-teens or their college years. For all health science schools, women tend to be higher utilizers of the psychiatric student health service than their male counterparts, with 72 percent of visits by women as opposed to 28 percent by men. These gender differences have been stable over the years.

Psychiatric services are underutilized by certain students. Ethnicity and race clearly affect the consultation rate. Again, at the author's institution, 80 percent of the consulting students are Caucasians, less than 20 percent are Asians, and African Americans and Hispanics together represent less than 7 percent. The dental school and the Graduate School of Arts & Science have a much higher proportion of Asian students than the proportion of Asian students who consult the psychiatric service, suggesting a barrier in utilization of psychiatric health services for this group. Hispanic students are also noted to underutilize the psychiatric service, while African American students consult in proportion to their student body representation. Psychological symptoms (60 percent), interpersonal difficulties (61 percent), and academic problems (22 percent) are the most common motives for students' initial consultations. In spite of the intense immersion in the curriculum, the primary focus for the presenting complaints of most medical students is in the context of the problem of human "closeness." Concern and conflict about education and work seem to be swept aside by these issues, although first-year students have greater uncertainty early on about meeting educational standards. Their primary complaints are almost always related to aspects of their romantic involvements. Depression, both major and minor, is common, as well as a wide range of anxiety disorders. The distribution of diagnoses has been remarkably stable, with mood disorders at 41 percent, anxiety disorders 20 percent, and adjustment disorders 17 percent.

A student mental health service performs a dual function. The manifest aspect of the work is, of course, the delivery of high-quality clinical care. However, because student-patients are, themselves, learning how to take care of patients, not just of themselves, counseling takes on a significant additional dimension, having to do with the modeling effect on the students; i.e., the counselor becomes the role model with whom the student can identify. It is precisely because of this mechanism of identification, especially at this time in these students' lives, that health service physicians and mental health clinicians play a role that is not only clinical in the ordinary sense of the word but to a significant degree a part of the educational process itself.[73]

Health science curricula shape students' professional development with the expectation that it will lead them to become "humanistic physicians" (in the case of medical students) who have an ideal of altruistic patient care.[74] However, our actual clinical experience is that the unfolding of this stressful process may produce feelings which affect or are antithetical to that ideal and therefore threaten to interfere with this goal. In fact, the conflicts arising from these disturbing psychological motivations are often an important component in the issues that bring students to treatment.[75,76] Helping students resolve these conflicts brings together the dual functions of the student mental health service; i.e., the therapeutic and educational dimensions of the work done by college health clinicians.

BENCHMARKS

Utilization data from most student health services at academic medical centers demonstrate high rates of use by medical, dental and nursing students. Data from the American College Health Association's Advisory Committee on Benchmarking illustrate the differences between the aggregate data from the 221 participating schools and those data available for health science students at the author's institution.[77] While it is not known how many respondents to the ACHA survey included data from health science students, seven benchmarks are comparable:

1. Percent of students "who were users" in the benchmark survey averaged approximately 55.1 percent of enrolled students, with the mean number of annual visits of 1.8 "per total student enrollment"; comparable figures for the author's institution for health science students are 91 percent utilization, with a mean number of visits per enrolled student of 6.8.
2. The "student patient visits per FTE health care provider" benchmarked at a mean of 2,222 as compared to 3,425 from the author's university.
3. The "number of students per FTE mental health provider" in the author's school is less than 400, the "minimum" level observed in the benchmark survey.
4. The average "percentage of female students who received a Pap smear" in the reported benchmark study was 12.9 percent, as compared to 60 percent; the author believes this reflects the high rate of contraceptive use requiring annual exams amongst health science students.
5. MMR compliance was found to be similar to the benchmark schools.
6. Hepatitis B immunity and/or immunization with hepatitis B vaccine in academic medical centers is generally greater than 90 percent; benchmark data varied between 11.2 percent and 37.8 percent.
7. 100 percent of international students with clinical contacts at the author's institution have current tuberculin testing as opposed to a much lower number in benchmark schools.

There is no question that higher numbers on most of the benchmarks noted above reflect the fact that compliance for certain of these is required in order to participate in a health care setting. In addition, the process of ascertaining appropriate immunizations and testing increases the number of visits made by health science students. Indeed, many of the unique issues previously discussed in this text likely account for increased health utilization by health science students. While specific documentation and more detailed data benchmarking are not available, it is important to emphasize that, whatever the reasons, it is clear that it is considerably more costly per student served to operate a health service for health science students than for students not involved in the healing arts.

CONCLUDING OBSERVATIONS

This chapter has presented discussion on those special issues which arise in the care of health science students. The contiguity of the health care setting to the academic program of these students presents service requirements that differ from those provided for other students. Not only are policies and procedures different, but in some cases the organizational structure of the health service may need to be modified to accommodate these services. It is inescapable that the overall cost per student of these services is higher than the average cost per student not in health science. Unless it is appropriate that health care of health science students be subsidized by other students or by the university, a broad-based method for financing must be implemented.

A focus upon health science students' unique clinical and administrative needs will require collaboration between individual health services and universities, the ACHA and national academic organizations (e.g., the Association of American Medical Colleges, the American Dental Education Association and others) with those establishing standards for prevention and treatment of health risks in students, e.g., CDC. Also required are adequate technological and conceptual frameworks for data management embodied in medical informatics. Stable funding sources for health science students' programs of services are not always available through individual institutions and, increasingly, it is more difficult for costs to be borne by individual students. Thus a broad-based insurance program designed for health science students or at least a partially self-funded program may be useful.

The management paradigm for a health service program that requires 100 percent of students to utilize health service facilities must be that of "managing care"; i.e., the health service must be the primary care provider for all clinical and preventive services. To accomplish this, six critical factors are essential:

1. university cooperation
2. close interaction of the health service staff with the medical community
3. providers who are both competent in primary care and also knowledgeable about the available specialty care
4. detailed utilization data, both historical and current, available in real time
5. financial management which allows at least the standard of care reflected in the local medical community
6. effective clinical and financial procedures for care out-of-area; i.e., sites where health service contracts and university policies do not exist

Clearly, there are both advantages and disadvantages to this paradigm of "managing" student health care. Advantages include, among others, responsibility and autonomy for student health policies and procedures; confidentiality and privacy for medical records; internal control ensuring accurate student enrollment, fee payment and utilization reviews; and direct involvement of students in the process of service evaluation, cost and revision. Conversely, disadvantages are related primarily to the increased expertise required of the staff to manage these programs and, as in any managed care program, to cost constraints which might potentially restrict access to, and quality of, services. Specific concerns include the complexity of local management procedures, particularly for a given institution; breadth of experience in health care management, budgeting and accounting required for staff; required access to care only through the student health service; and complex payment procedures for out-of-area care.

Articulation of the principles upon which the service is structured yields a series of quality assurance indicators by which effective clinical services can be measured, costs analyzed and programs improved. The most important principle is to obtain data that accurately describe what we do. The basic principles can be summarized:

*   enrollment procedures must be simple and accurate, contain complete demographic in-

formation and be available to providers through an internal, computerized information system

- access to information and care must be available 24 hours a day, 7 days a week
- a convenient facility must be available for easy access to care and must include educational materials regarding services and procedures
- access to primary care must be timely, appropriate, complete and coordinated with students' total health status
- ancillary data must be accurate, complete, accessible as needed, and integrated with all other clinical data
- specialty care must be accessible as needed, appropriate to the specific patient problem, and integrated with students' primary care
- procedures for approval, coordination, and negotiation of payment for care outside the health science campus must insure costs no greater than those *within,* if at all possible
- patient care data should be maintained in a medical record format, paper and/or electronic, which is easily available to those providing clinical care and to those performing utilization analysis
- direct access to a psychiatric service, structured to permit prompt appointments, maximum privacy and confidentiality, and appropriate duration of treatment without excessive costs
- integration of health risk surveillance, maintenance and education with ongoing primary care
- availability and access to health care resources within the university system
- patient care encounters viewed by students as timely, accurate, appropriate, sensitive and comfortable
- treatment plans including, where applicable, mechanisms to prevent transmission of disease from student to patient

Structuring a health service to respond to these principles may not be practical or easily achieved in all universities. However, such an effort will not only assure excellence in clinical care but will also enable us to examine more critically the outcomes of our efforts with these students who will become tomorrow's health care providers. As has often been stated by Dr. Margaret Bridwell of Maryland, "If we do our job correctly with health science students, we could change the face and quality of modern American medicine."[78] Agreeing, we must focus our efforts to meet the challenge of that presumption.

REFERENCES

1. Garrison, FH in "An Introduction to the History of Medicine", 4th Edition, WB Saunders, Phila, 1966, pp. 435-43.

2. Occupational Safety and Health Administration. Occupational exposures to blood borne pathogens: Final rule. Federal Reporter. 1991; 56: 4004-4183.

3. Pierog MB. Graduate Health Insurance: Why Graduate Students are Different from Undergraduates. Student Health Spectrum 2000; 4(1): 7-8.

4. Henning K. Ey S. Shaw D. Perfectionism, the imposter phenomenon and psychological adjustment in medical, dental, nursing and pharmacy students. Med Educ. 1998; 32(5): 456-464.

5. O'Connor PG. Spickard A Jr. Physician impairment by substance abuse. Med Clin North Am. 1997; 81(4): 1037-1052.

6. Hembree WC. Unique Health Care Needs of Health Sciences Students in "Principles and Practice of Student Health" Vol 3 College Health, Chapter 26. Third Party Publishing Co., Oakland CA, 1993; pp. 808-819.

7. Barzaksky B. Jones HS. Etzel SI. Educational Programs in US Medical Schools, 1999-2000. JAMA 2000; 284(9): 1114-1158.

8. American Association of Dental Schools. Admission Requirements of US and Canadian Dental Schools: Entering Class of 2001. 2000; 38th Edition: 6-22.

9. The American Occupational Therapy Association. OT Programs Accredited by the Accreditation Council for Occupational Therapy Education (ACOTE). September, 2000.

10. American Association of Nursing Education. Nursing School Academic Programs. 2000; 1-69.

11. American Physical Therapy Association. Accredited Programs for the Physical Therapist. 2000; 1-24.

12. AAMC Executive Council. Association of American Medical Colleges' Recommendations Regarding Health Services for Medical Students. June, 1992.

13. Patrick K. Student Health. Medical Care Within Institutions of Higher Education. JAMA 1988; 260: 3301-3305.

14. New York State Immunization Update, New York State Department of Health, Summer 2000, 1-11.

15. ACHA Guidelines. Recommendations for Institutional Prematriculation Immunizations. January 2000.

16. CDC. Measles, Mumps, and Rubella – Vaccine Use and Strategies for Elimination of Measles, Rubella, and Congenital Rubella Syndrome and Control of Mumps: Recommendations of the Advisory Committee on Immunization Practices (ACIP). MMWR. 1998; 47(RR-8): 1-50.

17. CDC. Hepatitis B Virus: a comprehensive strategy for eliminating transmission in the United States through universal childhood vaccination: recommendations of the Immunization Practices Advisory Committee (ACIP). MMWR 1991; 40 (No. RR-13): 1-38.

18. CDC. Prevention of Varicella: Recommendations of the Advisory Committee on Immunization Practices (ACIP). MMWR. 1996; 45(RR11): 1-25.

19. CDC. Core Curriculum in Tuberculosis. What the Clinical Should Know. 4th Edition, 2000.

20. CDC. Immunization of Health Care Workers. Recommendations of the Advisory Committee on Immunization Practices (ACIP) and the Hospital Infection Control Practices Advisory Committee (HICPAC) MMWR 1997; 46(RR-16): 1-42.

21. CDC. Immunizations of Adolescents. Recommendations of the Advisory Committee on Immunization Practices, the American Academy of Family Physicians, and the American Medical Association. MMWR 1996; 45(RR-13): 1-15.

22. AMA. Council on Scientific Affairs. Chemoprophylaxis for Health Care Workers and Medical Students. CSA Report 18 – A-99, pp. 1-12.

23. CDC. Public Health Service Guidelines for the Management of Health-Care Worker Exposure to HIV and Recommendations for Postexposure Prophylaxis, MMWR 1998; 47(RR-7): 1-28.

24. ACHA. Vaccine Preventable Disease January 2000 Institutional Prematriculation Immunization Policy Survey. Minutes VPDTF, June 2000.

25. Marinho RT. Moura MC. Pedro M. Ramalho FJ. Velosa JF. Hepatitis B vaccination in hospital personnel and medical students. J Clin Gastroenterol. 1999; 28(4): 317-322

26. Diekema DJ. Ferguson KJ. Doebbeling BN. Motivation for hepatitis B vaccine acceptance among medical and physician assistant students. J Gen Intern Med. 1995; 10(1): 1-6.

27. Marinho RT. Ramalho F. Velosa J. Low response to hepatitis B vaccine in health care workers and medical students in Lisbon, Portugal. Hepatology. 1998; 28(4): 1166.

28. CDC. Prevention and Control of Influenza. Recommendations of the Advisory Committee on Immunization Practices (ACIP). MMWR 1998; 47(RR-6): 1-33.

29. CDC. Recommendations for Prevention and Control of Tuberculosis Among Foreign-Born Persons. Report of the Working Group on Tuberculosis Among Foreign-Born Persons. MMWR 1998; 47(RR-16): 1-18.

30. CDC. Prevention of Hepatitis A Through Active or Passive Immunization: Recommendations of the Advisory Committee on Immunization Practices (ACIP). MMWR. 1999; 48(RR12): 1-37.

31. CDC. Prevention and Control of Meningococcal Disease and Meningococcal Disease and College Students. MMWR 2000; 49(RR-7): 1-20.

32. CDC. Poliomyelitis Prevention in the United States. Updated Recommendations of the Advisory Committee on Immunization Practices (ACIP). MMWR. 2000; 49(RR-5): 1-22.

33. CDC. Recommendations for Prevention of HIV Transmission in Health-Care Settings. MMWR 1987; 36(SU02): 1-16.

34. CDC. Public Health Service statement on management of occupational exposure to human immuno-deficiency virus, including considerations regarding zidovudine postexposure use. MMWR 1990; 39 (RR-1), 1-9.

35. CDC. Recommendations for Prevention and Control of Hepatitis C Virus (HCV) Infection and HCV-Related Chronic Disease. MMWR 1998; 47(RR-19): 1-39.

36. CDC Pamphlet. Exposure to Blood. What Health Care Workers Need to Know. P.1-8.

37. Henderson DK, Fahey, BJ, Willy M, Schmitt JM, Carey K, Kosiol DE, Lane HC, Fedio J, Saah AJ. Risk for Occupational Transmission of Human Immunodeficiency Virus Type 1 (HIV-1) Associated with Clinical Exposures. A Prospective Evaluation. Ann Int Med 1990; 113: 740-746.

38. Mangione CM, Gerberding JL, Cummings SR. Occupational Exposure to HIV: Frequency and Rates of Underreporting of Percutaneous and Mucocutaneous Exposures by Medical Housestaff. Am J Med 1991; 90: 85-90.

39. Jagger J, Hung EH, Brand-Elnaggar J, Pearson RD. Rates of Needle-Stick Injury Caused by Various Devices in a University Hospital. N Engl J Med 1988; 319: 284-288.

40. Fahey BJ, Koziol DE, Banks SM, Henderson DK. Frequency of Nonparenteral Occupational Exposures to Blood and Body Fluids Before and After Universal Precautions Training. Am J Med 1991; 90: 145-153.

41. Turner HS. Hurley JL. Butler KM. Holl J. Accidental exposures to blood and other body fluids in a large academic medical center. J Am Coll Health. 1999; 47(5): 199-206.

42. Sepkowitz KA. Occupational Acquired Infection in Health Care Workers. Part I. Ann Intern Med. 1996; 125: 826-834.

43. Sepkowitz KA. Occupationally Acquired Infections in Health Care Workers. Part II. Ann Intern Med. 1996; 125: 917-928.

44. Hembree, WC. Report of Health Sciences Students Task Force, ACHA, 1996.

45. Ganguly R, Holt DA, Sinnott JT. Exposure of Medical Students to Body Fluids. J Am Coll Health 1999; 47: 207-210.

46. Mercer/Foster Higgins. National Survey of Employer Sponsored Health Plans. February 2000.

47. Henderson DK. Postexposure Chemoprophylaxis for Occupational Exposures to the Human Immu-nodeficiency Virus. JAMA 1999; 281: 931-936.

48. Gerberding JL. Prophylaxis for Occupational Exposure to HIV. Ann Int Med 1996; 125: 497-501.

49. CDC. Surveillance of Health are Workers with HIV/AIDS. 2000. www.cdc.gov/hiv/pubs/facts/hcwsurv.html

50. CDC. Notice to Readers HIV Postexposure Prophylais Registry Closing. MMWR 1999; 48(09): 194-195.

51. Osborn EH. Papadakis MA. Gerberding JL. Occupational exposures to body fluids among medical students. A seven-year longitudinal study. Ann Intern Med. 1999; 130(1): 45-51.

52. CDC. Case-Control Study of HIV Seroconversion in Health Care Workers After Percutaneous Expo-sure to HIV-infected Blood – France, United Kingdom and United States, January 1988-August 1994. MMWR 1995; 44(50): 929-933.

53. AIDS/TB Committee of the Society for Healthcare Epidemiology of American (SHEA Position Pa-per). Management of Healthcare Workers Infected with Hepatitis B Virus, Hepatitis C Virus, Human Immu-nodeficiency Virus, or Other Bloodborne Pathogens. Infect Control Hosp Epidemiol 1997; 18: 349-363.

54. Members of the Student Health Services at Academic Medical Centers Task Force. Blood-Borne Pathogen Disease in Health Science Students: Recommendations from the Lexington Conference, Novem-ber 6–7, 2000. J Am Coll Health. 2001; 50-3: 107–120.

55. CDC. Management of Possible Sexual, Injecting-Drug-Use, or Other Nonoccupational Exposure to HIV, Including Considerations Related to Antiretroviral Therapy. MMWR 1998 47(RR-17): 1-11.

56. Lurie P, Miller S, Hecht F, Chesney M, Lo B. Postexposure Prophylaxis after Nonoccupational HIV Exposure. Clinical, Ethical and Policy Considerations. JAMA. 1998; 280: 1769-1773.

57. Hembree WC. Task Force of Health Sciences Students: Health Care Essentials for Health Sciences Students. American College Health Association Annual Meeting, Orlando FL, May 1996.

58. Clark KH, Clark AS, Hembree, WC. Analysis of Health Care Assisted by a Microcomputer. AAMSI 1983; 2: 129.

59. Hembree WC, Clark AS, Clark KH. Microcomputer-assisted utilization analysis: Changing Patterns of Health Care in a Health Sciences Student Health Program. SCAMC 1985; 6: 343.

60. Hembree WC, Gerberding AJ, Barnes M, Ferentz K. HIV Issues with Health Sciences Students. American College Health Association Annual Meeting. San Francisco CA, May, 1992.

61. Hembree WC. Just How Dangerous is the Study of Medicine to Today's Medical Student? Association of American Medical Colleges Annual Meeting, Washington DC, November, 1993.

62. Hembree WC. Self Funding. The Student Health Service Answer to Managed Care. American College Health Association Annual Meeting. 1998.

63. Hays LR. Cheever T. Patel P. Medical student suicide, 1989-1994. Am J Psychiatry. 1996; 153(4): 553-555.

64. Shapiro SL, Shapiro DE, Schwartz GER. Stress Management in Medical Education: A Review of the Literature. Acad Med 2000; 75: 748-759.

65. Guthrie E. Black D. Bagalkote H. Shaw C. Campbell M. Creed F. Psychological stress and burnout in medical students: a five-year prospective longitudinal study. J Roy Soc Med. 1998; 91(5): 237-243.

66. Toews JA. Lockyer JM. Dobson DJ. Simpson E. Brownell AK. Brenneis F. MacPherson KM. Cohen GS. Analysis of stress levels among medical students, residents, and graduate students at four Canadian schools of medicine. Acad Med. 1997; 72(11): 997-1002.

67. Stewart SM. Lam TH. Betson CL. Wong CM. Wong AM. A prospective analysis of stress and academic performance in the first two years of medical school. Med Educ. 1999; 33(4): 243-250.

68. Rosal MC. Ockene IS. Ockene JK. Barrett SV. Ma Y. Hebert JR. A longitudinal study of students' depression at one medical school. Acad Med. 1997; 72(6): 542-546.

69. Helmers KF. Danoff D. Steinert Y. Leyton M. Young SN. Stress and depressed mood in medical students, law students, and graduate students at McGill University. Acad Med. 1997; 72(8): 708-714.

70. Bramness JG. Fixdal TC. Vaglum P. Effect of medical school stress on the mental health of medical students in early and late clinical curriculum. Acta Psychiatr Scand. 1991; 84(4): 340-345.

71. Regier DA, Boyd JH, Burke Jr. JD, et al. One-month Prevalence of Mental Disorders in the United States Based on Five Epidemiologic Catchment Area Sites. Arch Gen Psychiatry 1998; 45: 977-986.

72. Kesslet RC, McGonagle KA, Zhao S, Nelson CB, Hughes CB, Eshleman S, Witchen HU, Kendler KS. Lifetime and 12-month Prevalence of DSM-III-R Psychiatric Disorders in the United States: Results from the National Comorbidity Survey. Arch Gen Psychiatry 1994;51: 8-10.

73. Freud S. The Ego and the Id. S.E., Volume XIX: 28-40.

74. Medical School Objectives Project (MSOP), http://wwww.aamc.org.

75. Lerner BA. Students' use of psychiatric services: the Columbia experience. JAMA. 1995; 274(17): 1398-1389.

76. Golinger RC. Reasons that medical students seek psychiatric assistance. Acad Med. 1991; 66(2): 121-122.

77. American College Health Association. 1998-1999 Benchmarking Datashare I. Overall Survey Results. Pp 1-26.

78. Bridwell M. Director, Student Health Service, University of Maryland, College Park, MD. Personal Communication.

CHAPTER 13

HEALTH CARE ISSUES
FOR THE INTERNATIONAL STUDENT

General Cultural Considerations
Mary Alice Serafini, MA, and Pornthip Chalungsooth, EdD, LCP

Medical Considerations
Christopher A. Sanford, MD, DTMH, and Elaine C. Jong, MD

GENERAL CULTURAL CONSIDERATIONS

The diversity of the student population in colleges and universities offers extraordinary opportunities and challenges to a student health service. International students represent a large group of diverse students encompassing special characteristics and exhibiting special needs. These students come to colleges and universities with a variety of backgrounds and experiences. The health provider's constant challenge is to recognize the uniqueness of each student patient and to develop a knowledge base of cultural information, which will allow successful interventions, diagnoses, and treatments.

THE POPULATION

During academic year 1999-2000, 465,002 international students studied in the United States.[1] Of this population, well over 50 percent of the students were from Asian countries, and significant numbers of students were from Europe, Central and South America, and Africa. The provision of health care services to students from these diverse areas of the world requires an appreciation and some understanding of the contrasts between the student's home culture and Western culture in their respective approaches to health and health care. These contrasts involve different socioeconomic backgrounds and educational experiences, differing approaches to religion, rural versus urban community experiences, as well as a variety of public and private health care systems and a variety (by Western standards) of traditional and non-traditional practitioners. In addition to these medical/sociological differences, unique psychological stresses affecting the lives of foreign students who choose to study in the United States must often be addressed during their encounters with health care personnel.

SOCIOECONOMIC ISSUES

On any college campus international students include those from very wealthy families to those from the poorest of circumstances. Some will have earned their way to the United States through outstanding scholarship, while others will be totally or partially funded by their families. Some students will use the stipends given for study in the United States to support their families at home as well as to support their own needs, while others may live comfortably with automobiles, apartments, and resources for active social lives. Many students from developing countries are skilled at subsistence living, a behavior that follows them to the United States. Other students, from fully developed countries, find the United States simply another life experience with a few variations from their home countries.

The educational backgrounds of the families of international students are as varied as the backgrounds of domestic students. While many are "first generation" students, others come from well-educated families with high expectations for success. Many of the latter are of elevated socioeconomic status in their home country and experience high personal regard in their home country's hierarchical structure; these students may be frustrated to discover their status in their home country makes no difference in their treatment on campus, in general, or by the student health service, specifically.

Finally, as has been true since the end of World War II when the number of international students coming to the United States to study began to increase, political and economic changes in the home country often impact the student studying in the United States. Destabilization of the currency of the government that is helping the student with financial support is a good example.

COMMUNITIES

International students, like their American counterparts, come from very rural to very urban living environments. Some are cosmopolitan, expecting all the advantages and lifestyles of urban life, while a campus of 15,000 in a small midwestern town may overwhelm others. Students also come from very close, collective communities or very individualistic communities. The variations in services and entertainment, the temporary loss of the home community, the loss of a familiar religious community, the loss of extended family, and above all, the loss of a social group can lead to significant mental and emotional stresses. While residence halls can provide an "instant community," international students may fail to appreciate the inherent support structure of on-campus housing; much depends upon the student's prior living circumstances.

HEALTH CARE SYSTEMS

Whether entering students are 18 years old, attending college for the first time, or older graduate students, they have some basic knowledge of health issues. While they are likely to be knowledgeable to some extent about their home country's health care system, they may be perceived as ignorant of health care by clinicians in the U.S. College health care providers must listen and learn about the student's health care perspective, which may be based on their traditional protocols, their high respect for the authority of a physician, and little or no knowledge of the value and skills of nurses, allied health care providers, or health educators. An international student may not be well prepared for a discussion which includes the collaborative decision-making that is typically afforded by college health care providers. Questions about treatment, medications, returning for follow-up care, home care, and the actual seriousness of an illness may be a new concept and, therefore, require a foreign student to develop a new set of skills to understand these issues. Often a student may experience disappointment with the United States health care system (often perceived by foreign students as the best in the world) when his/her expectations are not met.

Government subsidized health care is a reality in most countries of the world except the United States. Thus, accessing and using health care in the United States requires planning by the international student. Students must learn how to use an insurance plan (what is covered or not covered, deductibles and co-pays, how to file for benefits), when to use an ambulance, when (and when not) to access an emergency room, and when to use the college health service with its primary medical care, counseling and psychological services, and health education services. Particularly, they must learn to understand the economic savings that come from using the college health services as compared with using extramural facilities.

PSYCHOLOGICAL ISSUES

Health care providers must be alert for homesickness, isolation, alienation, and poor sleep patterns. Unfulfilled expectations and poor understanding of health care treatment may lead to difficulties in care management, lack of cooperation in treatment, and hopelessness regarding the healing process, all impeding full recovery. While these are issues for any student, they may be more serious for the international student, who is not only away from family and friends, but is also dealing with a new culture.

Psychological distress may create exaggeration and magnification of an illness. Psychological stresses may also be produced by perceptions (or the reality) of not being understood verbally or culturally, of distance or discrimination, or of invasion of "personal territory" by what may be viewed as only routine medical history taking or physical examination by a clinician.

Conversely, many international students share a common characteristic of being slightly more risk-taking than their peers, typified by having made a conscious decision to leave that which is familiar to live and to learn in an unfamiliar environment. This is a positive attribute that nurtures the quest for adventure, leads to opportunities, and may in fact be psychologically protective.

POTENTIAL RISK FACTORS

International students (as well as many domestic students) may suffer unnecessarily from an illness or injury because of inadequate knowledge about caring for oneself, particularly while studying in an alien environment. Further, health care providers may make an erroneous diagnosis or establish an erroneous treatment plan for students because of a misunderstanding through language or cultural differences between the provider and the student.

Several approaches may help to minimize these risk factors. These include:

- Providing educational programs regarding health care in the United States for international students before they enter the American educational system
- Providing staff training programs regarding transcultural issues and health care for campus health service personnel
- Offering consultation to providers with specific information on different cultural attributes
- Creating support groups for foreign and international students on health care topics such as stress reduction, time management, cross-cultural relationships, and dating
- Providing educational programs for staff in international program offices and teaching them how to appropriately refer students for physical or mental health care
- Recruiting a diverse health service staff

MEDICAL CONSIDERATIONS

MEDICAL ISSUES

The provision of health care to international students requires not only consideration of the usual common etiologies for illnesses found among peers of comparable age and gender in the host country but familiarity with the disease entities found in the international student's country of origin. Depending on prior access to health care and health care resources in the country of origin, newly arrived students may be susceptible to common vaccine-preventable diseases, or may have previously undiagnosed health conditions which may become manifest during their years of study in the United States. Thus, in addition to the usual "MASH" format used to elicit the patient's past medical history (medications, allergies, surgeries, hospitalizations), risk factors pertinent to a geographic medicine approach must be identified. Providers may need to inquire about living conditions in the country of origin: urban or rural, temperate or tropical, altitude, potable water sources and sanitation systems, predominant form of livelihood, and diseases or health problems commonly observed in the home community. Exposure to farm animals, proximity to bodies of fresh water, and dietary habits may also be pertinent. For example, some diseases are remarkably focal in their distribution (such as Bartonellosis, a bacterial disease that is found only in Peru, Ecuador, and Columbia in Andean valleys between 500 and 3200 meters), while others, such as tuberculosis and giardiasis, have worldwide distributions. (While details on specific tropical and imported diseases can be found in standard textbooks,[2,3,4] a useful resource for clinics that provide care to international students is the computer program "Gideon" [Global Infectious Diseases and Epidemiology Network, http://www.cyinfo.com].[5]) In addition, the immunization history of an international student may be difficult to interpret because of variations in generic and trade names for vaccines, vaccine availability in foreign countries, and language barriers with immunization reports.

It is not the intent of this discussion on unusual clinical syndromes seen in international students to be all-inclusive (discussions of specific diseases can be found in many excellent tropical medicine and infectious disease references). Rather, the information is presented in a manner which is more nearly akin to the presentation of an international student to an American university and to its health requirements and systems. The first interaction between these students and a student health service is commonly through immunization requirements, tuberculin testing, and in certain circumstances, chest X-rays. Thus, this material is briefly discussed first. The next point of contact usually involves visits related to illness, and the discussion in this text is designed to create awareness of common presenting symptoms which may reflect uncommon diseases and to alert the reader to these possibilities and, thus, the need to maintain a high index of suspicion for extraordinary diagnoses.

VACCINE-PREVENTABLE COMMUNICABLE ILLNESSES

Measles Vaccine

Documentation of two doses of measles vaccine or measles immunity is currently required for entry into many American colleges. Although measles is commonly given as a combination vaccine with mumps and rubella (MMR) in the United States, international students may have received only a monovalent measles vaccine, and thus may benefit from re-immunization with MMR.

Varicella Vaccine

Chickenpox (varicella) is usually a disease of childhood in the U.S. and other developed countries in temperate climate zones. However, the age of peak transmission of chickenpox is delayed until early adulthood among persons from tropical developing countries.[6] Thus, international students may be susceptible to varicella and could benefit from varicella immunization.

Hepatitis B Vaccine

Primary immunization with hepatitis B vaccine has been incorporated into the schedule of routine childhood immunizations in many countries. However, students from countries where hepatitis B is highly endemic and who were born before hepatitis B vaccine became widely available, may have a disproportionate risk for chronic hepatitis B infections (see section in this chapter on bloodborne pathogen infections). Completion of hepatitis B immunization followed by confirmation of protective levels of hepatitis B antibody is now an occupational health standard for health care workers in the United States. Health sciences students with asymptomatic chronic hepatitis B infections are, with increasing frequency, being detected by testing for hepatitis B antigens and antibodies when post-immunization testing shows a lack of protective hepatitis B antibodies.[7] Health sciences students born in areas highly endemic for hepatitis B who are shown to be hepatitis B surface antigen positive (particularly those that are hepatitis B e-antigen positive) may find limitation in their clinical training in the U.S., which may necessitate changes in career pathways. While most colleges and universities provide information on this issue to health sciences students before enrollment, international students may not receive the information in a timely manner or fully comprehend the implications of this policy.

Meningococcal Vaccine

Recent studies have shown that U.S. college freshmen living in residence halls have a higher risk of contracting meningococcal disease than other students.[8] Because of this increased risk, the American College Health Association (ACHA) and the Centers for Disease Control and Prevention (CDC) urge college students and their families to become informed about the meningococcal vaccine and consider immunization.[8] This recommendation may not be fully appreciated or understood by students coming from foreign countries.

The meningococcal vaccine available in the U.S. is a quadrivalent vaccine covering serogroups A, C, Y, and W-135, while abroad, a simpler A-plus-C vaccine is often the only available vaccine. Thus, even if there is a prior history of receiving the meningococcal vaccine, it may not be equivalent to the one used in the U.S. Newly arriving international students who will be living in residence halls need to be informed of the availability of meningococcal vaccine and offered immunization with the quadrivalent vaccine if they so desire and have not previously been immunized with this vaccine. Prior immunization with A-plus-C vaccine is not a contraindication to subsequent immunization with the quadrivalent vaccine.

TUBERCULOSIS SCREENING AND ABNORMAL CHEST X-RAYS

Tuberculosis Skin Tests

Tuberculosis (TB) is endemic in the developing world. It is estimated that between 19 percent and 43 percent of the world's population is infected with *Mycobacterium tuberculosis*; of those infected, 95 percent live in developing countries. While the number of reported cases of tuberculosis in the U.S. has declined steadily since 1992, the decrease has been limited to persons born in the U.S.[9,10,11]

A popular misconception among international students is that previous immunization with the BCG vaccine causes a positive PPD skin test for the remainder of the recipient's life, making PPD skin testing invalid and even contraindicated. In fact, BCG vaccine usually causes a positive PPD skin test only for four to five years in most recipients. And most importantly, PPD skin test reactivity following BCG vaccine does not correlate with degree of immune protection. Hence, a history of BCG vaccination in childhood is neither a barrier nor a contraindication to PPD skin test screening in adolescence and adulthood. If the PPD skin test is positive using standard criteria, the individual is considered at risk for having an active TB infection and needs appropriate further evaluation, treatment, and follow-up.[12,13]

If a chest radiograph is required for evaluation of an international student, the radiologist should be informed of the student's country of origin, since certain unusual (in the U.S.) disease processes may confuse X-ray interpretation. Paragonimiasis (infection with the lung fluke *Paragonimus westermani)* may present with chest X-ray findings that mimic tuberculosis. This entity should be high on the differential diagnosis of a patient with "tuberculosis" who fails to respond to an appropriate anti-tuberculosis regimen. Infection is acquired from ingesting the parasite in raw or undercooked crab or crayfish. The parasite may be acquired worldwide, but most infections in the U.S. are seen among persons from Southeast Asia. In patients from Southeast Asia, melioidosis, caused by the gram negative bacillus *Burkholderia* (formerly *Pseudomonas) pseudomallei* can cause chronic cavitary upper lobe lesions which may mimic tuberculosis. *B. pseudomallei* is a soil saprophyte endemic to this area, and is particularly prevalent in rice-growing regions. People raised on rice farms, and others exposed to soil (e.g., road construction crews) are at increased risk of infection. Most infections are asymptomatic and may remain latent for many years. The most common form of localized melioidosis is a subacute, cavitating pneumonia accompanied by profound weight loss. Activation of disease usually occurs at a time of decreased cellular immunity, such as another acute infection, trauma, malignancy, or diabetes.

A pulmonary echinococcal or hydatid cyst can be an unexpected finding on screening chest X-rays among people from any region of the world where humans live in close association with dogs and sheep. Humans become an accidental host when the parasite eggs are inadvertently ingested and the initial infection may have been subclinical and undiagnosed.

HEPATITIS

Hepatitis A

Hepatitis A virus infections are endemic in the developing world because of sanitary conditions which favor fecal-oral transmission. Most persons in developing countries display serologic evidence of past infection by the first decade of life. Infections in children are often sub-clinical; lifelong immunity results from natural infections. However, persons from higher socioeconomic backgrounds, even in areas where hepatitis A has a high rate of transmission, may still be susceptible to infection as young adults because of better sanitary conditions. This latter group of international students returning home to visit family and friends may contract hepatitis A during their trips unless they are immunized with hepatitis A vaccine or immune globulin.[25]

Hepatitis B

While the prevalence of hepatitis B is less than 0.5 percent in the U.S. and Europe,[14] it is over 10 percent in some regions of the Far East. In Asia about half of HBV transmission is vertical, between mother and infant. In sub-Saharan Africa and most other developing countries, heterosexual sex is the most common means of transmission. Acquisition of HBV from blood transfusion is rare in the U.S. (<1 in 100,000 units) but is a greater concern in developing countries due to inadequate screening.[15]

Hepatitis C

The highest prevalence of hepatitis C in the world is in North Africa with rates of 9 to 13 percent.[16] Any student from a developing country who has elevated liver function tests, or risk factors for hepatitis C (such as history of blood transfusion, intravenous therapy, intravenous drug use, and/or multiple sex partners) should be screened for hepatitis C antibodies. Anti-hepatitis C antibody is not protective and persists in chronic infection. The benefits of screening include a chance to educate the patient about healthy lifestyle practices, potential co-factors for progression of liver disease, and possible treatment with a-interferon and ribavirin.

Anemia

Worldwide, iron-deficiency anemia is a common nutritional disorder. Heme and non-heme iron in animal foods have high bioavailability, and hence diets with adequate animal protein usually provide adequate dietary iron. However, the non-heme iron of vegetable foods have poor bioavailability; absorption is inhibited by bulk, phytates, and fiber. Thus, populations that subsist on cereal staples such as wheat, maize, and rice have high rates of iron-deficiency anemia. Often families with sufficient funds to send a college student abroad consume a diet that is superior to the national standard, but it is worthwhile to inquire about past and present dietary patterns when an international student presents with anemia.

In addition to nutritional iron deficiency anemias, a variety of helminthic parasites can cause iron-deficiency anemia through chronic blood loss, hookworm being the most common. Worldwide, approximately 25 percent of the population is infected with hookworm (*Ancylostoma duodenale* and *Necator americanus*).[19] Hookworm infections cause chronic intestinal microscopic hemorrhages, leading to iron-deficiency anemia. Similarly, chronic infections with whipworm (*Trichuris trichiura*) and schistosomiasis (*Schistosoma mansoni* and *Schistosoma japonicum*) also can lead to iron-deficiency anemia; *Schistosoma haematobium*, by causing chronic bladder hemorrhage, also can contribute to an iron-deficiency anemia. Chronic infection with the fish tapeworm (*Diphyllobothrium latum*) can cause megaloblastic anemia due to vitamin B-12 deficiency.

In any anemic patient from a developing country, screening for tuberculosis (TB) and human immunodeficiency virus (HIV) is prudent; similarly, any patient who is found to be infected with either TB or HIV should be evaluated for the other. In Uganda, patients with active TB are six times as likely to be HIV-positive as those without active TB.[20]

Anemia can be caused by a number of genetically determined conditions, including the hemoglobinopathies causing sickle cell anemia, and alpha- and beta-thalassemia. A deficiency of the red cell enzyme glucose-6-phosphate-dehydrogenase (G6PD) is common among people from Africa and the Indian subcontinent. In G6PD-deficient individuals, severe hemolytic anemia may be triggered by certain oxidant drugs, including primaquine, sulfamethoxazole, dapsone, and nitrofurantoin.

PARASITIC INFECTIONS

A vast array of conditions, including allergies and malignancies, can cause eosinophilia, but in the international student, parasites are a common cause. In general, unicellular organisms (bacteria and protozoa) are not associated with eosinophilia. (Exceptions are *Toxoplasma gondii, Isospora belli,* and *Dientamoeba fragilis.*) More often it is the multicellular organisms or helminths (worms) that stimulate eosinophilia. Eosinophilia tends to correlate with the degree of tissue invasion by the parasite. Helminths that do not invade the intestinal mucosa, such as tapeworms and adult roundworms, cause little or no eosinophilia.

Migrating larval stages of several worms can cause a syndrome of cough, wheezing, and transient migratory infiltrates on chest x-rays. This syndrome is known as simple pulmonary eosinophilia and is accompanied by a striking peripheral blood eosinophilia. Many worms can cause this syndrome, but *Ascaris lumbricoides* is the most common. High levels of eosinophilia are seen during the initial larval migration phase through the lungs. The eosinophilia resolves when the adult worms are fully developed and take up residence in the intestinal lumen. Patients improve rapidly with appropriate antihelminthic treatment.

Parasite infections characterized by recurrent or persistent tissue-invasive stages, such as strongyloidiasis, trichinosis, filariasis, onchocerciasis, Loa Loa, and schistosomiasis, are associated with a more sustained eosinophilia. Tropical pulmonary eosinophilia is caused by filarial infection with *Wuchereria bancrofti* or *Brugia malayi.* Symptoms include cough and nocturnal wheezing. Peripheral blood eosinophils and the serum IgE are markedly elevated, and pulmonary infiltrates may be noted on chest x-rays. In refugees from Southeast Asia, the most common causes of cryptic eosinophilia have been found to be infections with *Strongyloides* and hookworm. Trichinosis is a worldwide risk when raw or undercooked pork is eaten. Cysticercosis (disseminated pork tapeworm) is not uncommon among immigrants from Latin America, and also is found among Asians. Filariasis is seen among individuals originating from tropical endemic areas in Africa, Asia, the Pacific, and Latin America. Onchocerciasis and Loa Loa are seen among persons originating from rural western Africa. Intestinal schistosomiasis can be acquired from contact with infected rivers and lakes in Africa, South America, and Asia, while urinary schistosomiasis is acquired in the Middle East and Africa.[21,22]

Chagas' disease, found in rural South and Central America, is caused by the flagellate protozoan *Trypanosoma cruzi.* Transmitted by the reduviid bug, *T. cruzi* infection leads to an acute phase lasting several weeks followed by a lifelong phase characterized by a positive serology and a low parasitemia. Clinically manifest chronic Chagas' disease develops in only 10 to 30 percent of patients with a positive serology. Years after the initial infection, chronic cardiomyopathy develops in 20 to 30 percent of patients; gastrointestinal megasyndromes develop in less than 10 percent. Although the majority of infections are transmitted by triatomine bugs in endemic areas, other modes of transmission include blood transfusion (in Los Angeles and Miami, one in 7,800 blood donors are positive for Chagas' Disease), and congenital transmission, which occurs in about 1 percent of deliveries of seropositive mothers.[17,18]

TROPICAL DISEASES PRESENTING WITH A FEVER

The presence of geographic risk factors make the consideration of malaria, dengue fever, hepatitis, typhoid fever, and tuberculosis compelling additions to the differential diagnosis of fever in international students. Fortunately, the scope can be narrowed by a knowledge of geographic distribution, incubation periods, usual modes of transmission, and organ system(s) most likely to be involved.

Malaria

Many people who are native to malaria endemic areas acquire partial immunity to malaria through repeated infections. This "semi-immunity" can also result in a prolonged incubation period or decreased severity of disease symptoms. Also, partial treatment (often self-treatment), and resistance of the malaria parasites to certain medications can prolong the incubation period.[23] Nonetheless, consideration of the diagnosis of malaria is mandatory in any febrile patient who is from a country which is endemic for malaria.

It is important to remember that treatment for malaria is based on the resistance pattern reported for malaria organisms in the region where the infection was acquired. The Centers for Disease Control and Prevention (CDC) publication Health Information for International Travel and the CDC web site are good sources for current information.[24]

Dengue Fever

Dengue fever is an emerging viral disease, with an increasing incidence reported in urban areas of tropical developing countries, where increasing numbers of infected humans and mosquito vectors are present. However, this disease is not likely to be seen among international students attending U.S. colleges or universities unless the student has only recently arrived in the U.S. or just returned from a visit home, because of its brief incubation period of three to eight days.

Hemorrhagic Fevers

Hemorrhagic fevers (HF) are not commonly seen in the U.S. in students from developed countries due to the brief incubation periods of these illnesses (four to ten days for the filoviruses, Ebola, and Marburg; one to two weeks for the South American HF's such as Argentinian hemorrhagic fever and Bolivian hemorrhagic fever). However, a bleeding diathesis in a formerly healthy student who has recently arrived from or visited an endemic area mandates patient isolation and appropriate serologic testing.

Bartonellosis

In students from Peru, Ecuador, or Columbia, fever, anemia, and jaundice suggest Bartonellosis, a bacterial disease that is found only in Andean valleys at elevations between 500 and 3200 meters.

ENTERIC INFECTIONS AND DIARRHEA

"Enteric infection" refers to a clinical syndrome with fever and gastrointestinal symptoms, particularly diarrhea. Etiologic agents include *Salmonella typhi* (typhoid fever); non-typhoidal *Salmonella* species, which yield a variety of illnesses collectively called Salmonellosis; *Yersinia enterocolitica*, which causes abdominal pain that can mimic acute appendicitis; and *Campylobacter jejuni*, which is typically associated with abdominal pain, fever, and diarrhea. Like hepatitis A, these diseases are endemic in the developing world in environments where fecal-oral contamination is prevalent.

Diarrhea, the most common ailment of travelers from developed to developing countries, can also be a problem in those arriving in the U.S. from developing countries. Diarrhea is usually defined as more than three unformed stools per day, or any number of unformed stools when accompanied by abdominal cramps, fever, nausea, or vomiting. Infectious etiologies probably account for most cases of diarrhea associated with foreign travel or residence. However, both infectious and non-infectious etiologies must be considered in international students with this complaint. Some tropical enteric infections cause more non-enteric symptoms than those specifically related to the gastrointestinal tract. For example, in infection with *Cyclospora cayetanenis,* fatigue, anorexia and weight loss may predominate, with minimal diarrhea. In people with risk factors for intestinal parasites, multiple parasites are more the rule than the exception. An initial approach to diagnosis includes stool culture for enteric bacterial pathogens (*Salmonella*, *Shigella*, *Campylobacter*, and *Yersinia*), ova and parasite examination, *Giardia* stool antibody testing, and special stool specimen stains for detection of *Cyclospora* and *Cryptosporidium.* A history of antecedent antibiotic necessitates a test for stool *C. difficile* toxin.[26,27]

ETHNIC REMEDIES

Practitioners caring for foreign-born students should inquire regarding their use of non-prescription, folk, or herbal remedies, since such practices are not uncommon in this group. For example, a number of folk remedies used by Hispanic communities on the West Coast have been found to contain toxic levels of lead. In many Southeast Asian cultures, "coining" is a common practice. A coin or other metal object is rubbed on the skin of an ill person until an abrasion or superficial irritation occurs. This is usually done in some sort of geometric pattern, most commonly on the back or chest. This harmless and well-intended practice should not be confused with child or domestic partner abuse.[28,29]

SPECIAL RISKS OF INTERNATIONAL STUDENT TRAVELERS

Students from developing countries who visit home fall into a category of travelers now recognized as a special travel health risk group: Visiting Friends and Relatives (VFRs). VFRs appear to be at higher risk for illness when they visit their native land compared with tourists from the United States and Canada who visit the same locale. There are several possible reasons for this: (1) VFRs are often less aware of the health risks posed by exposures in their country of origin; (2) expatriates often fail to seek travel clinic counseling, vaccinations and prophylactic medications before returning home; (3) the individual, his/her friends and relatives developed semi-immunity to malaria based on repeated infections over the years; this semi-immune state, which can decrease the severity of a life-threatening malaria infection to an ambulatory illness, is quickly lost once the semi-immune person is removed from the endemic area. International students from malaria endemic areas may not be aware of this phenomenon, and have the false belief that they are not at risk of serious or fatal malaria. They may think that malaria chemoprophylaxis drugs are necessary only for non-native visitors and tourists to their homeland and be unwilling to commit the time and resources necessary to obtain these drugs before travel home.[23,30]

CONCLUSION

The college health practitioner will often serve as the point of entry for foreign-born international students into the U.S. health care system. An attempt to understand the student's cultural background, assure appropriate vaccination, perform needed screening tests, and prompt diagnosis of illness will assist these students in reaching their full academic potential.

REFERENCES

1. The Chronicle of Higher Education, 2000-2001 Annual Issue, Sept. 1, 2000, Vol. XLVII, No. 1

2. Guerrant RL, Walker DH, Weller PF: Tropical Infectious Diseases: Principles, Pathogens and Practice. Philadelphia, Churchill Livingston, 1999.

3. Jong EC, McMullen R: The Travel and Tropical Medicine Manual, 3rd Edition. Philadelphia, WB Saunders, 2002.

4. Strickland GT: Hunter's Tropical Medicine and Emerging Infectious Diseases, 8th Edition. Philadelphia, WB Saunders, 2000.

5. Keystone JS. GIDEON computer program for diagnosing and teaching geographic medicine. J Travel Med 1999; 6:152-4.

6. Lee BW: Review of varicella zoster seroepidemiology in India and Southeast Asia. Trop Med Int Health 1998; 3:886-90.

7. Centers for Disease Control and Prevention: Immunization of health-care workers: recommendations of the Advisory Committee on Immunization Practices (ACIP) and the Hospital Infection Control Practices Advisory Committee (HICPAC).

8. Centers for Disease Control and Prevention: Meningococcal disease and college students. Recom-

mendations of the Advisory Committee on Immunization Practices (ACIP). MMWR 2000; 49 (RR07): 11-20.

9. SudreP, Dam GT, Kochi A: Tuberculosis: a global overview of the situation today. Bull. World Health Org 1992; 70: 149-150.

10. McKenna MT, McCray E, Onorato I: The epidemiology of tuberculosis among foreign-born persons in the United States, 1986-1993. N Engl J Med 1995; 332: 1071-1076.

11. Centers for Disease Control and Prevention: Progress towards the elimination of Tuberculosis: United States, 1998. MMWR 1999; 48:732-736.

12. Comstock, GW, Livesay VT, Woolpert SF: The prognosis of a positive tuberculin reaction in childhood and adolescence. Am J Epidemiol 1974;99: 131.

13. Centers for Disease Control and Prevention: Targeted tuberculin testing and treatment of latent tuberculosis infection. MMWR 2000; 49:12-18.

14. Hepatitis. The Merck Manual, 17th Edition, 1999. Merck Research Laboratories, White House Station, NJ, p. 381.

15. Moor AC, Dubbelman TM, VanSteveninck J et al.: Transfusion-transmitted diseases: risks, prevention and perspectives. Eur J Haematol 1999; 62:1-18.

16. Abdelaal M, Rowbottom D, Zawawi T, et al: Epidemiology of hepatitis C virus: A study of male blood donors in Saudi Arabia. Transfusion 1994; 34:135.

17. Leiby DA, Fucci MH, Stumpf RJ: Trypanosoma cruzi in low- to moderate-risk donor population: seroprevalence and possible congenital transmission. Transfusion 1999; 39:310-5.

18. Leiby DA: Present status of studies on Trypanosoma cruzi in U.S. blood donors. American Red Cross Medical and Scientific Updates, Number 99-1, May 5, 1999.

19. Parasitic Infections. The Merck Manual, 17th Edition, 1999. Merck Research Laboratories, White House Station, NJ, p. 1261.

20. Ravilgione M, Nunn PP, Kochi A, et al: The pandemic of HIV-associated tuberculosis. In Mann JM, Tarantola DJM (eds.): AIDS in the World II: Global Dimensions, Social Roots, and Responses. New York, Oxford University Press, 1996, p. 87.

21. Nutman TB, Ottesen EA, Leng S, et al: Eosinophilia in Southeast Asian refugees: Evaluation at a referral center. J Infect Dis 1987; 155:309.

22. Wolf MS: Eosinophilia in the returning traveler. Med Clin North Am 1999; 83:1019-32.

23. Kain KC, Harrington MA, Tennyson S, et al.: Imported malaria: prospective analysis of problems in diagnosis and management. Clin Infect Dis 1998; 27:142-9.

24. Centers for Disease Control and Prevention: Health Information for International Travel 1999-2000, DHHS, Atlanta, GA.

25. Jong EC: Risks of hepatitis A and B in the traveling public. J Trav Med 2001; 8 (Suppl 1). In press.

26. Herwaldt BL, de Arroyave KR, Roberts JM et al.: A multiyear prospective study of the risk factors for and incidence of diarrheal illness in a cohort of Peace Corps volunteers in Guatemala. Ann Intern Med 2000; 132:982-8.

27. Thielman NM, Guerrant RL: Persistent diarrhea in the returned traveler. Infect Dis Clin North Am 1998;12:489-501.

28. Center for Disease Control: Lead poisoning associate with use of traditional ethnic remedies: California, 1991-1992. MMWR 1993; 42:521-524.

29. Buchwald D, Panwala S, Hooton TM: Use of traditional health practices by Southeast Asian refugees in a primary care clinic. West J Med 1992; 156:507-11.

30. Dos Santos CC, Anvar A, Keystone JS et al.: Survey of use of malaria prevention measures by Canadians visiting India. CMAJ 1999; 160:195-200.

Chapter 14

Special Issues in Athletic Medicine

Mark Jenkins, MD

Introduction

College health care practitioners encounter an extensive range of sports related medical problems in the student population. This is true regardless of whether the clinician serves in a designated capacity of "team physician" for the university's athletic department or whether he/she sees students only when they seek care at the health center. Because students' involvement in athletics encompasses not only many types of sports but also levels of participation, the health care professional must be prepared to recognize and manage the wide variety of problems generated by sporting interests.

Thus, "athletic medicine" at the university level may be considered to include all forms of sports-related student activity. The importance of this field is emphasized by the large percentage of students involved in recreational, intramural, club, and varsity sports. These students may encounter an extensive spectrum of medical problems as a direct, or indirect, result of participation in sports.

In this chapter the terms *athlete, student,* and *student-athlete* are used interchangeably to denote any college student who regularly exercises or participates in sports. This broad definition is both necessary and practical. It acknowledges the full spectrum of college students' physical pursuits and, for the practitioner, facilitates consideration that exercise or sports participation may be involved in the clinical problem at hand. Thus, patients should not be restrictively funneled into "athlete" or "non-athlete" classifications based upon their membership in an athletic organization but evaluated and treated in the context of their clinical presentation with due consideration of their relative athletic activity and ability.

Although it is tempting to think of athletic medicine as simply a part of orthopedics, the range of medical conditions encountered encompasses many specialties. Since there is potential for all body systems to be affected by sports participation, it is useful to consider athletic medicine (sports medicine) as not belonging to any one medical specialty. In this light, a tripartite construct may be used to illustrate the overlapping relationship of sports medicine and the fields of family practice/internal medicine, orthopedics, and psychology (Figure 1). Although many specialties (e.g., dermatology, neurosurgery) have a role, or potential role, in the care of athletes, this simplified illustration contains the essential elements comprising athletic medicine.

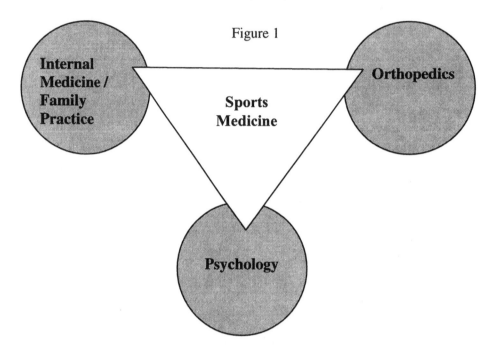

Figure 1

The "special issues" or topics chosen for this chapter are intentionally outside the arena of musculoskeletal injuries. There are already many excellent publications dealing with the diagnosis and management of orthopedic injuries. Instead, this chapter focuses attention on topics perhaps only briefly covered elsewhere. The specific issues discussed are selected to represent a wide spectrum of sports-related, non-orthopedic conditions and circumstances commonly encountered in a university setting. Arguably many other topics not included here are equally worthy of recognition, indeed enough to fill a comprehensive text. In this light, this chapter is a "snapshot" providing important detail but not fully representative of the entire scene. Hopefully, the reader will use this information both to gain an understanding of the diverse subject material covered and to serve as a launching point to further explore this fascinating area of college health.

PREPARTICIPATION ATHLETIC PHYSICAL EXAMINATION

Introduction

The preparticipation physical examination for student-athletes is a valued process for the vast majority of sports medicine programs in U.S. colleges. A recent survey indicated that 97 percent of National Collegiate Athletic Association (NCAA) participating schools require a preparticipation history and physical examination for their student-athletes,[1] although, as will be discussed later, there is considerable variation in the quality and depth of these examinations.

The purpose of the preparticipation exam is to ensure that students can participate in their sports without undue risk to their health, and to identify conditions that may become problematic, or require special accommodations, with sports activity. The first and foremost part of this goal is the identification of conditions representing an increased risk of morbidity or mortality. After initial identification such conditions must be thoroughly characterized, the risk assessed, and appropriate medical advice generated. Thus, initial screening is only the beginning; in-depth evaluation must follow for all those in whom a significant abnormality is diagnosed or suspected. This often necessitates specialist and/or sub-specialist consultation and appropriate diagnostic testing. After detailed scrutiny, the examining physician is better able to quantify the risk and make an informed and rational decision regarding athletic participation.

The essence of the rational decision process is to determine whether the disorder represents a significant enough risk to medically disqualify the athlete or, if not, the circumstances in which sports participation may be allowed. Deciding who should be allowed to train and compete, taking into consideration the sport, circumstances, and ethics, can be simple and straightforward or extremely challenging. In some cases (e.g., hypertrophic cardiomyopathy) the decision may be for outright disqualification. In others (e.g., absence of one testicle) it may mean acknowledgment and acceptance of the risk involved and the institution of specific steps to reduce that risk. Usually, the right decision is made by including a team of health professionals who then present and discuss the circumstances with the athlete and, in the case of a minor, his/her parents. This team should include the team (or health service) physician(s), the athlete's personal physician (if possible), specialty consultant(s) (e.g., cardiologist, bioethicist), and, for a varsity athlete, athletic department medical staff (e.g., the head athletic trainer).

Other representatives from the athletic department and/or the institution's risk management division should also be involved when needed. In all circumstances it is important to respect patient confidentiality. After the decision is made, the appropriate administrative office (e.g., athletic director, head athletic trainer) is able to coordinate any needed resources or reporting.

PREPARTICIPATION HISTORY AND PHYSICAL EXAM ELEMENTS

The preparticipation history and physical exam generally contains the following elements:

- Screen and evaluate for risk factors for sudden cardiac death
- Screen and evaluate for previous injury and related musculoskeletal conditions
- Screen and evaluate for other significant disease/health disorders

The first element will be discussed in detail below. The second and third elements, briefly summarized here, are an integral part of the examination process and are not to be over-looked.

Although there is necessary focus on the cardiovascular and musculoskeletal systems, an athletic preparticipation history and physical examination should include all of the components associated with a thorough physical. Inquiry regarding childhood illness, personal and family medical history, current medications, drug allergies, a menstrual history in women, immunization documentation, social factors and habits, and a review of systems should all be part of the examination. Significant current findings and/or past medical history should be pursued appropriately including the acquisition of previous medical records.

Screening for Sudden Death

Sudden cardiac death (SCD) in an athlete is defined as an unexpected, nontraumatic fatal event that occurs fewer than six hours after exercise in a previously healthy individual.[2] An analysis of 158 cases of sudden death in young athletes divided these events into two subcategories, *cardiovascular* and *noncardiovascular*.[3] In this series, noncardiovascular causes of SCD accounted for 15 percent of the total deaths and were due to circumstances such as hyperthermia and status asthmaticus. Eighty-five percent were attributable to cardiovascular sudden death, or *sudden cardiac death* (SCD). Many of these deaths are potentially preventable via a systematic screening process.

SCD in the young athlete (less than 35 years of age) is rare, affecting approximately 1/200,000 student-athletes per year.[4] However, these events are often highly publicized and generate considerable public concern. Young athletes are idolized for the model of health they portray, and thus, SCD is a tragedy that profoundly affects society.[5] In athletes over the age of 35, the most common cause of SCD is atherosclerotic coronary artery disease.[6,7,8] Although precise numbers are difficult to determine, SCD in the older athlete appears to be a more frequent occurrence than in younger athletes. Estimates in marathon runners are 1/50,000[9] and in joggers 1/15,000[6] annually.

SCD in young athletes is caused by a diverse spectrum of disorders (Figure 2). Approximately 90 percent of SCD cases occur in males and when adjusted for number of participants per year represents a five-fold increased risk as compared with female athletes.[10] Basketball and football are the most common sports in which SCD occurs. The most common cause in the U.S. is hypertrophic cardiomyopathy.[3]

Hypertrophic cardiomyopathy (HCM) has a prevalence of approximately 1/500 and is more common in men and African-Americans.[11] HCM is an inherited autosomal dominant disorder with variable, age-related penetrance.[12] To date, HCM can be caused by over 100 mutations on several genes.[12] The best noninvasive tool for identification of HCM is echocardiography. Due to the age-related penetrance, adolescents at high risk for the development of HCM need regular echocardiographic assessment. Thus, the athlete who presents for the preparticipation examination with a history of a prior normal echocardiogram should not lull an examiner into a false sense of security.

Commotio cordis is an interesting subcategory of SCD, despite the fact that it is induced by trauma. In this disorder, seemingly trivial blunt trauma to the chest results in ventricular fibrillation. Experimental evidence suggests that minor chest trauma causes

Figure 2. Causes of sudden cardiac death in young athletes

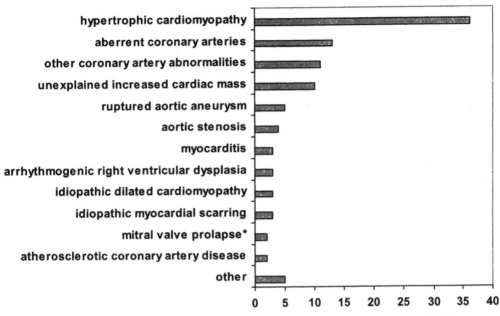

*Mitral valve prolapse has not been definitively established as a causative factor in SCD.

an electrical discharge, which if delivered during the vulnerable period of repolarization (T wave) results in lethal ventricular fibrillation.[13,14] This condition has a fatality rate of 90 percent[14] and can occur in virtually any sport but is primarily reported in sports involving relatively small, hard projectiles, such as baseball,[14,15] hockey,[16] and lacrosse.[17]

Cardiovascular Screening Recommendations

The catastrophic, high-profile nature of SCD and the potential for prevention command considerable medical interest. In 1996, the American Heart Association (AHA) proposed criteria for preparticipation cardiovascular screening in athletes.[18] The consensus panel recommendations took into consideration the benefits and limitations, cost-effectiveness, practicality, and medical and legal ramifications of preparticipation cardiovascular screening. They can be summarized as follows:

- Preparticipation screening is justified, based on moral, ethical, and legal considerations.
- Noninvasive testing can enhance diagnostic sensitivity, but routine use is not cost-effective and is not currently recommended.
- A complete and careful personal and family history, with appropriate physical examination, is the most practical screening approach.
- Screening should be done prior to competition in organized high school and college sports, and repeated every two years; an interim history should be done for intervening years.
- National standards for preparticipation screening should be established.

- The examination should be carried out by a health care worker—preferably a physician—with the requisite training, skills, and background in diagnosing cardiovascular disease.
- The screening exam should include and emphasize certain critical elements (Table 1).

Table 1. 1996 AHA cardiovascular preparticipation screening criteria[18]

Family history	Premature death
	Heart disease
Personal history	Previously detected heart murmur
	Increased systemic blood pressure
	Exertional chest pain
	Exertional syncope
	Excessive fatigue
	Exertional shortness of breath
Physical examination	Brachial artery blood pressure (sitting)
	Precordial auscultation (sitting and standing)
	Palpation of femoral pulses
	Stigmata of Marfan syndrome

A recent survey of NCAA institutions[19] evaluating the preparticipation cardiovascular screening process found that of the 879 schools surveyed, 855 (97 percent) required some form of preparticipation screening. The majority (85 percent) used team physicians to administer the screening. However, 75 percent of these physicians were orthopedists, a group that is arguably less skilled in cardiovascular evaluation than primary care physicians. Furthermore, some schools used nurse practitioners (19 percent) or athletic trainers (34 percent), either alone or supervised by a team physician. The 1996 AHA guidelines were used to judge completeness of preparticipation cardiovascular screening. Only 26 percent of the schools used 9 or more of the 12 recommended criteria (deemed adequate screening). More striking was that 24 percent utilized 4 or fewer criteria (deemed inadequate screening). Larger Division I schools were significantly more likely to perform adequate screening than Division II or Division III schools. Neglect in the performance of basic and necessary screening makes the inherently difficult task of identifying abnormalities associated with SCD even harder. Clearly, many institutions are failing in this responsibility.

Non-Invasive Screening Tests

The main drawback to routine use of noninvasive diagnostic testing (such as stress electrocardiography and echocardiography) to screen an athletic population is cost. The uncommon occurrence of clinically significant cardiovascular abnormalities, the large at-risk population, and the cost of diagnostic testing (e.g., echocardiography) mean routine noninvasive testing is not generally considered to be cost-effective. However, a few recent studies challenge this assertion. The use of 12-lead electrocardiography (ECG) in addition to a specific history and physical examination for preparticipation cardiovascular screening was evaluated by a 1998 study.[20] These authors prospectively analyzed 33,735 athletes from the Venetio region of Italy during 1979–1996. They evaluated reasons for disqualification and causes of SCD in athletes and in a similar group of nonathletes. Hypertrophic cardiomyopathy (HCM) was identified as a cause of death in only one athlete (2 percent of the cases of SCD) but in 16 deaths (7.3 percent) in the nonathletic comparison group. This is in distinct contrast to findings in the U.S., where HCM is responsible for approximately one-third of cases of SCD in athletes. Overall in the Italian study, the screening process resulted in 3016 athletes (8.9 percent) referred for further diagnostic evaluation (e.g., echocardiography, subspecialty workup). A total of 621 athletes were disqualified, with just over half due to cardiovascular abnormalities (22 specifically for HCM). The authors concluded that the screening process, which included a 12-lead ECG, was responsible for the low frequency of HCM in athletes who died suddenly. The direct applicability of these findings to the U.S. is not certain. One concern is that population-specific genetic differences may account for the relatively low prevalence of HCM in the Venetio region of Italy compared with findings in the U.S. This would be expected to make direct comparison of proposed screening methods problematic. (An interesting note is that, for over two decades, the Italian government has required a 12-lead ECG as part of the cardiovascular screening process for all athletes.)

A more recent investigation using high school athletes directly addressed the issue of cost-effectiveness of cardiovascular screening in the U.S.[21] This article found that, of the three recognized screening methods (2-D echocardiography, a specific cardiovascular history and physical examination, and 12-lead electrocardiography), the most cost-effective screening tool was the 12-lead ECG. The questions that this investigation raises have not been fully addressed at this time, and the reader is encouraged to evaluate future literature on this topic.

Additionally, beyond cost issues, routine use of noninvasive diagnostic testing for screening examinations has inherent limitations and may generate another set of problems, i.e., the issue of sensitivity and specificity. For the 12-lead ECG, specificity is limited by abnormalities which are largely due to the cardiovascular adaptations to strenuous exercise ("athlete's heart"), which are frequently found in young, healthy athletes.[22] Similarly, echocardiography may detect increased ventricular wall thickness representing normal exercise-related adaptation that may be confused with HCM. Athletes may potentially experience significant anxiety or inappropriate limitations on participation, or on health care insurance, as a result of false-positive testing.[18] Similarly, the sensitivity of noninvasive diagnostic testing is not 100 percent. Some coronary artery anomalies are notoriously difficult to detect with either the 12-lead ECG or echocardiography. As noted previously, the age-related penetrance of HCM means that it may be missed by echocardiography until growth is complete. Additionally, the 12-lead ECG does not typically identify congenital cardiac structural abnormalities.

Future Direction

The reader is encouraged to follow closely this evolving topic. Because of the inherent limitations of the preparticipation cardiovascular history and physical examination a need exists for better diagnostic tools. It is hoped that the application of existing technology and/or development of new technology will ultimately generate cost-effective methods possessing adequate sensitivity and specificity to diagnose cardiovascular disease, particularly HCM. Until better methods are formulated it is vital to emphasize proper and thorough implementation of the preparticipation cardiovascular history and physical examination. Additionally, sports medicine practitioners should continue to stress to both athletes and coaches the importance of prompt reporting of cardiovascular symptoms.

NUTRITION AND SUPPLEMENTS

The prevailing wisdom in athletics is that excellence is achieved by a combination of physical and mental hard work, rest, and nutrition. College athletes nearly always receive significant and specific instruction in the construction and implementation of a training program. However, there is often little guidance on proper nutrition. Therefore, it is important for sports medicine professionals not only to teach athletes about proper nutrition but to encourage a framework for athletes to learn on their own.

Complicating the acquisition of nutritional knowledge are myths and misinformation. The former represents lore handed down over time. The latter includes published or broadcast "information" from a variety of sources such as TV, radio, newspapers, magazines, books, and the Internet (e.g., web sites, newsgroups). These "misinformation" sources both perpetuate old myths and produce new erroneous material. The inquisitive college student is saturated with a constant parade of new diets—diets to lose weight, diets to gain weight, diets to build muscle, diets to enhance the immune system, diets to combat depression, diets to provide "energy," and more. Additionally, bewildering arrays of nutritional "supplements" appear on store shelves and web sites in ever increasing numbers. The 1994 Dietary Supplement Act has been largely responsible for the generation of a multi-billion-dollar-a-year industry. For the college athlete the plethora of nutritional "information" has made "separating the wheat from the chaff" very difficult ("low signal-to-noise ratio," to cite a more modern colloquialism).

It is well beyond the scope of this section to fully discuss nutrition and dietary supplements. However, a review of nutritional science essentials will provide useful groundwork and aid clinicians who provide care and advice to college athletes. Additionally, a few myths will be exploded and a few commonly used nutritional supplements discussed. However, it must be remembered that supplement fads evolve rapidly. New supplements become popular almost overnight as old ones are discarded, and this cycle is in constant flux and never-ending. Therefore, it is quite likely that between the writing and publishing of this text unanticipated new nutritional or supplement fads will be popularized, while "old ones" have disappeared.

Nutrition basics

Virtually everyone who has worked with athletes for more than a few months has heard dietary myths. This nutritional lore can be quite powerful and may affect, to variable degrees, almost all student athletes. Three common nutritional are that high-protein diets build muscle mass, all fat is bad and should be avoided, and vitamin and mineral supplements enhance performance.

In the mid-nineteenth century noted German scientist von Liebig postulated that muscles consume protein as fuel.[23] Manual laborers were thus encouraged to consume high amounts of protein, primarily in the form of animal flesh. The "eat muscle to build muscle" theorem has fundamental appeal. However, before the turn of the century it was proven that protein is not the prime fuel for muscular activity. Unfortunately, the fact that muscles primarily utilize carbohydrate and fat has not completely penetrated today's strength training community. The myth has been modified over time, and one now sees an array of purported "muscle building" amino acids,[24] but it still represents nutritional fallacy.

Protein requirements in athletes are only slightly higher than in sedentary individuals and range from 1.2 to 1.8 g/kg/d.[23,25] This amounts to approximately 12 to 15 percent of total caloric intake. Due to their overall greater caloric consumption, athletes easily meet requirements in nearly all cases. Protein consumption greater than 2 g/kg/d does not improve athletic performance or confer an anabolic effect. Thus, use of protein supplements does not result in lean body-mass (weight) gain as many athletes mistakenly assume. Additionally, excess protein intake due to the high nitrogenous load may have adverse effects on renal or hepatic function.

The high-protein myth is annoyingly persistent. However, dispensing sound nutritional advice, especially at the collegiate level, may ultimately help the athletic community overall shrug this "dead weight."

Few words carry such negative connotation as "fat." Yet fat is an essential dietary component, without which disease will occur. The typical Western diet is overly rich in saturated fats. But a diet in which fat is completely excluded is not compatible with a healthy existence. Linoleic acid is an essential fatty acid that must be included in the diet since it is not manufactured by the body, and is critical for the construction of cell membranes and nerves. Student-athletes should not view dietary fat as only contributing to unwanted body stores. They should be instructed that fat has vital functions and that there are "good" and "bad" types of dietary fat. (Generally, unsaturated fats represent the former, and saturated fats the latter.) The ideal percentage of macronutrient intake of fat by athletes is not known. Most college health practitioners agree, though, that dietary fat should not comprise more than 30 percent of total caloric intake[26] and that two-thirds of this should be unsaturated.

The discovery that the dietary absence of certain organic compounds results in disease is one of the most important discoveries in the history of medicine. For both the general public and the medical community, the concept that administration of a specific vitamin, normally supplied by a healthy diet, reverses the corresponding deficiency-induced disease-state is understandably powerful. It is, thus, a logical extension to suppose that doses higher than those physiologically required by the body will result in an enhanced mental or physical state. Despite the fact that decades of research have proven the futility of excess vitamin intake, the practice remains popular.

In athletes there is the belief, without basis in fact, that strenuous training may generate an increased need for certain vitamins. The lure of vitamins as "natural" performance-enhancers is strong, and it is not surprising that they have been consistently popular with athletes.

Mineral supplementation presents a somewhat different concern, and two commonly encountered deficiencies deserve further discussion. Iron is a metallic element required for the production of hemoglobin and myoglobin. Additionally, it is a component of several cytochromes which facilitate mitochondrial electron transport. Iron balance is determined by losses and dietary intake. The body can lose iron via blood, urine, or sweat, although only blood loss appears to be an important consideration. Some circumstances may predispose athletes to iron loss. It has been shown that a significant percentage of runners experience a small amount of gastrointestinal bleeding after runs longer than 10 km. Another phenomenon, referred to as "foot-strike hemolysis," occurs when red blood cells burst in the vessels of the feet due to intermittent compressive forces experienced during running, especially running on a hard surface. Most of the iron in free hemoglobin can be reclaimed, but some is filtered into the urine. Arguably the most important consideration is menstrual iron loss in female athletes.

Iron deficiency affects athletic performance proportional to severity. If significant enough to deplete body stores, production of hemoglobin declines and the resulting anemia impairs oxygen delivery to exercising muscle. Iron deficiency without anemia has not been proven to reduce exercise performance.

There are a variety of sources for dietary iron and several factors that influence how well dietary iron is absorbed. In general dietary iron is absorbed poorly. Animal sources (heme-iron) are about 10 to 25 percent absorbed. Plant sources (non-heme iron) are only 2 to 5 percent absorbed. Ascorbic acid (vitamin C) increases iron absorption, whereas tannic acid, found in tea and coffee, decreases it. Women have a dietary iron requirement of approximately 15 mg/day; and men, 10 mg/day. Although iron deficiency may potentially occur in anyone, it is not surprising that the largest group at risk is vegetarian women.

Calcium is another metallic element in which inadequate intake may occur in an otherwise healthy population. Many young women do not ingest recommended amounts of calcium, with long-term implications for developing osteoporosis. Dairy products are the chief source of dietary calcium; thus diets that exclude dairy products represent an increased risk of deficiency. Green plant sources contain calcium but the amount is small. For example, it takes 5 servings of broccoli or 16 servings of spinach to equal the calcium found in 1 serving of milk (servings are considered ½ cup). Current daily recommendations for calcium intake are 1300 mg for adolescents and 1000 mg for pre-menopausal women.[27] College female athletes should be educated about calcium, especially to understand that inadequate consumption may place them at increased risk for stress fractures during their youth and osteoporosis later in life.

Optimum macronutrient requirements for athletes

An athlete's nutritional practice has important ramifications for performance. Prolonged inadequate caloric intake will eventually deplete energy stores, resulting in declining exercise capacity. Similarly, poor protein intake results in reduced repair and recovery from exercise. Coaches and athletes have long been interested in the role of the diet in sports performance. It is reported that the distance runner Stymphalos attributed his Olympic victories in the fifth century B.C. to a meat-rich diet, differing from the primarily vegetarian diet traditionally consumed.[28] Since that time many dietary fads have come and gone. A recent example is the so-called Zone Diet forwarded by Barry Sears, Ph.D. Although the diet is in vogue as a performance-enhancing and weight-loss diet, and the subject of several popular books by Dr. Sears, there is no valid scientific support and there are considerable contrary data in the medical literature.[29] The Zone diet highlights both the pervasive appeal of "new" dietary strategies to improve exercise performance and the faux science that often underlies them.

For athletes, most of the scientific literature supports a diet in which the total caloric composition is derived from 55 percent to 60 percent carbohydrate, up to 30 percent fat, and 10 to 15 percent protein. Approximately one-half of the carbohydrate content should be from complex carbohydrates, and two-thirds of the fat content should be unsaturated. During heavy training and pre-competition, and for certain sports, carbohydrate requirements are increased (e.g., 60 percent to 70 percent of total calories). The recommended protein intake ranges from 1.2–1.8 g/kg/day,[30] which is approximately 10 percent–15 percent of the total calories ingested.[31,32] Total caloric needs of anaerobic and aerobic athletes are similar and are dictated by total energy requirements.

Special risk groups

Certain groups of athletes are at increased risk for nutritional deficiency. Deficits may be due to inadequate macronutrients, vitamins, or minerals. Insufficient total caloric intake may occur in athletes with eating disorders, vegetarians, those in whom competition is segregated by weight classifications (e.g., wrestling), or those in whom a lighter body weight is desirable (e.g., distance running). Similarly, vitamin and/or mineral intake may also be inadequate.

Nutritional supplements

In 1994 the U.S. Congress passed the Congressional Dietary Supplemental Health and Education Act (DSHEA). This action allowed for a wide variety of substances to be sold as "nutritional supplements" and not as drugs, thus bypassing regulatory oversight by the Food and Drug Administration (FDA). Provided these substances do not claim to diagnose, treat, or cure a particular disease, they can be marketed without having to submit to the same requirements as those for medications, such as quality control, efficacy, and safety.[33]

It is very important for the practitioner treating college athletes to realize that a number of nutritional supplements (e.g., androstenedione) appear on the NCAA list of banned substances. For the athlete and physician, product labeling may cause confusion as to what is actually contained within. This is especially true for herbal supplements comprised of multiple ingredients listed by botanical name and may result in the inadvertent ingestion of a banned substance. Because many do not consider nutritional supplements as "medications," use of these substances may not be apparent to the clinician. Thus, it is essential to ask direct questions regarding supplement use and make this inquiry a routine part of the patient history.

Supplements may be classified by type, or by their so-called mechanism of action. Vitamins, minerals, botanicals (herbs), and ergogenics (energy generating) are terms generally used to characterize nutritional supplements. Some of these substances (e.g., vitamin C) have a well-defined role in human biochemistry, and their absence results in disease, whereas others have no known requirement or function. With respect to performance enhancement, the mechanism of action, known or reputed, is a useful functional description of supplements. Such a functional classification includes:

- Energy substrate or intermediate (e.g., creatine)
- Anabolic (steroid) function (e.g., androstenedione)
- Anabolic (non-steroid) function (e.g., chromium picolinate)
- Mitochondrial catalyst (e.g., coenzyme Q-10)
- Delay of fatigue (e.g., caffeine)
- Enhanced recovery/repair (e.g., vitamin E)

Chromium is a metallic element that functions as a co-factor to augment the action of insulin. Picolinate is an organic ligand that has been shown to enhance absorption of chromium, in contrast with inorganic salts (e.g., chromium chloride), which are poorly absorbed. Chromium supplementation has been shown to improve insulin sensitivity in some patients with diabetes mellitus.[34,35,36] Thus the question arises as to whether chromium, due to this insulin-assisting (anabolic) effect, could function to increase muscle mass and strength. An initial study reporting increased lean body mass has been criticized for methodology flaws related to body composition testing, and subsequent research has not demonstrated an anabolic effect in young healthy adults.[37,38,39] All were double-blind, placebo-controlled trials that, in addition to testing body composition, also evaluated muscular strength of the subjects before and after the supplementation period.

The recommended daily dietary allowance of chromium is 50–200 micrograms and is supposedly safe. However, there are not enough data to reach conclusions regarding long term safety. A few isolated case reports raise concern. One such report describes suspected chromium picolinate induced rhabdomyolysis in a 24-year-old woman body builder who took 1200 micrograms over a 48-hour period,[40] and another describes severe toxicity from chronic ingestion.[41] The 33-year-old woman in this latter report presented with weight loss, anemia, thrombocytopenia, hepatic dysfunction, and renal failure due to chromium picolinate ingestion of 1200–2400 micrograms per day for four to five months.

Supraphysiological doses of anabolic-androgenic steroids (e.g., testosterone), in combination with a strength training program, result in increases in muscle size and strength.[42] However, the side effects of these substances can be severe and include immunosuppression, hypercholesterolemia, hypertension, infertility, testicular atrophy, premature epiphyseal closure, and liver abnormalities (e.g., peliosis hepatis). Concern about public safety was the driving force for the Anabolic Steroid Control Act. Passed by the U.S.

Congress in 1990, this act classified these drugs as Schedule III controlled substances. Despite what is known about anabolic steroids, the lure of the muscle-building properties continues to fuel the search for a "safe" steroid.

Androstenedione first appeared on the shelves in the U.S. in the 1990s and has been marketed as a "safe, natural" muscle builder. Androstenedione is an androgenic steroid produced by the adrenal gland, testis, and ovary. It is also found in several plants (e.g., yams). Androstenedione is converted to testosterone by the action of 5-alpha-reductase, although other pathways enable its conversion into estrone and estradiol. Androstenedione was first synthesized in the 1970s in former East Germany and was reportedly given to athletes en masse as part of their government-controlled sports program.

The supposition that androstenedione supplementation is safe and effective is suspect, because there are no data to support this claim. A recent placebo-controlled, double-blind study on young men investigated androstenedione supplementation combined with strength training.[43] The authors found no difference in muscular strength, muscle fiber type, body composition (lean body mass), serum free and total testosterone, serum LH, or serum FSH in the androstenedione-supplemented group. However, in this same group they did find a significantly reduced serum HDL concentration, and significantly increased serum estradiol and estrone concentrations. There have been similar findings in other published studies. To date, androstenedione has not been shown to increase serum testosterone,[43,44,45,46] increase lean body mass,[46] or increase strength.[43,46]

These findings suggest that young men who take androstenedione will not only fail to benefit, but, in fact, may experience harm. Adverse effects such as increased risk of atherosclerotic disease, gynecomastia, and possibly, malignancies (e.g., breast cancer) are, over time, at least theoretical considerations. There has been no investigation into safety or efficacy in women.

Creatine is a nitrogenous compound found predominantly in muscle. A 70 kg adult has about 120 g of creatine in muscle tissue; the daily turnover is roughly 2 g. Approximately 50 percent of this is replaced by the diet, and 50 percent is synthesized by the liver and kidneys from glycine, arginine, and methionine. Creatine is eliminated from the body by the kidneys either as creatine or as creatinine, which is formed from the metabolism of creatine.

In muscle most of the total creatine pool is in a phosphorlyated state (creatine phosphate) and functions as an energy reserve. Creatine phosphate is capable of donating a high-energy phosphate group to ADP to quickly regenerate ATP in a step catalyzed by the enzyme creatine kinase. Creatine phosphate is present in concentrations that are about four- to five-fold greater than ATP.

At rest, ATP, which is the ultimate energy supply for muscle, is present only in limited supply, usually only enough for 2 to 3 seconds of high intensity work (e.g., putting the shot). By utilizing the high-energy phosphate reservoir in creatine phosphate, high-intensity work can be sustained for approximately 10 seconds. As exercise persists for longer periods of time, anaerobic glycolysis and then, finally, aerobic glycolysis are utilized to generate ATP. The ATP-creatine system is the fastest component of the anaerobic system and is used by power athletes (e.g., football). During rest creatine can be regenerated back to creatine phosphate, but this takes approximately 30 to 60 seconds. Aerobic glycolysis is the primary system used by endurance (distance) athletes. In these athletes ATP levels remain remarkably unchanged during exercise, because ATP is generated at the same rate it is used. Aerobic glycolysis is a much more energy-efficient system, but the generation of ATP is considerably slower than with the anaerobic system. The utilization of energy during exercise is represented in Figure 3.

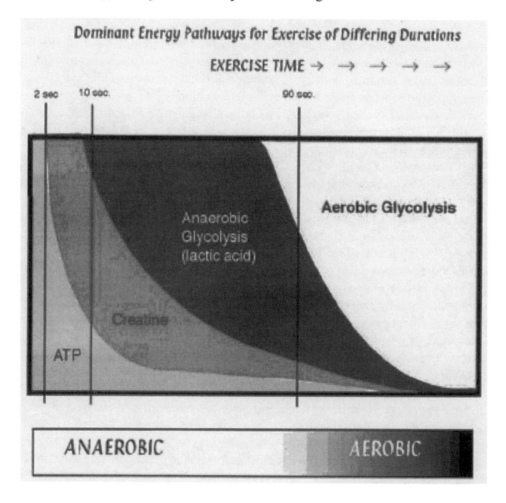

Considering the pathways of energy utilization during exercise, it might be expected that for short-term high-intensity exercise higher concentrations of intramuscular creatine phosphate would result in improved performance. Higher muscular creatine content can be achieved by increased creatine ingestion. Subjects fed 20 g of creatine per day for several days demonstrated a 20 percent increase in total creatine stores, of which approximately 30 to 40 percent was in the phosphorylated form.[47] In individuals thus supplemented a number of placebo-controlled investigations have documented performance enhancement for specific tasks:

- Five sets of 30 maximum voluntary knee extensions, with 60 seconds rest between sets[47]
- Ten 6-second bouts, with 30 seconds rest. High-intensity work on a bicycle ergometer[49]
- Bench press; five sets to failure (predetermined 10 rep maximum), with 2-minute rest periods. Jump squats; five sets of 10, with 2-minute rest periods, using 30 percent of each subjects predetermined 1 rep maximum[50]
- Maximum continuous jumping exercise; 45 seconds. All-out treadmill running (approximately 60 seconds) at 20 km/hr, 5 degree incline[51]
- Cycling to exhaustion at 150 percent peak VO2 at several different protocols; (a) nonstop, (b) 60 seconds work / 120 seconds rest, (c) 20 seconds work / 40 seconds rest, and (d) 10 seconds work / 20 seconds rest. (Group d showed the greatest improvement with creatine supplementation[52])
- Gains in bench-press lifting volume, the sum of bench press, squat, and power clean-lifting volume, and total work performed during 6-second running in NCAA division 1A football players[53]
- Three maximal kayak ergometer tests of 90, 150, and 300 s duration on a wind-braked kayak ergometer. (Improvement seen in all three tests[54])

In short, the available literature indicates that creatine supplementation improves performance of high-intensity intermittent exercise.

No studies have yet demonstrated improvement during endurance activities, and from the understanding of energy pathways used during these sports, benefit would not be expected. An additional, potentially negative factor for distance sports is the weight gain associated with creatine use.[53,54] Increased body mass, which averages 1 to 2kg in supplemented athletes,[55] is generally detrimental to athletes engaged in sports such as distance running and cycling.

Given the performance enhancement in athletes supplemented with creatine, use by college students is understandably popular. A recent anonymous survey of NCAA Division I athletes found that just over 40 percent reported using creatine.[56] In addition, male athletes use creatine more often than female athletes.[56,57]

Considering the only recent popularity of creatine use, there are no long-term studies documenting safety. Initially there was concern regarding dehydration, increased risk of heat-related illness, gastrointestinal disturbance, muscle cramping, and renal and hepatic toxicity, the latter being potentially mediated by increased nitrogenous load and increased solute concentration in the urine. Reports of toxicity have been anecdotal, and recent investigations and reviews have not found definitive evidence of adverse effects.[58,59,60,61] There is still concern, however, due to the lack of the same quality standards that are applied to pharmaceuticals and because the manufacture of creatine may introduce contaminants into the commercially distributed product. (Such was the case in the 1980s when a contaminant present in batches of tryptophan, a supplement widely used as a sleep aid, resulted in an epidemic of eosinophilia-myalgia syndrome.)[62]

In short there are no documented short-term adverse effects associated with creatine use, but long-term studies have not been conducted. Although creatine use is apparently safe, there is still rational concern regarding quality control standards in manufacturing, potential idiosyncratic reactions in creatine consumers, and the possibility of long-term side effects.

DRUGS IN SPORTS

Athletic competition conjures up noble ideals in the minds of many people. Dedication, valor, honor, purity, sportsmanship, and heroism are concepts often forwarded as representing "what is right" in sports. Unfortunately, the drive to win, especially considering the potential monetary gains and the "big business" side of modern sports, has yielded a dark side. Although the use of reputed performance-enhancing drugs is not a new phenomenon in athletics, the advent of modern nutritional biochemistry and the spread of "information" via the Internet have enabled penetration on a scale never imagined just a few decades ago. Equally disheartening is the diversion of new legitimate medical treatments to the athletic population (e.g., erythropoietin and human growth hormone). The ever-increasing number of substances appearing on the banned list of many governing bodies (e.g., NCAA, International Olympic Committee) is alarming. Thus, it is important to examine why athletes take performance-enhancing drugs, to review some of the current compounds and their associated morbidity and mortality, and to discuss what the sports governing bodies are doing to prevent the problem.

The simple question of why athletes use performance-enhancing drugs has complex answers. Several common considerations are listed below.[63]

- Everybody else is doing it
- Financial rewards
- Limited access to proper training, nutritional knowledge, and/or psychological methods to enhance performance
- Pressure from coaches, peers, and/or parents
- The drive to win at all costs
- Attitudes and expectations in the community
- The role of the media in perpetuating some, or all, of the above

The specifics are frequently dictated by individual characteristics, the particular sport, and the drug in question.

Banning and testing for the use of specific chemical compounds by athletes is a much discussed ethical issue.[64,65,66] Although it may be argued that use of performance-enhancing drugs, regardless of known side effects, should be determined by autonomy only and not legislated by the various sports associations, high-profile adversities and subsequent public outcry have been very influential. An additional consideration is the prevailing public opinion that sports should be "pure" and free of the taint of drug use. For governing bodies, the chief concern is that unrestricted policies would apply an inordinate amount of pressure on athletes to use performance-enhancing drugs and thus cause substantial harm. These arguments are used to justify orchestrated drug testing.

On the negative side of testing are personal invasion (e.g., blood drawing) and the limitations of sensitivity and specificity, and potential harm to an individual as a result of false positive testing.

The current state of affairs represents a blend of medical science, specific athletic team and organizational goals, politics, public opinion, and legislation. For each banned substance there may be significant arguments for or against prohibition. One complicating factor is that valid evidence regarding both efficacy and harm often lags behind popular use and/or governing-body legislative decisions. Regardless, for the health professional who deals with athletes, it is of paramount importance to practice and prescribe in a manner that does no harm and does not violate the specific sporting association's current rules and/or the laws of the state, province, or country.

Banned substances and banned procedures currently include the following: narcotics, stimulants, anabolic agents, diuretics, masking agents/methods, street drugs, peptide hormones and analogues, and blood doping. (See Table 2)

The prospect for increasingly sophisticated "doping" is of great concern to many sporting organizations. The mapping of the human genome and related research will expand the current array of hormones, polypeptides, and factors already available and will yield enormous benefit for many areas of medicine. However, as has already been seen with erythropoietin, these advances can be misdirected from curing disease towards altering physiology to enhance performance in sports. The new frontier of advances in human biochemistry and genetics will undoubtedly lead to a new frontier for artificial sports performance enhancement.

For sports organizations trying to insure a "level playing field," keeping pace with the anticipated wave of new "doping" methods will be very challenging. For example, the lack of testing methods for erythropoietin makes detection of users very difficult, if not impossible. In the infamous scandal in the 1998 Tour de France, several teams' medical personnel were caught with hundreds of doses of erythropoietin. Thus "doping" was detected through possession, not through blood or urine testing of cyclists.

The willingness of governments and private organizations to cheat and the advent of new technologies may herald a dark future. What was once science fiction may become reality. Will sports turn to in vitro genetic manipulation? Will athletic attributes become encoded in the lab? Winning in international sports competition may be determined by who has the best laboratory and is willing to use it. Of course this is all conjecture, but given the dark chapters past it does give pause for concern.

SPECIFIC MEDICAL ISSUES IN SPORTS

Concussion

Concussion is a frequently encountered clinical problem in sports, with more than 300,000 occurrences per year in the U.S.[67] In NCAA football alone there are approximately 1500 concussions annually.[67] In collegiate soccer the incidence is 0.6 per 1000 athlete-exposures for men (0.4 per 1000 for women) per season.[67] While contact sports would be expected to have a greater incidence of concussion, concussion may occur in any sport.

Table 2. NCAA Banned Substances for the Year 2001–2002

Stimulants

Amiphenazole	Dimethylamphetamine	Nikethamide
Amphetamine	Doxapram	Pemoline
Bemegride	Ephedrine	Pentetrazol
Benzphetamine	Ethamivan	Phendimetrazine
Bromantan	Ethylamphetamine	Phenmetrazine
Caffeine (a)	Fencamfamine	Phentermine
Chlorphentermine	Meclofenoxate	Picrotoxine
Cocaine	Methamphetamine	Pipradol
Cropropamide	Methylene-dioxy methamphetaminie	Prolintane
Crothetamide	(MDMA) (Ecstasy)	Strychnine
Diethylpropion	Methylphenidate	and related compounds *

Anabolic Agents

Anabolic steroids	Fluoxymesterone	Norethandrolone
Androstenediol	Mesterolone	Oxandrolone
Androstenedione	Methandienone	Oxymesterone
Boldenone	Methenolone	Oxymetholone
Clostebol	Methyltestosterone	Stanozolol
Dehydrochlormethyltestosterone	Nandrolone	Testosterone (b)
Dehydroepiandrosterone (DHEA)	Norandrostenediol	and related compounds *
Dihydrotestosterone (DHT)	Norandrostenedione	*Other anabolic agents*
Dromostanolone		Clenbuterol

Substances Banned for Specific Sports

Rifle

Alcohol	Nadolol	Timolol
Atenolol	Pindolol	
Metoprolol	Propranolol	and related compounds*

Diuretics

Acetazolamide	Flumethiazide	Quinethazone
Bendroflumethiazide	Furosemide	Spironolactone
Benzthiazide	Hydrochlorothiazide	Triamterene
Bumetanide	Hydroflumethiazide	Trichlormethiazide
Chlorothiazide	Methyclothiazide	
Chlorthalidone	Metolazone	and related compounds *
Ethacrynic acid	Polythiazide	

Street Drugs

Heroin	Marijuana (3)	THC
		(tetrahydrocannabinol) (3)

Peptide Hormones and Analogues

Chorionic gonadotrophin (HCG - human chorionic gonadotrophin) (d)	Growth hormone (HGH, somatotrophin) (d)	Erythropoietin (EPO) Sermorelin
Corticotrophin (ACTH) (d)		

*The term "related compounds" comprises substances that are included in the class by their pharmacological action and/or chemical structure. No substance belonging to the prohibited class may be used, regardless of whether it is specifically listed as an example.

The definitions of positive depend on the following:
(a) for caffeine—if the concentration in urine exceeds 15 micrograms/ml.; (b) for testosterone—if the administration of testosterone or the use of any other manipulation has the result of increasing the ratio of the total concentration of testosterone to that of epitestosterone in the urine to greater than 6:1, unless there is evidence that this ratio is due to a physiological or pathological condition. (c) for marijuana and THC—if the concentration in the urine of THC metabolite exceeds 15 nanograms/ml. (d) All the respective releasing factors of the above-mentioned substances also are banned.

*"Reprint permission granted by the NCAA. This material is subject to annual review and change."

Difficulties encountered with the careful study of sports related concussions are problems in reporting and a lack of objective criteria for grading and management. In the mid-1990s, in an attempt to develop more uniform and descriptive terminology, the term "mild traumatic brain injury" (MTBI) was adopted. *Concussion* and *MTBI* are still used interchangeably in the medical literature and will be similarly used in this chapter. MTBI (concussion) is defined as a trauma-induced alteration in mental status that may or may not be accompanied by a loss of consciousness. A concise denotation of concussion used by the NCAA is "post-traumatic impairment of neural status."[68] Neither definition includes a requirement for loss of consciousness or amnesia. Milder forms of concussion may have only subtle symptoms. These milder occurrences contribute to underreporting because they may go unrecognized by teammates, coaches, athletic trainers, or team physicians.

Signs and Symptoms

The athlete who has sustained a concussion may be observed to be unresponsive when initially evaluated by the training staff. All athletes who are unconscious should be assumed to have a cervical spine injury until proven otherwise and should be treated accordingly. The majority of concussions, however, do not result in a loss of consciousness. The athlete may appear dazed, confused, or "out of it" (Table 3). He may have trouble recalling plays and processing information related to the game. The player may repeatedly ask the same question(s), display inappropriate behavior, or appear unsteady.

Table 3.

Symptoms of concussion	Signs of concussion
Headache	Dazed
Blurry or double vision	Inappropriate emotional state (laughing, crying)
Vertigo	Unusual behavior
Tinnitus	Confusion
Difficulty concentrating	Disorientation
Memory impairment	Amnesia (retrograde and/or anterograde)
Irritability	Balance difficulties
Nausea	

The athlete who has suffered a concussion should undergo examination by a skilled sports medicine professional immediately after the injury if possible but ideally no later than within five to ten minutes of the injury. Serial examinations should follow at regular intervals. Any athlete with prolonged loss of consciousness, deteriorating mental status, or neurological examination suggestive of a more serious intracranial injury should be immediately transported to a trauma center and neurosurgical consultation should be obtained. It is, understandably, best to err on the side of caution in the management of head injuries.

To facilitate initial and serial assessment of an athlete with a concussion, a Standardized Assessment of Concussion (SAC) test has been developed.[69,70] This test is easily administered by athletic trainers and physicians, takes approximately five minutes, and can provide more objective data on the severity of a concussion. An ever-present problem is the tendency of players to downplay or underreport their symptoms so that they can return to play. Furthermore, impairment from concussion may be subtle. Therefore, standardized testing of memory, attention, orientation, and concentration is needed to properly assess and follow deficits. This evaluation is important for the determination of return to sports.

Pathophysiology of Concussion

There are two basic mechanisms through which external force may be applied to the skull with resultant cerebral injury. In one, the athlete is motionless and a moving object impacts the cranium. In the other, the athlete is moving and collides with a fixed object or an object with a different trajectory. This causes relative motion of the brain within the cranium. Neuronal injury may result from compression, traction, or shearing forces acting on brain tissue. Shearing forces are very poorly tolerated by neural tissue.

Concussion is diagnosed by a collection of signs and symptoms. There is no clinical pathological correlate in athletes who have suffered a concussion. Radiographic imaging studies (e.g., CT, MR) in concussed athletes are usually normal except in circumstances where there is additional injury (e.g., subdural hematoma). Thus, concussion is a clinical diagnosis which relies on observations by medical staff and the athlete's subjective complaints. The unanswered question for concussions is, What do the observations and symptoms actually represent within the central nervous system (CNS)? In practical terms this concern may be divided into short- and long-term considerations.

On-the-Field Evaluation

The most immediate and important clinical consideration in concussion is the rapid assessment for the presence of a life-threatening injury. When assessing an unconscious athlete on the field, the ABCs (airway, breathing, circulation) should be quickly determined by the sports medicine staff. The next step is to determine the level of CNS functioning using the Glasgow Coma Scale. It is essential to assume that all athletes have a cervical spine injury until proven otherwise and to evaluate accordingly. The sports medicine staff must decide if immediate transportation to a hospital is indicated or if further evaluation on the sideline is appropriate. An emergency care plan, with backup contingencies, should be developed by all involved sports medicine staff prior to the start of the season.

Catastrophic CNS injury may become manifest quickly after the traumatic episode or may be delayed. Thus, evaluation by a physician immediately after injury, followed by repeated serial examinations at short intervals, has been recommended.[71] Careful examination for the presence of skull, facial, and cervical spine fractures and a neurological examination should be performed on all athletes who have sustained a concussion.[71] This should be done regardless of whether or not there was a loss of consciousness. Neuropsychological testing should be performed on the sideline and again at 24 hours and at 5 days after the injury.[72] The previously mentioned SAC[73] test is useful in this setting.

A rare but frequently fatal complication of a seemingly mild TBI is the so-called second impact syndrome (SIS). Although the exact initiating mechanism is not understood, the final pathway appears to be loss of autoregulation of cerebral blood flow, leading to progressive cerebral edema, and ultimately, death from brain stem herniation. SIS derives its name from the belief that it occurs following a second mild TBI in an athlete who is still symptomatic or has not completely recovered from a previous mild TBI. A recent review of published case reports, however, has led to doubt regarding the validity of this assumption.[74] Regardless of whether this devastating injury results from a primary concussion or a secondary insult in someone who has not fully recovered from a prior concussion, it is important to be cognizant of, and watchful for, this malignant process.

There is concern that repeated episodes of MTBI may result in long-term neurological impairment. A recent investigation involving collegiate football players found that having two or more concussions is significantly associated with long-term deficits in speed of information processing and executive functioning (Trail Making Test).[75] Similarly, a study of amateur soccer players found an inverse correlation between concussions and performance on several neuropsychological tests.[76] Further study into the remote sequelae of concussions has important implications for the management of concussion and for sports organizations in general.

Guidelines for Management and Return to Sport

To address the clinical concerns surrounding concussion and establish a standardized approach to its management, many authors and organizations have proposed a number of different guidelines. The shortcoming of all of these recommendations is that they are arbitrary and not evidence-based.[77] Guidelines for the management of concussion are constructed from the clinical experiences of an expert or a consensus panel of experts, in conjunction with the available medical literature. Thus, while they are practical for clinicians caring for injured athletes, there has not yet been prospective analysis to validate the return-to-play recommendations. Therefore, the guidelines should be considered rough approximations and not replacements for clinical judgment. Any number of circumstances may occur in which deviation from the published guidelines is entirely appropriate. Accordingly, the NCAA does not currently endorse any one set of guidelines. It must be emphasized that every episode of concussion should be evaluated based on individual circumstances and managed by an experienced physician exercising independent clinical judgment. Neurosurgical consultation and further testing should be obtained as needed.

One set of guidelines for concussion grading and return-to-play recommendations developed by Cantu[78] is presented here to provide a framework for management.

Grading Scale for Concussion

Grade 1—No loss of consciousness. Post-traumatic amnesia lasting less than 30 minutes.

Grade 2—Loss of consciousness lasting less than 5 minutes, or post-traumatic amnesia lasting longer than 30 minutes.

Grade 3—Loss of consciousness lasting longer than 5 minutes, or post-traumatic amnesia lasting longer than 24 hours.

Return to Play Recommendations for First and Subsequent Concussion(s)

Grade 1—May return to play if asymptomatic for one week. Athlete may return to play that day in a small number of select circumstances if normal clinical examination at rest and exertion.
- 2nd concussion—Return to play in two weeks if asymptomatic for prior seven days.
- 3rd concussion—Terminate season. May return to play next season if asymptomatic.

Grade 2—May return to play within two weeks if asymptomatic for prior seven days at rest and exertion.
- 2nd concussion—Minimum of one month. May return to play if asymptomatic for one week. Consider termination of season.
- 3rd concussion—Terminate season. May return to play next season if asymptomatic.

Grade 3—Minimum of one month. May then return to play if asymptomatic for one week at rest and exertion.
- 2nd concussion—Terminate season. May return to play next season if asymptomatic.

Although there are differences among the various concussion guidelines regarding grading and return to play, there is universal agreement that no player should return to participation while still symptomatic, and no athlete rendered unconscious for any length of time should return to play in the same game or practice in which the injury occurred.[71,72] Athletes who return to play while still symptomatic may be at risk for the second impact syndrome. Furthermore, these individuals have altered reaction times[79] and difficulty rapidly processing information,[80] which puts them at risk for further injury.

Prevention of Concussion

Strategies for prevention of concussion involve four main areas: equipment, neck strengthening exercises, technique, and competitive rules.

The equipment used for a particular sport is important in preventing injury, particularly in contact sports, and proper fit, use, and maintenance should be assured. For example, in football correct inflation of the air bladders in a helmet and use of shock-absorbing mouthpieces can help safeguard against concussion. The evolution of the modern football helmet makes an interesting historical review and gives perspective on how safety equipment changes over time. Undoubtedly, as new substances and methods in material science are developed safety equipment will continue to evolve and improve.

The athlete can actively participate in prevention of concussion through neck strengthening exercises and use of proper techniques in their sport. Improved neck strength is beneficial because it dampens the acceleration and deceleration forces applied to the head. Proper tackling techniques should be taught by coaches and utilized by athletes to help avoid circumstances in which head injury is likely to occur. Finally, the rules of a particular sport can minimize the chances of head injury. An example is the rule in football banning "spearing."

Final Thought on Concussion

Sports-related MTBI is a challenging area for sports medicine. The high prevalence, acute complications (including life-threatening cerebral edema), and potential long-term sequelae make this an important issue for athletes, coaches, and sports medicine practitioners. Management difficulties derive from the lack of evidence-based criteria for severity categorization and return-to-activity guidelines. Neuropsychological testing has emerged as the primary clinical and investigative tool for concussion, and future prospective analysis should help delineate current shortcomings in management and answer questions regarding long-term sequelae.

THE FEMALE ATHLETE TRIAD

Disordered eating, amenorrhea, and osteoporosis are the three components of a syndrome termed the *female athlete triad*.[81] The exact prevalence of this triad is not completely known, because of poor recognition and presence of strong denial. The terminology *disordered eating* is used in distinction to *eating disorders* and refers to a range of behaviors, including bingeing and/or purging, food restriction, prolonged fasting, use of certain medications (diuretics, diet pills, and/or laxatives), and thought patterns relating to food or body image.[82] It is important to note that the term *disordered eating* is not restricted to individuals who fulfill the DSM-IV criteria for anorexia nervosa or bulimia nervosa. Disordered eating and the addition of a new category to DSM-IV, *eating disorder not otherwise specified (NOS)*, are useful in diagnosing the triad by including athletes who partially, but not completely, fulfill the criteria for anorexia or bulimia nervosa.[83] Importantly, disordered eating may be unintentional. An athlete may be consuming a diet that would otherwise be healthy for a sedentary woman but is inadequate to meet the added requirements of exercise.

Amenorrhea is a direct result of disordered eating. Abnormal eating patterns lead to insufficient total caloric, protein, and/or fat intake for the athlete's energy expenditures. One currently proposed hypothesis is that the physiologic stress of an "energy deficit" alters hypothalamic and, subsequently, ovarian function.[83] From a clinical perspective, the evaluation of an athlete with amenorrhea is focused on defined causes (e.g., pregnancy), since "athletic amenorrhea" is, essentially, a diagnosis of exclusion.

The third part of the triad is osteoporosis. Despite the fact that some athletes may enjoy the apparent training convenience of amenorrhea, it is a warning sign that a serious health problem is developing. The hypogonadal state in these athletes results in inadequate bone formation and/or premature bone loss, which in turn leads to fragility and increased risk of fracture. This is especially concerning, because young adulthood is a time when a woman's maximum bone mineral density (BMD) is achieved. The impaired bone mineralization carries increased risk of training-related injuries (e.g., stress fractures) in young women[84,85] and may predispose to osteoporosis later in life.[86]

The World Health Organization has adopted criteria for the classification of osteoporosis which compares bone mineral density (BMD) based on standard deviation (SD) departure from the mean for young healthy adults. However, these criteria may not be sensitive enough to identify the full scope of the problem of abnormal bone mineralization in amenorrheic athletes. For example, a 17-year-old amenorrheic athlete may prematurely stop increasing her BMD but yet not meet WHO criteria for osteopenia. Nonetheless, premature arrest in BMD growth clearly represents an abnormal state.

WHO criteria are defined as:

- Normal—BMD up to 1 SD below the mean
- Osteopenia—BMD 1–2.5 SD below the mean
- Osteoporosis—BMD more than 2.5 SD below the mean
- Severe osteoporosis—BMD more than 2.5 SD below the mean plus one or more fragility fractures

The main goals of treatment are to normalize caloric intake, reestablish a normal menstrual cycle, increase bone mineral density, and employ methods to prevent recurrence. Reduction of training volume and intensity, coupled with increased caloric intake, is a practical approach.[83] In the course of exercise counseling, the sports medicine specialist must consider total physical activity, not just sport-specific activity. Nutritional assessment is essential, as is psychological evaluation for the presence of an eating disorder (e.g., anorexia), or co-morbid conditions such as substance abuse or depression. As previously noted, in some cases the inadequate calorie intake is inadvertent and not due to an eating disorder. Educating the athlete about proper nutrition,[87] the pathophysiology of triad development, and the medical complications, both short- and long-term, is an important part of treatment. Oral contraceptives have been shown to help increase bone mineral density,[88] but the ensuing resumption of menses may mask the underlying disordered eating.[83]

Frank eating disorders are notoriously difficult to treat and are best managed by a combination of psychotherapy, nutrition and exercise counseling, and general medical care,[89] preferably by practitioners with skill in this area. Treatment should be stepped up in intensity as dictated by clinical severity.

THE FATIGUED ATHLETE

Few problems are as frustrating for student-athletes or as challenging to sports medicine physicians as prolonged fatigue. Short-term, post exercise fatigue is, of course, a natural and expected consequence of training. However, fatigue that persists for longer periods of time—days or weeks—is an abnormality that requires intervention. Recent reviews[90,91,92] have highlighted this clinical problem and suggested a diagnostic framework, but because of the heterogeneity of potential diseases, there is no standardized approach or set laboratory evaluation.

In addition, there is no consensus for what constitutes prolonged or unusual fatigue. In working with athletes and coaches it is wise to avoid the use of the term "chronic fatigue," because of the implied reference, however unintentional, to "chronic fatigue syndrome." Even if instructed otherwise, students or coaches may erroneously associate the latter syndrome with the athlete's condition. This self-labeling is ultimately counterproductive in the diagnostic approach, generates unwarranted fear and anxiety, and is potentially damaging to an athlete's psyche.

For this discussion the term "prolonged fatigue" is used and is defined as a decrease in mental and/or physical performance associated with weariness, altered mood, or somatic symptoms that occurs for two or more weeks.

Clinical Presentation and Considerations

The fatigued student-athlete comes to the attention of the sports medicine professional in one of several ways. The athlete may be referred by the coach and/or athletic trainer because of observation and discussion, or the individual will directly seek medical attention because symptoms have become too significant to ignore. Parents, peers, or teammates may have a role in this "referral" process as well. Often by the time the athlete presents, he/she has had several suggestions as to the possible etiology of the fatigue. The athlete may state that he/she is there simply to get his/her "iron level" or "blood count" checked. Although it may be tempting, especially in a busy clinical setting, to order the requested laboratory test(s) it is best to ask a few open-ended questions (e.g., How have workouts and competition been going?). The answers to these questions will help outline the actual clinical problem and ensure that the athlete gets access to the appropriate venue of care.

A full history and physical examination for the athlete with fatigue is best performed by an experienced sports medicine diagnostician (e.g., a general internist). Although extensive prior contact with athletes is not a requirement, it is beneficial because it enables better communication and understanding on the part of the clinician. Athletes use idiomatic language to describe training and problems experienced. For example, the athlete may complain of "going anaerobic" prematurely in an easy workout. Appropriate communication and empathy are of significant advantage in the determination of the exact diagnostic framework to utilize. Furthermore, communication with the coach to obtain additional information is facilitated.

At times it may be difficult for the athlete to "open up" and feel comfortable discussing his/her situation. This is especially true if there is conflict with the coach, outside personal stressors, or disenchantment with his/her sport. Acknowledging these potential difficulties and informing the athlete that what gets reported to the coach is only what the clinician and athlete agree upon can be helpful.

Diagnosis

The history and physical examination should include all the elements normally found in a thorough exam. An important element for the history of present illness is *when* the fatigue occurs. Is it present all the time, outside of exercise and with day-to-day activities, or does it occur only during exertion? This may help isolate conditions that would be expected to diminish only exercise performance (e.g., mild anemia) from those conditions that would be expected to occur pervasively throughout the day (e.g., infectious mononucleosis). For fatigue that is solely exercise-related, it is helpful to determine the circumstances under which it is likely to occur. For example, does the fatigue occur at the very end of a hard "set," or at the end of a difficult workout session, or does it become manifest very early during an easy warm-up routine?

Standard questions regarding past medical history, medication use, social activities and habits (including tobacco, alcohol, and other drug use), class work and academic standing, peer relationships, family medical history, and, specifically, dietary supplement use (herbal remedies, vitamins, performance-enhancing substances, etc.) are all vital parts of the history. Additionally, questions regarding current team dynamics, individual athletic goals, and long-term plans can occasionally reveal important clues. Finally, there should be a complete review of systems documenting pertinent positives and negatives.

The physical examination should include all relevant organ systems, with more extensive scrutiny of a particular system performed as needed based upon historical elements. A partial list of diagnostic considerations is given in Table 4. The listed elements are by no means comprehensive, and the clinician should not limit the differential diagnosis to the diseases presented here.

There are no evidence-based guidelines regarding appropriate laboratory testing, but some basic screening is probably justified. Generally, a complete blood count, urinalysis, and determinations of serum electrolytes, creatinine, and liver function is a reasonable approach. More specialized testing should be guided by clinical judgment and results of the preliminary screening tests.

Treatment and return to sport

Once the diagnosis is determined, appropriate treatment can be instituted. Return to sport depends upon the clinical entity and severity. There are no specific guidelines, and clinicians should avoid a "cookbook" approach. In general, athletes and coaches tend to push for early return, especially if the competitive season is underway. The team physician must have ultimate authority and responsibility for the safe return of the athlete to his/her sport and should not be unduly influenced by external forces. Depending on the diagnosis, prognosis, and the specific sport involved, return may be done on a graded scale (e.g., workouts every other day at a reduced level, limited game participation) and the athlete's progress monitored clinically. For some circumstances follow-up laboratory testing is needed, but the physician should not rely solely on "numbers" to guide return-to-competition recommendations. The athlete's symptomatology and clinical exam provide the most important and relevant information.

OVERTRAINING

The benefits of exercise are well documented; however, excess training can lead to a number of health problems. While coaches and athletes understand that achievement in sports is rooted in hard work, the concept of appropriate and necessary rest is less deeply rooted. Athletes, coached or self-directed, have a tendency to train too much, resulting in injury, illness, and/or poor performance. A well-designed training program balances training stress and recovery and is the optimal way to enhance performance while minimizing the risks of excess.

Overtraining describes a situation in which excess training has resulted in poor ath-

Table 4. Diagnostic considerations in the fatigued athlete

Endocrine / Metabolic	Hypo- and hyperthyroidism
	Hypo- and hyperparathyroidism
	Diabetes Mellitus
	Hyponatremia
	Hypokalemia
Cardiovascular	Myocarditis
	Pericarditis
	Ischemic heart disease
	Hypertrophic cardiomyopathy
	Dilated cardiomyopathy
	Arrhythmias and conduction disturbances
	Valvular disease (e.g., aortic stenosis)
Hematologic	Anemia (iron deficiency, macrocytic, etc.)
Toxic	Alcohol, tobacco, and other drugs
	Medication (iatrogenic)
	Dietary supplements
Nutritional	Inadequate protein and/or caloric intake
	"Fad" dieting
	Insufficient or inappropriate macronutrients
	Insufficient or inappropriate micronutrients
Neoplastic	Leukemia
	Lymphoma
	Testicular cancer
	Breast cancer
Renal	Glomerulonephritis
	Acute tubular necrosis (e.g., NSAID-induced)
	Renal insufficiency
Respiratory	Asthma
	Allergies
Neurological	Multiple sclerosis
Gastrointestinal	Malabsorption syndromes (e.g., celiac disease)
	Inflammatory bowel disease
Infectious	Infectious mononucleosis
	Hepatitis
	Post-viral syndrome
	Cytomegalovirus
Psychiatric	Depression
	Eating disorder
	Bipolar disorder
Psychological	Interpersonal relationship difficulties
	Academic stress
	Poor sleep hygiene (e.g., REM deficit)
	Failure to achieve goals or meet expectations
Miscellaneous	Pregnancy
	Overtraining syndrome

letic performance. The short-term state of excess resulting in declining performance is termed *overreaching*. Overreaching may be an intentional, temporary component of the training program. If overreaching is followed by appropriate rest, then performance enhancement occurs. However, if overreaching is extended with inadequate rest, then the overtraining syndrome (OS) will likely develop. The hallmark of OS is poor athletic performance but often involves additional signs and symptoms such as depression, mood changes, insomnia, irritability, loss of appetite, menstrual irregularities, difficulty concentrating, and frequent injury or illness. There are several biochemical abnormalities that have been observed in overtrained athletes, but none have yet proven useful diagnostically or prognostically. No single lab abnormality is consistently found in OS, and a number of biochemical derangements may be found in athletes who are not overtrained. Thus OS is a clinical diagnosis. Laboratory testing should be interpreted with caution. Abnormal tests should alert the clinician to the potential presence of an undiagnosed medical condition and not be simply attributed to OS.

Diagnosis

There are no set criteria for the diagnosis of OS. The one requirement, by definition, is a decline in athletic performance. Impaired performance may potentially be due to any number of diseases and conditions and is thus not unique to OS. The practical implication is that OS is a diagnosis of exclusion.

A careful history and physical examination with appropriate laboratory testing is warranted on all athletes with persistent symptoms suggestive of OS. Usually, "persistent" is defined as underperformance that continues despite two or more weeks of relative rest.

OS should be considered in an underperforming athlete when:

- There is poor athletic performance, and a thorough history and physical examination, with appropriate laboratory testing, has failed to identify a defined medical condition
- A review of the athlete's training schedule, with consideration of social and psychological stressors and overall workload (e.g., academics, extracurricular activities) has identified a scenario that is consistent, or potentially consistent, with overextension

Mechanism

It is widely accepted that the normal, adaptive response to training is a cycle of damage followed by repair. Appropriately applied strenuous exercise causes microtrauma to the musculoskeletal system. The subsequent inflammatory response not only heals this damage but provides a little extra "buildup." This is termed *supercompensation* and explains the observed gradual improvement in strength or performance that occurs when an athlete consistently trains (training effect). In the case of OS, excessive training and/or inadequate recovery progressively undermine the repair process resulting in *decompensation*.

The life of a student revolves around many factors and is in an almost constant state of flux. There are schedules to juggle, social activities, exams and papers, and training and competition. The sum total of these stressors ultimately influences a central mechanism and impairs the ability to recover from exercise. The hypothalamic-pituitary-adrenal axis seems the most likely mechanism through which overtraining is expressed. This concept is graphically depicted in Figure 4.

Figure 4

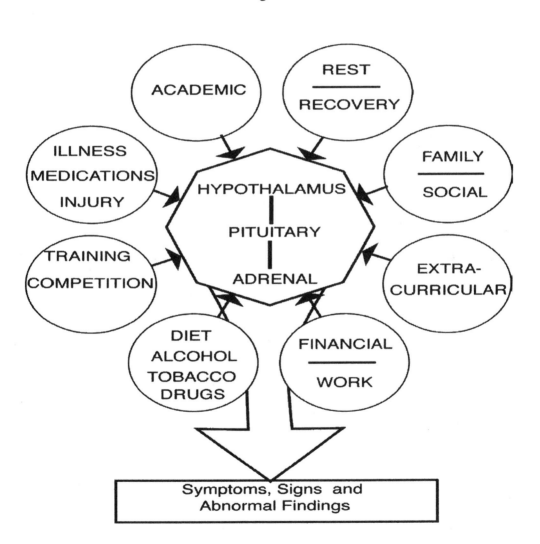

The *exact* pathways through which overtraining brings about the signs, symptoms, and various biochemical perturbations observed in OS are not known. A variety of hypotheses have been suggested,[93,94,95,96] but none have yet been proven or enjoy universal support. Recently, an intriguing theory has proposed a central role for cytokines in the expression of OS.[97] Cytokines, originally isolated from B and T lymphocytes, are proteins produced by immune system cells from a variety of tissues (e.g., liver, brain), and are an essential part of inflammation and repair. This hypothesis forwards the concept of a systemic immune response as a plausible mechanism through which OS manifests. However, further research is needed to fully characterize the syndrome.

Treatment of OS

The only effective treatment for OS is rest. With respect to training, rest may be absolute or relative. In the former, no athletic activity is permitted for a specified time frame. In the latter, exercise occurs but with reduced total volume and intensity. Often absolute rest followed by relative rest is used to bring about proper recovery. The duration of each type of rest cannot be prospectively determined. The same is true for the timing, frequency, intensity, and duration of training sessions during the relative rest phase. Specifics must be determined on a case-by-case basis and are influenced by individual factors, the presence of external stressors, duration of OS, the athlete's sport, concurrent illness or injury, the athlete's support group, and the coaching staff. The extensive variability of these determining factors currently negates the prospect of meaningful recommendations based on a preconceived set of criteria. Proper implementation of a recovery plan, therefore, requires continuous monitoring, feedback, and adjustments to the training schedule. It is important that the athlete, coach, and physician work together in a coordinated fashion to facilitate the recovery process.

Once the athlete has recovered, attention should be directed towards prevention of recurrence. The concept of periodized training is perhaps one of the most useful methods for the prevention of OS.[98] This very practical strategy utilizes construction of a training regimen characterized by exercise load buildup followed by reduced load in alternating cycles. Periodization makes full use of the manner in which the human body adapts. The programmed periods of relative rest allow for recovery and facilitate supercompensation. In summary, this process enhances improvement and minimizes risk of overtraining, illness, and/or injury.

ATHLETES WITH PERSISTENT INJURY OR UNRELENTING FATIGUE

Scholarship athletes have the opportunity to obtain both a valuable college education and a memorable and enriching sports experience. Although only a small percentage ultimately pursue a career in professional sports, many former college athletes feel that the time spent training and competing provided a very valuable "outside the classroom" education. Values such as teamwork, camaraderie, and leadership, as well as experiences in achieving goals and learning how to handle adversity, are some of the aspects valuable to the student, no matter what career is pursued.

The college athletic experience entails a great deal of hard work, and athletes face a challenging task of balancing academics and sports participation. A further strain can be the scholarship itself. At its simplest level the athletic scholarship is a contract between the student and the institution. Scholarships reward the student through several possible arrangements which essentially differ in the degree of funding. The gain for the institution is name recognition and media attention, which can translate into support and funding, not only for athletics, but for the institution as a whole. Unlike in some professional sports, the student-athlete's "contract" has no contingencies for performance statistics or "wins." University athletic programs expect, as part of the contract, the student to fully participate in all practices, meetings, and competitions under the direction of the head coach for the particular sport. Furthermore, adherence is expected to all codes of conduct for the particular school and NCAA and team rules. Violations of rules are grounds for disciplinary actions, including dismissal.

To help protect the student and preserve the student-institution relationship (contract) the NCAA has an extensive set of rules backed by sanctions. These rules help ensure equality in intercollegiate competition, safety of training and competition, and a quality education for the student-athlete. For example, if a student-athlete becomes permanently injured and can no longer safely compete in his/her sport, there are provisions for continuation of the same level of financial support for the duration of his/her college education. This designation, in scholarship jargon, is referred to as a "medical." The athlete who obtains a "medical" may be expected to fulfill other duties for the team, such as managing equipment, but the continuation of the scholarship means the athlete is not required to face a potentially large and unexpected financial burden. Without this rule some athletes would undoubtedly have to withdraw from school and thus lose their opportunity to obtain a college degree.

The "medical" rule is fair, ethical, and needed; however, there is an unintended consequence. The medical may become a sought-after "prize" for the athlete who no longer wishes to participate in his/her sport. The reasons for this include academic and other external stressors, ongoing conflict with the coach, and a change in interest/loss of pleasure. If the athlete voluntarily withdraws, then scholarship funding for subsequent years is lost. However, as previously noted, if the athlete is disqualified for medical reasons (involuntarily withdraws), then funding continues.

No rational individual would truly make it a goal to become seriously injured or self-inflict an injury. Thus, the student will often manifest the desire to discontinue athletic participation through different means. Examples include an injury that won't heal, persistent fatigue, and pain that chronically impairs his/her ability to perform. This is *not* to say that the majority of student-athletes in this circumstance are being factitious or malingering. The athlete accurately reports what he/she experiences; however, insight is often lacking. It is not apparent to him/her that the "injury" may be strongly influenced by his/her disenchantment with the sport. This scenario presents unusual difficulty for the athlete and the sports medicine team.

The exact incidence of this situation is not known, and understandably, it is a difficult area for which to obtain valid information or achieve controlled scientific scrutiny. Most of the information for this discussion is derived from direct experience and long-term follow-up and, thus, is admittedly anecdotal. The descriptive term used by the author is *psychologically enhanced injury or illness* syndrome (PEI).*

Presentation of the athlete with PEI

There is considerable variation in the manner in which athletes with PEI encounter the sports medicine team. Development of this syndrome may occur at any time in the season, in any sport, in any year of study, and in both men and women. There may or may not be an identifiable preceding precipitating event or conflict. The athlete may initially present to the training-room staff with a series of seemingly unrelated injuries or may present repeatedly with the same injury. The training-room staff may, after a period of time, become frustrated and express this to the athlete (verbally or by body language). The coaching staff may become involved out of concerns for the athlete's health, performance that is not up to par, or absenteeism from practice and/or competition.

Approach to the athlete with PEI

Team physicians may encounter the athlete early or late in the course of PEI. Late-stage findings may reveal considerable anger on the part of the athlete and training-room staff. The former may feel that the training-room staff or coaches are not taking the "injury" seriously. The latter may feel that the athlete is malingering. The team doctor is often faced with the challenge of sorting out a series of injuries or extensively pursuing a single injury.

　　If PEI is suspected, then nonthreatening questions about potential stressors in the athlete's life may prove useful. Gentle probing of such factors as academic course work, major area of study, career plans, peer relationships, and other aspects of the student's life should be done. However, the athlete will often emphatically deny, and sometimes resent, the suggestion that there may be psychological or external issues involved. Nevertheless, team physicians should continue to maintain a caring, non-accusatory approach for all students, because there will be the occasional athlete who is willing to explore potential psychological contributors. Even if there are not identifiable external issues, the clinician has conveyed consideration of the athlete as a complete individual and not just a "cog" in the team hierarchy. Not to be overlooked is the fact that in some circumstances there will be an undiagnosed medical condition that is responsible for all of the athlete's symptoms. Thus, in all circumstances of chronic illness or injury a thorough medical evaluation should be done.

Outcomes

There are four potential outcomes for PEI. The athlete may accomplish the desired "medical" status, or he/she may continue to progress from one injury to the next throughout

---

* Very few references are available in the literature on this subject. The term "PEI" is one coined by the author, based on observation and clinical evaluation of athletes.

his/her entire collegiate career, never competing or training to any significant degree, which is effectively the same result. The athlete may "recover," either spontaneously or with the aid of medical and psychological assistance. In this case a certain period of sports disability occurs, but he/she is then able to resume full participation. Often there is no open admission of potential psychological issues, and the athlete has a strong desire to move forward and may not wish to discuss what has happened. The fourth outcome is that the athlete will decide that he/she no longer wishes to pursue his/her sport, even though there is no definitive diagnosis to qualify for a medical. He/she will express this desire to his/her coach and withdraw. In these latter cases this may entail transfer to another school, acquisition of alternate financial support, or withdrawal from pursuit of a college degree. This final situation is an unfortunate reality of participation in college athletics and one that all institutions should strive to avoid.

SPECIAL STUDENT-ATHLETE CONSIDERATIONS

Sickle-cell trait

Sickle-cell trait (SCT) is characterized by the presence of one normal gene for hemoglobin A and one abnormal gene coding for hemoglobin S. Approximately 9 percent of African-Americans have sickle-cell trait.[99] Individuals with SCT have a normal life expectancy, and the primary consideration is genetic counseling regarding family planning. There are, however, certain potential concerns for athletes.

SCT is associated with splenic infarction during exercise at altitudes greater then 5000 ft (1500 m) in non-altitude-adapted individuals and is more common in Caucasians.[100] SCT has also been associated with hematuria and hyposthenuria. The latter may increase susceptibility to dehydration during exercise in hot or humid conditions. Exercise-associated sudden death has been reported in military recruits with SCT.[101,102] The risk of sudden death in this population represents a 40-fold increase.[103] The mechanism is thought to be due to acute complications of vaso-occlusion-induced rhabdomyolysis.[99,104] These clinical consequences are rare, and SCT is still regarded as a benign hereditary condition. Accordingly, the NCAA does not currently recommend routine screening for SCT or restrictions on training or competition in those with known SCT.[105]

Disabled student-athletes

As a result of improved access, the Americans with Disabilities Act (ADA 1992) and changing societal perceptions, more handicapped individuals are participating in sports than ever before. The NCAA has taken a supportive position for those impaired students wishing to compete in collegiate sports, as evidenced in this excerpt from the NCAA Sports Medicine Handbook: ". . . the NCAA recognizes the right of impaired athletes to an equal opportunity to participate in high-quality sport or recreational programs. These individuals should be eligible for intercollegiate programs if they qualify for a team without any lowering of standards for achievement, attendance or completion of required tasks, and if their participation does not put others or themselves at significant risk of substantial harm. Medical exclusion of an impaired student from an athletics program should occur only when the impairment presents significant risk of substantial harm to the health or safety of the individual and/or other participants that cannot be eliminated or reduced by reasonable accommodations."[106]

Thus, team physicians must carefully consider the desire of an impaired student to participate in sports so that the student is neither inappropriately excluded nor placed in a situation which could potentially jeopardize his/her health. Considerations include the specific sport or activity in question, the nature of the handicap and current medical status, established medical information on the risks involved with that handicap, availability of protective equipment, and the ability of the student and/or parents to fully understand the risks involved.[106]

Athletes recovering from infectious mononucleosis

Infectious mononucleosis (IM) is a commonly encountered clinical problem in the college health care setting. This illness—characterized by fatigue, fever, tonsillitis, and adenopathy—requires special consideration in a student-athlete. The natural clinical course of IM entails, in some patients, waxing and waning symptomatology. The duration of the illness and the lack of any effective treatment make IM a frustrating experience for many athletes. For the clinician, the main objective is to guide a safe recovery and a timely return to sports participation. Stress of vigorous exercise early in convalescence may contribute to recurrence of symptoms; thus clinicians are often hesitant to permit an early return to sports. The variability in severity and duration of clinical symptoms in IM means there is large variability in the correct time frame for resumption of exercise. The reflexive use of an arbitrary number of days (e.g., one month) may be easy for the clinician, but it is not useful in caring for the student. This approach will restrict activity for some athletes inappropriately, while in others will lead to a premature return. Each case should be individualized, according to the following considerations.

- The specific sport
- Competitive season or off-season
- Is reduced or limited participation possible?
- With splenomegaly, contact vs. non-contact sport (see below)
- Severity of clinical course, including associated complications of IM
- Duration of illness
- Presence of other stressors (e.g., academic)
- Concurrent medical conditions or injuries.
- Availability of an experienced physician to monitor and adjust the degree of sports participation.

Particular consideration of the risk of traumatic rupture of the spleen is important for contact sports. Athletes should be held from contact until it can be determined that splenomegaly is not present.

AN AFTERWORD

No discussion of athletic medicine programs in a textbook on college health would be complete without some comment on the overall responsibility of the college health service in athletic medicine programs. It is ironic, to say the least, that those physical activities which through the years developed into intercollegiate athletic programs which exist today actually began in college health services as part of an effort to improve physical health, thereby increasing fitness for academic intellectual pursuits. It would be naïve to assume by any stretch of the imagination that intercollegiate athletics today have little if any relationship to their original purpose. Because of this, there may be those who think it naïve for a modern day college health service to be responsible for a medical program for student athletes. We suggest, however, that the very opposite may be true; that, in fact, it is essential for a college health service to be prepared to meet unique and special primary care needs of all its students, including student athletes. A similar comment could be made for any number of groups of students—international students, health science students, and many more. We believe that students can get the best care consistently, and particularly within the legal constraints of various sports organizations such as the National Collegiate Athletic Association (NCAA), through well-prepared and well-managed college health services.

There is no place in the medical care of college student athletes for the "bidding wars" which occur, particularly at NCAA Division I schools, nor for the emphasis on being a "team physician" for a large school because the "title" publicizes an individual or a private practice. While it is evident that expert specialist care and consultation are essential in certain aspects of sports medicine, just as they are in many other areas of practice, it is inappropriate to separate the medical care of the college athlete from the care received by other students who may also have unique and special needs. To the contrary, if the unique and special needs of many groups of students, including athletes, cannot be met by the student health service, then the fault lies within the health service itself, either structurally, organizationally, or with the extent of—or lack thereof—its practice.

REFERENCES

1. Pfister GC, Puffer JC, Maron BJ. Preparticipation cardiovascular screening for US collegiate student-athletes. JAMA 2000; 283(12):1597–1599.

2. Maron BJ, Epstein SE, Roberts WC. Causes of sudden cardiac death in competitive athletes. J Am Coll Cardio 1986; 7:204–214.

3. Maron BJ, Shirani J, Poliac LC, Mathenge R, Roberts WC, Mueller FO. Sudden death in young competitive athletes. Clinical, demographic, and pathological profiles [see comments]. JAMA 1996; 276(3):199–204.

4. Maron BJ, Gohman TE, Aeppli D. Prevalence of sudden cardiac death during competitive sports activities in Minnesota high school athletes. J Am Coll Cardiol 1998; 32(7):1881–1884.

5. Maron BJ. Sudden death in young athletes: Lessons from the Hank Gathers affair [see comments]. N Engl J Med 1993; 329(1):55–57.

6. Thompson PD, Funk EJ, Carleton RA, Sturner WQ. Incidence of death during jogging in Rhode Island from 1975–1980. JAMA 1982; 247:2535–2538.

7. Waller BF, Roberts WC. Sudden death while running in conditioned runners aged 40 years or over. Am J Cardiol 1980; 45:1292–1300.

8. Tabib A, Miras A, Taniere P, Loire R. Undetected cardiac lesions cause unexpected sudden cardiac death during occasional sport activity. A report of 80 cases. Eur Heart J 1999; 20(12): 900–903.

9. Maron BJ, Poliac LC, Roberts WO. Risk for sudden cardiac death associated with marathon running [see comments]. J Am Coll Cardiol 1996; 28(2): 428–431.

10. Van CSP, Bloor CM, Mueller FO, Cantu RC, Olson HG. Nontraumatic sports death in high school and college athletes. Med Sci Sports Exerc 1995; 27(5): 641–647.

11. Maron BJ, Gardin JM, Flack JM, Gidding SS, Kurosaki TT, Bild DE. Prevalence of hypertrophic cardiomyopathy in a general population of young adults: Echocardiographic analysis of 4111 subjects in the CARDIA Study [see comments]. Circulation 1995; 92(4):785–789.

12. Burch M, Blair E. The inheritance of hypertrophic cardiomyopathy. Pediatr Cardiol 1999; 20(5): 313–316.

13. Link MS, Wang PJ, VanderBrink BA, et al. Selective activation of the K(+)(ATP) channel is a mechanism by which sudden death is produced by low-energy chest-wall impact (Commotio cordis). Circulation 1999; 100(4): 413–418.

14. Maron BJ, Link MS, Wang PJ, Estes NA. Clinical profile of commotio cordis: An under appreciated cause of sudden death in the young during sports and other activities. J Cardiovasc Electrophysiol 1999; 10(1): 114–120.

15. Abrunzo TJ. Commotio cordis. The single, most common cause of traumatic death in youth baseball. Am J Dis Child 1991; 145(11): 1279–1282.

16. Deady B, Innes G. Sudden death of a young hockey player: Case report of commotio cordis. J Emerg Med 1999; 17(3): 459–462.

17. Edlich RFJ, Mayer NE, Fariss BL, et al. Commotio cordis in a lacrosse goalie. J Emerg Med 1987; 5(3): 181–184.

18. American Heart Association. Cardiovascular preparticipation screening of competitive athletes. Med Sci Sports Exerc 1996; 28(12): 1445–1452.

19. Pfister GC, Puffer JC, Maron BJ. Preparticipation cardiovascular screening for US collegiate student-athletes. JAMA 2000; 283(12): 1597–1599.

20. Corrado D, Basso C, Schiavon M, Thiene G. Screening for hypertrophic cardiomyopathy in young athletes. N Engl J Med 1998; 339(6): 364–369.

21. Fuller CM. Cost effectiveness analysis of screening of high school athletes for risk of sudden cardiac death. Med Sci Sports Exerc 2000; 32(5): 887–890.

22. Holly RG, Shaffrath JD, Amsterdam EA. Electrocardiographic alterations associated with the hearts of athletes. Sports Med 1998; 25(3): 139–148.

23. Biochemical and physiological aspects of human nutrition. 2000; 898.

24. Williams MH. Facts and fallacies of purported ergogenic amino acid supplements. Clin Sports Med 1999; 18(3): 633–649.

25. Rankin JW. Role of protein in exercise. Clin Sports Med 1999; 18:499–511.

26. Krauss RM, Eckel RH, Howard B, et al. AHA Dietary Guidelines. Revision 2000: A Statement for Healthcare Professionals from the Nutrition Committee of the American Heart Association. Circulation 2000. [web page] http://circ.ahajournals.org/cgi/content/full [Accessed 10 Aug 2001].

27. Calcium and Osteoporosis Prevention [web page] http://www.eatright.org/feature/0501.html [Accessed 10 Aug 2001].

28. Simopoulos AP. Opening address. Nutrition and fitness from the first Olympiad in 776 B.C. to 393 A.D. and the concept of positive health. Am J Clin Nutr 1989; 49, supplement: 921–926.

29. Cheuvront SN. The Zone diet and athletic performance. Sports Med 1999; 27:213–228.

30. Economos CD, Bortz SS, Nelson ME. Nutritional practices of elite athletes. Sports Med 1993; 16:381–399.

31. Singh A, Pelletier PA, Deuster PA. Dietary requirements for ultra-endurance exercise. Sports Med 1994; 15:301–308.

32. Exercise Physiology: Energy, Nutrition, and Human Performance. 1991; 71.

33. Angell M, Kassirer JP. Alternative medicine—the risks of untested and unregulated remedies. N Engl J Med 1998; 339(12):839–841.

34. Mertz W. Chromium in human nutrition: a review [see comments]. J Nutr 1993; 123(4):626–633.

35. Anderson RA, Cheng N, Bryden NA, et al. Elevated intakes of supplemental chromium improve glucose and insulin variables in individuals with type 2 diabetes. Diabetes 1997; 46(11):1786–1791.

36. Fox GN, Sabovic Z. Chromium picolinate supplementation for diabetes mellitus. J Fam Pract 1998; 46(1):83–86.

37. Walker LS, Bemben MG, Bemben DA, Knehans AW. Chromium picolinate effects on body composition and muscular performance in wrestlers. Med Sci Sports Exerc 1998; 30(12):1730–1737.

38. Hallmark MA, Reynolds TH, DeSouza CA, Dotson CO, Anderson RA, Rogers MA. Effects of chromium and resistive training on muscle strength and body composition. Med Sci Sports Exerc 1996; 28(1):139–144.

39. Lukaski HC, Bolonchuk WW, Siders WA, Milne DB. Chromium supplementation and resistance training: Effects on body composition, strength, and trace element status of men [see comments]. Am J Clin Nutr 1996; 63(6):954–965.

40. Martin WR, Fuller RE. Suspected chromium picolinate-induced rhabdomyolysis. Pharmacotherapy 1998; 18(4):860–862.

41. Cerulli J, Grabe DW, Gauthier I, Malone M, McGoldrick MD. Chromium picolinate toxicity. Ann Pharmacother 1998; 32(4):428–431.

42. Bhasin S, Storer TW, Berman N, et al. The effects of supraphysiologic doses of testosterone on muscle size and strength in normal men [see comments]. N Engl J Med 1996; 335(1):1–7.

43. King DS, Sharp RL, Vukovich MD, et al. Effect of oral androstenedione on serum testosterone and adaptations to resistance training in young men: A randomized controlled trial [see comments]. JAMA 1999; 281(21):2020–2028.

44. Rasmussen BB, Volpi E, Gore DC, Wolfe RR. Androstenedione does not stimulate muscle protein anabolism in young healthy men. J Clin Endocrinol Metab 2000; 85(1):55–59.

45. Ballantyne CS, Phillips SM, MacDonald JR, Tarnopolsky MA, MacDougall JD. The acute effects of androstenedione supplementation in healthy young males. Can J Appl Physiol 2000; 25(1):68–78.

46. Wallace MB, Lim J, Cutler A, Bucci L. Effects of dehydroepiandrosterone vs androstenedione supplementation in men. Med Sci Sports Exerc 1999; 31(12):1788–1792.

47. Harris RC, Soderlund K, Hultman E. Elevation of creatine in resting and exercised muscle of normal subjects by creatine supplementation. Clin Sci (Colch) 1992; 83(3):367–374.

48. Greenhaff PL, Casey A, Short AH, Harris R, Soderlund K, Hultman E. Influence of oral creatine supplementation of muscle torque during repeated bouts of maximal voluntary exercise in man. Clin Sci (Colch) 1993; 84(5):565–571.

49. Balsom PD, Soderlund K, Sjodin B, Ekblom B. Skeletal muscle metabolism during short duration high-intensity exercise: Influence of creatine supplementation. Acta Physiol Scand 1995; 154(3):303–310.

50. Volek JS, Kraemer WJ, Bush JA, et al. Creatine supplementation enhances muscular performance during high-intensity resistance exercise. J Am Diet Assoc 1997; 97(7):765–770.

51. Bosco C, Tihanyi J, Pucspk J, et al. Effect of oral creatine supplementation on jumping and running performance. Int J Sports Med 1997; 18(5):369–372.

52. Prevost MC, Nelson AG, Morris GS. Creatine supplementation enhances intermittent work performance. Res Q Exerc Sport 1997; 68(3):233–240.

53. Kreider RB, Ferreira M, Wilson M, et al. Effects of creatine supplementation on body composition, strength, and sprint performance. Med Sci Sports Exerc 1998; 30(1):73–82.

54. McNaughton LR, Dalton B, Tarr J. The effects of creatine supplementation on high-intensity exercise performance in elite performers. Eur J Appl Physiol 1998; 78(3):236–240.

55. Biochemical and physiological aspects of human nutrition. 2000; 888–889.

56. Greenwood M, Farris J, Kreider R, Greenwood L, Byars A. Creatine supplementation patterns and perceived effects in select Division I collegiate athletes [In Process Citation]. Clin J Sport Med 2000; 10(3):191–194.

57. LaBotz M, Smith BW. Creatine supplement use in an NCAA Division I athletic program. Clin J Sport Med 1999; 9(3):167–169.

58. Poortmans JR, Francaux M. Adverse effects of creatine supplementation: Fact or fiction? [In Process Citation]. Sports Med 2000; 30(3):155–170.

59. Robinson TM, Sewell DA, Casey A, Steenge G, Greenhaff PL. Dietary creatine supplementation

does not affect some haematological indices, or indices of muscle damage and hepatic and renal function [In Process Citation]. Br J Sports Med 2000; 34(4):284–288.

60. Volek JS, Duncan ND, Mazzetti SA, Putukian M, Gomez AL, Kraemer WJ. No effect of heavy resistance training and creatine supplementation on blood lipids. Int J Sport Nutr Exerc Metab 2000; 10(2):144–156.

61. Terjung RL, Clarkson P, Eichner ER, et al. American College of Sports Medicine Roundtable. The physiological and health effects of oral creatine supplementation. Med Sci Sports Exerc 2000; 32(3):706–717.

62. Kilbourne EM, Philen RM, Kamb ML, Falk H. Tryptophan produced by Showa Denko and epidemic eosinophilia-myalgia syndrome [comment]. J Rheumatol Suppl 1996; 4681-4688; discussion 89–91.

63. Brukner P, Khan K. Clinical Sports Medicine.

64. Oliver S. Drugs in sports. Justifying paternalism on the grounds of harm. Am J Sports Med 1996; 24S:43–45.

65. Catlin DH, Murray TH. Performance-enhancing drugs, fair competition, and Olympic sport. JAMA 1996; 276:231–237.

66. Frost N. Drug screening for athletes: Do the means justify the ends? [comment]. Curr Probl Pediatr 1994; 24(10):334.

67. Sports-related recurrent brain injuries—United States. Morb Mortal Wkly Rep 1997; 46:224–227.

68. Guideline 20: Concussion and second impact syndrome. NCAA Sports Medicine Handbook 2000-2001 2000; 52.

69. Kelly JP, Rosenberg J. The management of concussion in sport: Report of the quality standards subcommittee. Neurology 1997; 48:575–580.

70. Wojtys EM, Hovda D, Landry G, et al. Current concepts: Concussion in sports. Am J Sports Med 1999; 27(5):676–687.

71. Cantu RC. Return to play guidelines after a head injury. Clin Sports Med 1998; 17:145–60.

72. Cantu RC. Cerebral concussion in sport. Management and prevention. Sports Med 1992; 14(1):64–74.

73. Kelly JP, Rosenberg J. The management of concussion in sport: Report of the quality standards subcommittee. Neurology 1997; 48:581–585.

74. McCrory PR, Berkovic SF. Second impact syndrome. Neurology 1998; 50:677–683.

75. Collins MW, Grindel SH, Lovell MR, et al. Relationship between concussion and neuropsychological performance in college football players [see comments]. JAMA 1999; 282(10):964–970.

76. Matser EJT, Kessels AG, Lezak MD, Jordan BD, Troost J. Neuropsychological impairment in amateur soccer players. JAMA 1999; 282:971–973.

77. Collins MW, Lovell MR, McKeag DB. Current issues in managing sports-related concussion. JAMA 1999; 282:2283–2285.

78. Cantu RC. When to return to contact sports after a cerebral concussion. Sports Med Digest 1988; 101-102.

79. Bleiberg J, Halpern EL, Reeves D, Daniel JC. Future directions for the neuropsychological assessment of sports concussion. J Head Trauma Rehabil 1998; 13(2):36–44.

80. Gronwall D, Wrightson P. Memory and information processing capacity after closed head injury. J Neurol Neurosurg Psychiatry 1981; 44:889–895.

81. Yeager KK, Agostini R, Nattiv A, Drinkwater B. The female athlete triad: disordered eating, amenorrhea, osteoporosis. Med Sci Sports Exerc 1993; 25(7):775–777.

82. Nattiv A, Agostini R, Drinkwater B, Yeager KK. The female athlete triad: The inter-relatedness of disordered eating, amenorrhea, and osteoporosis. Clin Sports Med 1994; 13(2):405–418.

83. Sanborn CF, Horea M, Siemers BJ, Dieringer KI. Disordered eating and the female athlete triad. Clin Sports Med 2000; 19(2):199–213.

84. Reeder MT, Dick BH, Atkins JK, Pribis AB, Martinez JM. Stress fractures: Current concepts of diagnosis and treatment. Sports Med 1996; 22(3):198–212.

85. Benson JE, Engelbert-Fenton KA, Eisenman PA. Nutritional aspects of amenorrhea in the female athlete triad. Int J Sport Nutr 1996; 6(2):134–145.

86. White CM, Hergenroeder AC. Amenorrhea, osteopenia, and the female athlete. Pediatr Clin North Am 1990; 37(5):1125–1141.

87. Manore MM. Nutritional needs of the female athlete. Clin Sports Med 1999; 18(3):549–563.

88. Hergenroeder AC, Smith EO, Shypailo R, Jones LA, Klish WJ, Ellis K. Bone mineral changes in young women with hypothalamic amenorrhea treated with oral contraceptives, medroxyprogesterone, or placebo over 12 months. Am J Obstet Gynecol 1997; 176(5):1017–1025.

89. Walsh JM, Wheat ME, Freund K. Detection, evaluation, and treatment of eating disorders: The role of the primary care physician [In Process Citation]. J Gen Intern Med 2000; 15(8):577–590.

90. Puffer JC, McShane JM. Depression and chronic fatigue in athletes. Clin Sports Med 1992; 11(2):327–338.

91. Puffer JC, McShane JM. Depression and chronic fatigue in the college student-athlete. Prim Care 1991; 18(2):297–308.

92. Derman W, Schwellnus MP, Lambert MI, et al. The "worn-out athlete": A clinical approach to chronic fatigue in athletes. J Sports Sci 1997; 15(3):341–351.

93. Gastmann UA, Lehmann MJ. Overtraining and the BCAA hypothesis. Med Sci Sports Exerc 1998; 30(7):1173–1178.

94. Snyder AC. Overtraining and glycogen depletion hypothesis. Med Sci Sports Exerc 1998; 30(7):1146–1150.

95. Walsh NP, Blannin AK, Robson PJ, Gleeson M. Glutamine, exercise and immune function: Links and possible mechanisms. Sports Med 1998; 26(3):177–191.

96. Kentta G, Hassmen P. Overtraining and recovery: A conceptual model. Sports Med 1998; 26(1):1–16.

97. Smith LL. Cytokine hypothesis of overtraining: A physiological adaptation to excessive stress? Med Sci Sports Exerc 2000; 32(2):317–331.

98. Fry RW, Morton AR, Keast D. Periodisation and the prevention of overtraining. Can J Sport Sci 1992; 17(3):241–248.

99. Cecil Textbook of Medicine. 1996; 889.

100. Franklin QJ, Compeggie M. Splenic syndrome in sickle cell trait: Four case presentations and a review of the literature. Mil Med 1999; 164(3):230–233.

101. Diggs LW. The sickle cell trait in relation to the training and assignment of duties in the armed forces: III. Hyposthenuria, hematuria, sudden death, rhabdomyolysis, and acute tubular necrosis. Aviat Space Environ Med 1984; 55(5):358–364.

102. Sateriale M, Hart P. Unexpected death in a black military recruit with sickle cell trait: case report. Mil Med 1985; 150(11):602–605.

103. Kark JA, Posey DM, Schumacher HR, Ruehle CJ. Sickle-cell trait as a risk factor for sudden death in physical training. N Engl J Med 1987; 317(13):781–787.

104. Le GD, Bile A, Mercier J, Paschel M, Tonellot JL, Dauverchain J. Exercise-induced death in sickle cell trait: Role of aging, training, and deconditioning. Med Sci Sports Exerc 1996; 28(5):541–544.

105. NCAA Sports Medicine Handbook. 2000; 59–60.

106. NCAA Sports Medicine Handbook. 2000; 56–57.

CHAPTER 15

HEALTH SERVICES FOR STUDENTS
WITH DISABILITIES

Marlene Belew Huff, LCSW, PhD, and Joyce B. Meder, RNP, MPA

INTRODUCTION

In the 1995–96 academic year, as part of the National Postsecondary Student Aid Study (NPSAS), 6% of a nationally representative sample of 21,000 undergraduates indicated having a disability such as a hearing or speech disorder, a mobility impairment, or vision problems not correctable with glasses. Twenty-nine percent indicated a learning disability, 23% an orthopedic impediment, 16% non-correctable low vision, 6% decreased hearing or deafness, and 3% a speech impediment. Twenty-one percent reported "some other health-related" disability.[1] And, while some disabilities are obvious, like most of those just described, other disabilities are "hidden," such as learning disorders and mental illness.

Disabilities notwithstanding, there are more similarities than differences in the characteristics of students with disabilities when compared to their non-disabled peers. For example, in 1998, about the same proportions of both groups:[2]

- were students of color (about one in five);
- had spent about four hours per week on homework while in high school;
- listed similar reasons why they had decided to attend college;
- were attending the college that had been their first choice;
- traveled about the same distances to attend college, and;
- were living off campus with parents, relatives, or in an apartment.

With regard to differences, first year college students who self-reported disabilities were more likely than their peers to:[2]

- be male;
- be 20 years or older;

- come from families with slightly higher median incomes;
- have spent more time between high school graduation and entry into college;
- be attending two-year colleges, and;
- predict they would need extra time to complete their educational goals.

THE AMERICANS WITH DISABILITIES ACT

The Americans with Disabilities Act (ADA) and Section 504 of the Rehabilitation Act of 1973 have implications for all colleges and universities. Key language from Section 504 states:

> No otherwise qualified individual with a disability in the United States shall solely by reason of his or her disability, be excluded from the participation in, be denied the benefits of, or be subjected to discrimination under any program or activity receiving federal financial assistance.[3]

Title II of the ADA states:

> Subject to the provisions of this title, no qualified individual shall, by reason of such disability, be excluded from participation or be denied the benefit of the services, programs, or activities of a public entity, or be subjected to discrimination by such entity.[3]

Signed into law on July 26, 1990, the ADA is wide-ranging legislation intended to make society more accessible to people with disabilities.

It is divided into five titles:

1. **Employment (Title I):** Businesses must provide reasonable accommodations to protect the rights of individuals with disabilities in all aspects of employment.
2. **Public Service (Title II):** Public services, which include state and local government instrumentalities, the National Railroad Passenger Corporation, and other commuter authorities, cannot deny services to individuals with disabilities participation in programs or activities which are available to people without disabilities.
3. **Public Accommodations (Title III):** All new construction and modifications must be accessible to individuals with disabilities. For existing facilities, barriers to services must be removed if readily achievable.
4. **Telecommunications (Title IV):** Telecommunication companies offering telephone service to the general public must have telephone relay services to individuals who use telecommunication devices for the Deaf (TTYs) or similar devices.
5. **Miscellaneous (Title V):** This title includes a provision prohibiting either (a) coercing or threatening or (b) retaliating against persons with disabilities or those attempting to aid people with disabilities in asserting their rights under the ADA.

An individual with a disability may be covered under the ADA if at least one of the following conditions is met:

- the presence of a physical or mental impairment that substantially limits one or more major life activities;
- the presence of a record of such an impairment;
- the individual is regarded as having such an impairment.

Other individuals who are protected by ADA in certain circumstances include those who have an association with an individual known to have a disability (such as parents), and those who are coerced or subjected to retaliation for assisting individuals with disabilities in asserting their rights under the ADA.

When a student with a disability presents to a college health service and requests a specific disability-related service, it may not be clear whether the service being requested is one that must be provided under the ADA/Section 504. Generally speaking, if students without disabilities are eligible for a particular service, then students with disabilities can expect the same level of service. Most institutions have an "ADA/Section 504" compliance officer, who should be contacted for specific questions regarding the law as well as to clarify the services expected to be available to all students—including those with disabilities. Since accommodations required under the ADA are made on an individual basis, it is important to individualize the services needed. Student health personnel, the ADA/Section 504 compliance office staff, and the individual with the disability should all be included in deciding on accommodations.

The institution and/or the student health service may provide services *beyond* those required by the ADA/Section 504, but it is important to understand the differences between services mandated by these acts and those provided voluntarily. On occasion, an individual with a disability will request an accommodation that could cause an undue burden on the institution. In these cases, the spirit of the ADA/Section 504 encourages all involved parties (students, administrators, and student health personnel) to agree to a compromise as to the most appropriate way to reasonably accommodate the individual, given the resources of the institution.

Student health professionals also need to be aware of the requirement for facility accessibility. The institutional office responsible for facility accessibility can assist in determining whether the student health service clinic facility meets state and/or federal architectural standards.

COMMUNICATION

Students with disabilities are particularly sensitive to "person-first language."[4] Person first language refers to the "person first" and the disability second. This distinction is important because it emphasizes what a student can do, focusing on ability rather than disability,[6] and distinguishes the person from the condition.[5,6]

Attitudes towards people with disabilities are complex, and some disabilities seem to be consistently "evaluated positively," whereas others tend to be "evaluated negatively," depending on the situational context.[5,6] Thus, increasingly, many health services encourage "person first" language, since language affects—perhaps even determines—attitudes. More specifically, these health services believe that "person first" language has a positive effect on the campus's attitudes toward students with disabilities or, at the least, promotes a less negative effect than more traditional forms of address.[7]

Language that tends to increase attitudinal barriers includes language that:

- perpetuates myths about and stereotypes of people with disabilities;
- uses nouns instead of adjectives to describe people with disabilities;
- uses demeaning or outdated words or phrases in reference to persons with disabilities.[6]

Incorporating person first language into student health service communication may not be as difficult as it initially seems. Staff who are skeptical about the value of eliminating language bias may respond more positively when it is presented in conjunction with examples of bias in other areas. For example, language that reflects a student's disability may be compared with language that reflects sexism or racism.[5,6]

Table 1 shows examples of "person first" language.

Table 1

Labels not to use ...	Person First Language ...
The handicapped or the disabled	Students with disabilities
The mentally retarded or he's retarded	Students with mental retardation
She's a Down's; she's a mongoloid	She has Down Syndrome
Birth defect	Has a congenital disability
Epileptic	A person with epilepsy
Wheelchair bound or confined to a wheelchair	Uses a wheelchair
She is developmentally delayed	She has a developmental delay
He's crippled; lame	He has an orthopedic disability
She's a dwarf (or midget)	She has short stature
Mute	Is nonverbal
Is learning-disabled or LD	Has a learning disability
Afflicted with, suffers from, victim of	Person who has . . .
She's emotionally disturbed; she's crazy	She has an emotional disability
Normal and/or healthy	A person without a disability
Quadriplegic, paraplegic, etc . . .	He has quadriplegia, paraplegia, etc . . .

Communication is also impeded at times by the discomfort felt when one has had little interaction with students with disabilities; feelings of awkwardness and uncertainty are not unusual. Interacting can be more comfortable with certain guidelines.[8]

- Speak directly to a student with a disability, just as you would with any other student. If appropriate, sit down and speak at eye level.
- Don't think that you need to avoid words such as "walking," "standing," "seeing," or "running." People with disabilities use the same language as persons without disabilities.
- When it appears that an individual might need assistance, ask if you can help. If your help is needed, the individual will accept it.

- Accept the fact that a disability exists. Ignoring the disability is a sign of disrespect for the person. It is denying the person's existence as a total human being and communicates that the disability somehow indicates that he or she is "less than."
- If an individual's speech is difficult to understand, don't hesitate to ask him/her to repeat the sentence(s).
- Always speak directly to the individual with a disability. Don't assume that a companion needs to be informed of the conversation that is taking place.

Special considerations for interacting with students who have low vision may be helpful.[8]

- Continue to use words that refer directly to vision (e.g., "see" and "look"). Students who are blind or have low vision use these words as well.
- Identify yourself by name. Do not assume that blind students or students with low vision will recognize the sound of a voice, even if you have met before.
- Speak directly to the person, maintain eye contact even if blind students or students with low vision do not look back at you. There should be no change in the tone of voice.
- Remember that all animals used for assistance are "working" animals. Do not distract the animal in any way unless the owner allows it.

There are also special considerations for interacting with students who are deaf or hard of hearing.[8]

1. Deafness and being hard of hearing are examples of a hidden disability.
2. Speak clearly and directly. Do not exaggerate; shouting is not necessary. Do not cover your mouth as the student may depend on reading your lips in order to understand the conversation.
3. Practice good communication skills. If you do not understand the conversation, say so.
4. Be visual—use your hands and body to make gestures and expressions that communicate the essence of your verbal message.
5. When appropriate, arrange for a sign language interpreter to maximize communication with those who primarily use sign language.
6. If you are not communicating as effectively as you would like, write the message down and communicate in writing. This will avoid any mistakes that might occur verbally.

COMMON SPECIFIC MEDICAL CONCERNS OF THE STUDENT WITH A DISABILITY

Skin Concerns

The process of skin pressure relief in an individual *without* a disability is a continuous dynamic activity, with a recognized chain of events. Pressure leads to tissue ischemia that in turn leads to pain. As a consequence, the individual moves to relieve the pressure, blood supply is restored, and the ischemic pain disappears.[9] On average, a person without a disability alters body position during sleep every 11.6 minutes.[9] For students with mobility or sensory disabilities, such frequent levels of movement to prevent skin breakdown may be difficult or impossible.

Pressure spots/decubiti develop as a result of two processes—occlusion of blood vessels by external pressure, and endothelial damage of arterioles and micro-circulation by application of friction and shearing forces.[9] Pressures spots/decubitus ulcers are a major concern for those students with disabilities who sit or lie in one position for long periods or use equipment (i.e., crutches) that may cause skin damage. Students with decreased sensation and/or circulation are at particular risk for experiencing some type of skin breakdown. Since most students with disabilities are well aware of the risks involved for the development of pressure spots/decubitus ulcers, the treatment required from student health personnel most likely includes monitoring and prevention rather than advanced skin care or repair.

Urinary tract Infections

Frequent urinary tract infections (UTI) are common among students with specific types of disabilities. The higher risk of urinary stasis is compounded by the tendency to have insufficient fluid intake because of inability to easily access fluids in certain situations. Other concerns related to bladder care include inaccessible restroom facilities, the need to follow catheterization schedules, and infrequent voiding.

Pyuria should be treated only when the student with a disability has a documented infection and not strictly on the basis of the results of a routine urinalysis. The urine of a student who requires self-catheterization is rarely sterile. Annual referrals to a urologist may be important for a regular evaluation of overall renal function, since these students are predisposed to the formation of renal calculi.

Respiratory Concerns

Regular movement enhances the reduction of the frequency of pulmonary infections and the development of sepsis.[10] Thus, regular body position changes are essential for students at risk of developing pulmonary difficulties, or for those already suffering from chest complaints. Body position changes enhance oxygen transport due to the effect on the distribution of ventilation and perfusion throughout the lungs,[9] and affords preventive and treatment advantages as well. Altering chest position, for example, redistributes and mobilizes mucus and interstitial fluid from dependent lung areas, thereby helping to prevent the development of localized atelectasis.[9]

Musculoskeletal Issues

Students with orthopedic limitations are at particular risk of developing osteoporosis, flexion contractures, and postural impairment, leading to diminished proprioception and altered balance mechanisms.[10] Further concerns include stasis edema and deep vein thromboses, and the risk of pulmonary embolism.

PRACTICAL SUGGESTIONS FOR PROVIDING STUDENT HEALTH SERVICES TO STUDENTS WITH DISABILITIES

Making an Appointment

When scheduling an appointment in the student health service, the student should indicate that she/he has a disability, as it may affect the services needed during the visit. What accommodations, if any, the student will require should be discussed. The person making the appointment needs to be aware of the importance of the issues. Some of these include:

- How much time should be allocated for the appointment;
- Is the clinic and/or exam room physically accessible to students who use wheelchairs or have other mobility impairments?;
- Will one or more assistants be needed to aid in transferring and positioning during the examination?;
- Will a sign language interpreter be needed during the visit?;
- If available, will the client need to use any special equipment (i.e., high/low table, obstetrical stirrups)?

Access

A common barrier to students with disabilities receiving student health care is the inability to transfer to a treatment table without assistance. Often, it is to the benefit of the health service to create a "transfer team" that can be called upon to assist students who need physical assistance in order to receive services. Transfer methods to help staff in physically assisting students with disabilities seeking health service(s) include:

- **Pivot Transfer.** Standing in front of the student, the assistant takes the student's knees between her/his knees, grasps the student around the back and under the arms, raises her/him to a vertical position and then pivots the student from the wheelchair to the table. The exam table must be low enough for the student to sit; therefore, a hydraulic high-low table may be needed when using this transfer method.
- **Cradle Transfer.** Bending or squatting beside the student, the assistant puts one arm under both of the student's knees and puts the other arm around her/his back and under the armpit. The assistant stands and carries the student to the table. Two assistants can be used if they grasp each other's arms behind the student's back and under her/his knees, if one assistant cannot do it alone.
- **Two-Person Transfer.** In all two-person transfers, the assistants must be careful to work together to lift the student over the arms of the wheelchair from a sitting position onto the exam table. A stronger, taller person should always lift the upper half of the student's body. There are two ways to perform a two-person transfer. Method 1 requires the student to fold her/his arms across her/his chest. The assistant standing behind the student kneels down, putting her/his elbows under the student's armpits, and grasps the student's

opposite wrists. The second assistant lifts and supports the student under the knees. Method 2 can be used if the student cannot fold his/her arms. The assistant standing behind the student puts her/his hands together if possible, so there is less likelihood of losing hold of the student. The second assistant lifts and supports the student under the knees.

Some students with disabilities use a "slide board," which forms a bridge from the wheelchair to the exam table for the student to slide across. In order to use this method, the table and chair must be approximately the same height. Most exam tables are higher than wheelchairs; thus, many student health services have acquired high/low exam tables. These tables can be adjusted to the height that will facilitate the safest and easiest transfer. A wider table can also make transfer and positioning easier even, if it is not adjustable in height.

Physical Examinations

There are a number of things the student with a disability and the clinic staff can do to enhance the physical examination:

- Each disability affects each person differently. The sensitivity of student health personnel in asking only pertinent questions about the disability increases the comfort and cooperation of the student.
- Speak directly to the student, not to his/her friend, attendant, or interpreter.
- The communication system used by a student with decreased hearing or a speech impediment (e.g., a sign language interpreter, word board, or talk box) should be discussed at the onset of the clinic visit.
- It is not necessary to remove all clothes for all exams; clothing removed should be only that which is necessary for the exam.
- Remove or rearrange furnishings in an exam room to provide space to negotiate a wheelchair or for an interpreter to accompany the student.
- Paper covering can be removed from the exam table if it is an impediment during transfers and positioning.
- A student with a mobility-related disability (i.e., spinal cord injury, polio, or cerebral palsy) should be given the option of bringing a urine sample (if needed) to the student health clinic.
- Use specialized educational materials (i.e., Braille or taped information or three-dimensional anatomical models) to make information accessible to students with visual impairments.

In short, these few, simple steps markedly improve the experience of both the health care provider and the disabled student in health care encounters.

REFERENCES

1. U.S. Department of Education, National Center for Education Statistics, National Education Longitudinal Study of 1988, Third Follow-up Survey, 1994 (NELS: 88/94), Data Analysis System.

2. American Council on Education. (1998) Health Resource Center. Unpublished data from the Cooperative Institutional Research Program, UCLA, selected years.

3. *ADA Handbook: Basic Resource document.* (1993) U.S. Equal Opportunity Commission and U.S. Department of Justice.

4. Hadley, R.G. & Brodwin, M.G. Language about people with disabilities. *J Counsel and Dev.* 1988;67(3):147–149.

5. Patterson, J.B. & Witten, B.J. Disabling language and attitudes toward persons with disabilities. *Rehabil Psychol.* 1987;32(4):245–248.

6. LaForge, J. Preferred language practice in professional rehabilitation journals. *J Rehabil* 1991:49–51.

7. Cook, D. (1992). Psychosocial impact of disability. In R.M. Parker & E.M. Szymanski (Eds.), *Rehabilitation Counseling: Basics and Beyond* (2nd ed.). Austin, TX: PRO-ED.

8. International Association of Business Communicators (1982). *Without Bias: a Guidebook For Nondiscriminatory Communication* (2nd ed.). New York: Wiley.

9. Dean, E. & Ross, J. Oxygen transport: The basis for contemporary cardiopulmonary physical therapy and its optimization with body positioning and mobilization. *Phys Ther Prac. 1992*;1(4):34–44.

10. Colin, D. Comparison of 90° and 30° laterally inclined positions in the prevention of pressure ulcers using transcutaneous oxygen and carbon dioxide pressures. *Adv Wound Care* 1996;9(3):35-38.

CHAPTER 16

HEALTH PROMOTION IN HIGHER EDUCATION

Christine G. Zimmer, MA, CHES

Over the past two decades, institutions of higher education have been recognized as integral partners in the quest for achieving national health priorities. These priorities focus on the prevention of unnecessary disease, disability, and human suffering and on access to preventive health services for all.[1,2] Higher education will be held accountable for leading and shaping these health priorities for learning communities. This will require a fuller definition and understanding of the characteristics, risk perceptions and risk behaviors of students, faculty, and staff. It will also involve the assessment of community dynamics affecting health, learning, community connection, and citizenship. Institutions of higher education will be expected to strengthen upon environmental determinants of health, learning, retention, and productivity within their campus cultures and to a make a full commitment to support community standards and resources that protect the health and human potential of learning community members.

Colleges and universities have traditionally represented one of the few constituencies outside the military through which large numbers of 18–24-year-olds can be reached with consistent health education messages. Over the past decade, however, a more complex student body has emerged, including a broadened diversity of age, ethnicity, culture ,and socioeconomic status. Enrollments now include increasing numbers of older students, women, and part-time students, along with traditionally underrepresented populations, each with its unique health needs and risks.[3] These students bring with them more complex family histories, emotional needs, learning motivations, and learning styles than previous generations.[4] They often juggle work and family obligations in addition to

---

This chapter is not intended to be a "cookbook" of programming for health promotion activities. Rather, it is to provide an overview of the growth and recent development of health promotion in university communities and insight into future direction.

their studies. Many lack adequate health insurance coverage.[5] Homogeneous student populations have given way to a more complex matrix of smaller student communities, with students more likely to define their "community" as a residence hall, an athletic team, a sorority or fraternity system, an international student community, or a fragmented population of evening and distance learners. They may also identify with others through a shared academic major, shared extracurricular activities, or shared age, gender, or sexual orientation. Protecting individual and community health status within higher education requires engagement of these diverse student communities as active health partners and problem solvers.

Running parallel to changes in student demographics is a changing public health agenda. This agenda includes a stronger emphasis on the socioeconomic determinants of health, propelled by widespread psychological and physiological dependence on mood-altering substances, an epidemic of interpersonal violence, and the prevalence of social injustice. To enhance individual capacity for health, responsible citizenship, and learning, colleges and universities will need to address not only individual health behaviors, but also the institutional culture and context that may enable, support or encourage high-risk behavior.[1,2]

A shift has also occurred in the paradigm of college health. This new paradigm places greater emphasis on health imperatives that support the institutional mission, with a focus on defining and measuring the relationship between health and learning outcomes. This new paradigm requires data-driven decision-making accompanied by individual and community needs assessment, health resource mapping, and strategic planning designed to protect and improve the health of all members of a learning community. It acknowledges the need to impact the psychosocial determinants that influence health behaviors, learning, and retention. It measures best practice by quality improvement indicators, accreditation standards, and data-driven evaluation of individual and community health improvement. While this paradigm retains a focus on clinical medicine and recovery from illness, it places increasing attention on prevention of disease and promotion of health from a clinical, environmental, and community perspective.

The new college health paradigm also includes a broader definition of "community," embracing employees as stable and influential carriers of a campus culture. Supporting and enhancing the physical and psychological health of employees is integral to healthy adult role-modeling and to the coaching, mentoring, and referral functions which employees need to provide for students. In addition, building health partnerships with faculty and staff affords the opportunity to strengthen their capacities and increase their motivation to join us as assessors, nurturers, and supporters of student and community health. This new paradigm also offers opportunities to create a systems-wide approach to curriculum infusion of health messages and skills essential to reducing unnecessary disease, disability, and human suffering. Strengthening the physical and emotional well-being of employees and their dependents also enhances an institution's capabilities for professional recruitment, retention, and productivity, and for financial stability related to employee health-care cost containment.

OUR BEGINNINGS

Visionary leaders have played key roles in the development of student health initiatives over the last century and a half. In the early 1800s, the health care and health education of college students were assigned to a local physician who saw to the medical concerns of students and taught short courses in anatomy and hygiene.[6,7] In 1836, Mt. Holyoke, America's first higher education institution for women, became the first institution to offer a course on hygiene and physiology.[8] In 1856, William Stearns, president of Amherst College noted:

> Students of our colleges have bodies which need care and culture as well as intellectual and moral powers. . . . The breakdown of the health of students . . . which is exceedingly common, involving the necessity of leaving college in many instances . . . is in my opinion wholly unnecessary if proper measures could be taken to prevent it.[9]

Four years later, President Stearns appointed Edward Hitchcock, MD, to serve as Professor of Hygiene at Amherst College (see Chapter 1).[10] Dr. Hitchcock became a prominent pioneer of health and physical education for students through his ongoing attempts to identify a link between health education and improved health status.[11]

Over the next several decades, health programs for students evolved from an emphasis on physical education to the introduction of classes that concentrated on personal hygiene and factors contributing to healthful living or environmental hygiene.[12] The primary focus of this education was still the development of the body. Issues of lifestyle, including alcohol use, nutrition, or reproductive concerns, were only sporadically integrated into lectures. College health officials rarely had a mandate (and often, not even permission) for open discussion regarding personal health issues.[13]

The discovery of microorganisms in the late nineteenth century and their relationship to disease led to the expansion of public health initiatives in the early 1900s, with parents advocating for more effective health education programs at colleges and universities.[14] During this time, organized efforts to improve the health of students increased, with financial support from the federal government.[13] Congress provided limited funding for colleges to establish a department coordinating the teaching of hygiene, health examinations, and sanitary supervision of the institution, aimed at controlling infectious disease.[15]

This federal funding stimulated more expansive thinking regarding the role and scope of public health activities. Thomas Denison Wood, a physical education theorist, proposed a new definition of health education, describing it as "the sum of experiences, in school and elsewhere, which favorably influence habits, attitudes and knowledge relating to individual, community and racial health."[7,16] Thus, for the first time, Wood's paradigm separated health and physical education, with physical education becoming only one component of a more comprehensive approach to individual and community health. Subsequently, Wood became the first professor of health education at Columbia Teachers College, which awarded its first degree in health education in 1922.[13]

By 1934, most major colleges and universities had a student health service that was separate from their department of physical education.[17] However, these health services were focused primarily on clinical care. Health education initiatives remained suspended between physical education programs and academic departments of health and hygiene.

In 1920, the American Student Health Association (subsequently renamed the American College Health Association) was formed to promote the health of college students through health education, preventive and therapeutic medical care, and attention to a healthful environment in the campus community.[9] This association was composed primarily of physicians and professors who shared a common interest in the health of students. Later, during the 1950s, the association created special-interest sections to provide professionals with an opportunity to develop programs on topics of mutual concern. It was at this time that the Health Education Section was created.[18] But the section remained small, even into the early 1970s, when its membership consisted of fewer than a dozen physicians and professors of health education and just one health educator.[19]

THE DEVELOPMENT AND EXPANSION OF HEALTH EDUCATION PROGRAMS

In 1954, Dr. Ruth Boynton, University of Minnesota health service director, and the first dean of the University of Minnesota School of Public Health, hired the nation's first college health educator.[14] This visionary appointment was one of Dr. Boynton's many pioneering contributions to the field of college health. Her commitment to community health in higher education was followed in the early sixties by Dr. Robert Gage's appointment of a health educator to develop a community model of health education for the University of Massachusetts Amherst campus health service. These health educators were lone pioneers until the late 1970s.

Healthy People: The Surgeon General's Report on Health Promotion and Disease Prevention was published in 1979.[20] This revolutionary document followed large-scale epidemiologic studies of the early 1970s that established smoking as the source of most lung cancers and identified the link between smoking, elevated serum cholesterol, and high blood pressure and the development of heart disease. It further identified a shift in patterns of disease causation, from infectious disease to preventable causes of premature death and disability and provided data linking lifestyle and environmental risk factors with unnecessary death, disease, human suffering, and health care costs. *Healthy People* was the first federal document to describe a national commitment to improving the health of U.S. citizens through the prevention of disease and the promotion of positive health behaviors. It focused on goals for health education and promotion that could profoundly influence the health of Americans.

In 1980, the U.S. Public Health Service published a second document *Promoting Health, Preventing Disease: Objectives for the Nation.*[21] Based on findings summarized in *Healthy People,* it established a national health agenda and strategic plan, targeting fifteen priority areas for risk reduction, accompanied by 226 measurable objectives for improving individual and community health status over the following decade.

This new health agenda was accompanied by a growing social consciousness focused on consumerism, women's equality, social justice, concerns regarding sexual risk-taking, and the use of alcohol and other drugs on college campuses. It was also during this period that the emergence of HIV infection and AIDS legitimized health education as the only vehicle for stemming an epidemic for which the nation had no cure. These changes triggered a subtle shift in the role of the college health service, now challenged by an emerging social mandate to focus on the promotion of health and the prevention of disease for student populations.[10]

By the mid 1980s, larger college health services began to employ health educators to lead the development of programs targeted to individual and community health improvement for their campuses. Most health services typically hired a single person to plan and provide all health education services. A handful of larger institutions, however, invested in teams of health educators specializing in health risk appraisals, the management of stress, nutrition, sexuality, substance abuse, and cost-effective strategies for helping students manage self-limiting conditions. During this time, the number of health educators employed in higher education increased to sixty to eighty nationwide. These early practitioners initiated the development of many innovative programs and services, including the use of trained peer educators.[19]

During this era, health education strategies were initiated with limited resources, limited research on best practice models, limited understanding of effective teaching and learning strategies, and limited understanding of individual and community change. In an attempt to keep pace with the emerging national health promotion agenda, many smaller institutions placed responsibility for campus health education activities in the hands of health service nursing staff whose training was focused on clinical practice rather than population-based prevention strategies. Thus, many programs evolved without the benefit of competencies needed by health promotion planners to assess, develop, implement, and evaluate the quality or effectiveness of prevention and intervention strategies targeted to perceptual or behavioral change. In addition, there were no measurable standards of practice by which to evaluate or benchmark either processes or outcomes. Awareness activities, written information, and didactic presentations were the primary tools employed. The goal was to reach as many students as possible with protective health information.

Further, most health service directors saw little need for dedicating resources to needs assessment or for measuring the effectiveness of health education programs. The field of college health had not yet created a tracking system for assessing health risks or identifying health needs of college students, both essential for data-driven decision-making and for providing feedback to key stakeholders. During the last two decades of the century, however, mechanisms and resources to fill these gaps have been initiated, leading to a more defined approach to health promotion and education planning, implementation, and evaluation.

INCLUSION IN THE NATIONAL HEALTH OBJECTIVES PLANNING PROCESS

During the nineties, the U.S. Department of Health and Human Services partnered with the Institute of Medicine, National Academy of Sciences to continue the national prevention agenda and to initiate the strategic planning process for the last decade of the century. For the 1980s, national priorities had been established by a limited number of invited experts. These priorities had not received the broad ownership and visibility needed to improve the health of Americans. Thus, in developing the 1990 health objectives, the federal government called upon health practitioners, health advocates, private organizations, public agencies and consumers to contribute to the objectives-setting process.[1] Public hearings were scheduled throughout the country, during which health care providers and concerned citizens could contribute their perspectives regarding what they believed to be key risks to health.

In 1985, leaders of the Health Education Section of the American College Health Association (ACHA) petitioned the ACHA Board of Directors to appoint a Task Force on Achieving the National Health Objectives in Higher Education. This task force was charged with reviewing the emerging health objectives for the Year 2000 and identifying the capacity and effectiveness of college health in meeting pertinent health objectives for the (then) 12 million students enrolled in institutions of higher education.[22] In pursuit of this goal, the Task Force initiated a dialogue with the Office of Disease Prevention and Health Promotion (ODPHP), the Centers for Disease Control and Prevention (CDC), and other lead agencies involved in setting the health objectives for the Year 2000. Through these partnerships, the Task Force learned the federal government did not recognize college students as an at-risk population. Further, they had not considered college campuses as communities or work settings. Additional data was needed regarding the health needs and behaviors of college students and the extent of services and resources dedicated to prevention of disease and promotion of health for the college population. While nationally based statistics on selected aspects of health behavior could be gleaned from surveys conducted by the National Center for Health Statistics, baseline data on the health of traditional college-age students did not exist.[23] Furthermore, no system of data collection was in place for linking college students to any national health monitoring process. It also became apparent that many health professionals working in college and university health services were unaware of the existence and potential role of the national health objectives in strengthening the college health model.

With the support and leadership of ODPHP, the Task Force organized one of the first national public hearings at which individuals working in the field of college health had an opportunity to speak about student health priorities. Held at the 1987 ACHA annual meeting in Chicago, this public hearing elicited wide participation from leaders in college health, who provided testimonies regarding the key risks to health for college students.

Ultimately, the Task Force proposed that college students be identified by the federal government as a specific population at risk. They also recommended to both the federal government and the ACHA Board of Directors that a national system be created to gather baseline data describing the health of college students and to track and measure the health of students in higher education against relevant health objectives.[22]

In 1990, *Healthy People 2000: National Health Promotion and Disease Prevention Objectives* was published. It called for an integrated approach supported by individuals, families, communities, health professionals, schools, worksites, media, and government to increase the span of healthy life, reduce health disparities, and achieve access to preventive services for all Americans.[1] *Healthy People 2000* established twenty-two targeted prevention priorities, with 298 measurable objectives categorized under three main headings: lifestyle decisions, environmental protection, and preventive services. These priorities provided a framework for establishing a campus health promotion focus for the 1990s.

Through the leadership of the Task Force, college students were included in the federal agenda as a national population at risk. This inclusion recognized institutions of higher education as a national partner in the promotion of health, linking them with the federal government, state health departments, community leaders, school systems, businesses, hospitals, and the media in a leadership role of health protection. Although many of the national health objectives were relevant in some way to the health of college students and to higher education communities, the national objectives specifically identified higher education as responsible for improving student health in four priority areas: reduction of heavy alcohol use; institutionalization of health promotion programs for students, faculty, and staff; broad-based HIV education for students and employees; and increased immunization levels for students.

Subsequently, the Task Force authored *Healthy Campus 2000: Making It Happen.*[25] This publication provided a succinct overview of relevant national health objectives for higher education communities. It was designed to serve as a guide for assessing campus and student health problems and suggested a process by which campus constituencies could select and prioritize health objectives to improve individual and community health status on their respective campuses.

PROFESSIONAL CERTIFICATION

Spurred by the national prevention agenda, the profession of health education was strengthened through a newly formed National Commission for Health Education Credentialing (NCHEC). The commission initiated a certification process defining responsibilities and competencies for entry-level health education specialists.[26] This skill-based certification was subsequently integrated into the development of competency-based curricula for undergraduate education leading to a bachelor's degree in community health education. Seven areas of responsibilities were outlined including individual and community needs assessment; planning, implementing, and evaluating health education programs; coordinating the provision of health education services and resources; and communicating health information. Certification was attained by completion of a bachelor's degree in community health education and successful validation of competencies by examination. Credentialing was maintained by the completion of continuing education contact hours over a five-year period. By the 1900s, health education was recognized as a specific health occupation by the Department of Labor "Standards Occupation Classification," achieving recognition of certification for health educators both within and outside the profession.

STRENGTHENING THEORY-BASED PRACTICE

Throughout the 1980s and 1990s, the ability to apply theories of health behavior to programs and services designed to address defined health needs became increasingly critical for health promotion practitioners. Planning models emerged that provided guidelines for addressing educational, organizational, environmental, epidemiological, behavioral, socioeconomic, and cultural assessment and diagnosis. These models offered a structure for applying theory-based practice to identification, selection, and implementation of appropriate and effective interventions and strategies. Planning models like PRECEDE-PROCEED defined new direction for individual, organizational, and community health improvement.[27,28,29] These models afforded theoretical application to school, community, health care, and occupational settings, all of which were relevant to higher education communities. They allowed practitioners to explore health risk behaviors in a socioeconomic context and to prioritize services based on severity, prevalence, and the capacity to respond to specific health needs.

Meanwhile, theories of learning and of individual and community health status improvement continued to evolve, contributing new understandings regarding the effectiveness of health promotion and education interventions. Among the more significant theories were those growing out of the field of psychotherapy and addiction behavior. The "transtheoretical model of stages of change" was one such model.[30] Using a comparative analysis of the leading theories of psychotherapy and behavior change, the transtheoretical model integrated ten key processes of behavior change unfolding through a sequence of predictable stages, with specific processes needed at each stage to effect success. The model was augmented by motivational interviewing techniques that prepared people for changing unhealthy behaviors and stimulated their progress through each stage of change.[31] The transtheoretical model was initially applied to an analysis of self-change strategies used by persons attempting to stop smoking. It rapidly expanded to include investigations and applications to a broad range of health behaviors. These studies empirically supported intervention strategies matched to each individual stage of change as most likely to result in adoption and maintenance of new behaviors.[32]

A second empirical application of best practice occurred with "diffusion of innovations theory."[33] This theory defined a process by which a new behavior is communicated and adopted among members of a social system. It demonstrated that successful behavior change and maintenance involves a variety of strategies applied to various settings and systems using formal and informal media and communication channels.[34,35]

Models of social marketing evolved, applying behavior change theory to population-based settings.[36] Social marketing employed commercial marketing approaches to analyze, plan, implement, and evaluate programs designed to effect behavior changes that support improved community health status. These models used a systems approach to bring about adoption or acceptability of ideas or practices to enhance community welfare.

Environmental approaches also emerged, encompassing an ecological approach to campus health. With environmental management, the concept of reaching a critical mass of campus leaders and community members took on greater relevance. Most recently, grant funding has supported the analysis of environmental strategies using social norms theory to reduce high risk alcohol use and its negative impact on learning communities.[37,38]

Theories of learning, educational psychology, and moral development have also contributed to effective individual change strategies. Engaged learning formats, process learning, and service learning have been more fully integrated into health promotion planning.

In addition, there has been a shift from fear-based education to a focus on positive protective options and skill-building. Finally, interdisciplinary partnerships have emerged involving artists, educators, health professionals, and even sociologists in the integration of theories that expand our ability to influence individual and community health status.

With the link between theory, research, and practice now established as a cost-effective quality improvement indicator for benchmarking, the next step was to create standards to define best practice processes and competencies for health promotion in higher education.

NATIONAL STANDARD-SETTING FOR HEALTH PROMOTION IN HIGHER EDUCATION

Despite the identification of competencies for health promotion planners and the development of theories of best practice for improving individual and community health status, health promotion programs in higher education continued to evolve without the benefit of measurable standards of performance for evaluating process and outcomes. This deficit prompted the American College Health Association, in May of 1996, to create a Task Force on Health Promotion in Higher Education.[39] The Task Force was charged with the development of standards for health promotion and education programs within the context of the college health model, linking the critical role of college health and the mission of higher education with national health priorities. Task Force members were asked to review and analyze the current role and the scope of practice of health promotion and education in higher education and to draft standards of practice for this setting. Standards were needed to provide post-secondary institutional leaders with guidelines for building capacities within their campus communities to increase health and to improve learning outcomes. Standards were also needed to ensure that both institutional and health service leaders would have benchmarks for assessing the scope and effectiveness of their health promotion services and to guide health promotion planners in improving and measuring the effectiveness of their efforts.

The Task Force initiated its analysis of the scope of practice with the development of the national Survey on Health Promotion and Education in Institutions of Higher Education.[40] It was designed to identify:

- the process by which program planners establish health promotion priorities and create strategic plans that meet program mission and goals;
- current strategies, networks, and resources for implementing health promotion within institutions of higher education;
- performance measures, indicators of best practice, outcome measures, and evaluation tools currently used for health promotion evaluation;
- gaps and deficiencies in the delivery of health promotion services, as well as barriers to implementing health promotion and preventive services goals;
- the range of professionals involved in health promotion planning and delivery.[41]

A list of health promotion and education definitions designed to aid respondents in survey completion was also created to accompany the survey (see glossary at end of chapter for an updated definitions list).[42]

In 1997, the survey was mailed to a stratified random sample of 600 ACHA Member Institutions. Sampling was randomized by region of the country and level of institutional resources, identified by level of ACHA membership. Response rate was 75.3%.[43] In 1998, a second survey targeting 95 key leaders from the Nurse-Directed and Health Education sections of ACHA and from the National Association for Student Personnel Administrators (NASPA) was initiated. These key informants, selected for their nationally recognized efforts in health promotion and representing diverse institutions of higher education, gave a response rate of 90.5%.

Survey analysis offered comparisons between the larger random sample and key informants.[*]

Selected summary data included the following:

- 82.8% of random sample respondents came from four-year institutions;
- 62.4% came from institutions with less than 10,000 students; 47.6% from institutions with less than 5,000 students;
- less than half of both the random sample and key informants reported having institutional mission statements that included concepts of health or quality of life;
- 79.4% of the larger sample identified some level of funding for student health promotion; 37.8% identified some level of funding for faculty/staff health promotion and education services; funding percentages for key informant respondents were higher than for random sample recipients;
- the vast majority of primary health promotion planners were located within the campus health service; campus counseling services and student affairs/campus recreation programs represented distant second and third locations;
- over half of random sample respondents indicated they had no formal name for their health promotion services, leading to conjecture that health promotion services may be integrated into clinical nursing responsibilities or shared between several offices across campus;
- key informants were more likely to have a mission statement that guided planning of their health promotion services;
- credentials of primary health promotion planners differed significantly between key informants and random sample respondents, with key informant planners more likely to hold a masters degree or doctorate in community, school, or public health;
- health promotion staffing patterns differed, with one-fifth of the random sample respondents indicating no health education professional on their campus, while a third of key informants indicated four or more full-time employees responsible for health promotion planning, implementation, and evaluation;
- in addition, nearly twice as many key informants had three or more professional health promotion staff compared to random sample respondents;

---

*For all data, the adjusted percentage of valid responses was used. Test of significance used was a z-test for proportions. Level of significance was set at P>.05.

- there also appeared to be a clear difference in health promotion staffing patterns depending on the size of an institution; over 30% of institutions with less than 10,000 students reported having no health education specialist; institutions of 5,000–9,999 students were more likely to report having at least one health educator (39.3% of the random sample and 66.7% of key informants); institutions of 10,000–20,000 students were most likely to have two or more health education professionals to lead their health promotion services;
- funding for professional health promotion staff and program budgets came from a variety of resources; for both key informants and random sample respondents, primary funding sources were similar—student fees and/or direct health service budget allocation; other funding sources included general university funds; funding from an institution's division of student affairs; grants; state funding; and innovative funding ventures;
- the larger the size of the institution, the greater the use of student fees for health promotion and the greater the likelihood of a dedicated budget for health promotion.

Information was also collected regarding health promotion needs assessment practices, use of theoretical program planning and behavior change models, time invested in a variety of health promotion functions, information on campus health promotion networks, and evaluation strategies employed to measure quality and outcome of programs and services. Respondents were offered twenty-four health promotion functions and asked to identify the amount of time invested in each function. Key informants were more likely to use behavior change and education theories as well as community organization models. Key informants were also significantly more likely to invest time with peer education and service learning. Over 80% of key informants conducted evaluation activities for services and resources provided. They were also more likely to use outcome evaluation than random sample respondents.

Survey outcomes as reported above provided preliminary answers regarding credentials of primary health promotion planners, methodologies of health promotion services, current resource commitment, and evaluation and benchmarking strategies. They furnished a data-driven snapshot of the role and scope of health promotion services in higher education at the close of the twentieth century. The intent of the survey was to capture a perspective on health promotion practices that would guide the development of core standards and best-practice outcomes for the coming decade.

At the American College Health Association annual meetings of 1998 and 1999, the Task Force sponsored four working sessions to identify core functions and performance measures for creating professional standards, using literature review and survey outcomes. Working sessions invited broad-based professional review and discussion that resulted in a progressive refinement of a core standards draft. Public comment was then widely sought through the American College Health Association website. The resulting product, entitled "National Core Standards for Health Promotion in Higher Education," was approved in May 2000 by the American College Health Association Board of Directors. These standards provided measurable guidelines for quality assurance and a framework for the accreditation of health promotion services in post-secondary institutions. The standards identified five interdependent characteristics of effective practice, shown below.

1. Leaders who demonstrate competency in community-based health promotion.
2. Integration with and commitment to the academic mission of the institution.
3. Use of a collaborative process to ensure appropriate campus community participation in planning, implementing and evaluating health-related initiatives.
4. Demonstration of cultural competence and inclusiveness in working with populations of diverse cultures and identifies in addressing issues of diversity and health.
5. Competency in using appropriate resources and quantity and quality of research.[44]

The Task Force also drafted a self-assessment tool to be used by those responsible for health promotion planning and evaluation in a higher education community, giving vice presidents for student affairs, health service directors, and campus health promotion planners a tool for evaluating and improving the outcomes of programs and services based on defined core standards for health promotion planners.[45]

DEVELOPING A NATIONAL DATA BASE FOR HEALTH IN HIGHER EDUCATION

Responding to the need for a national database to track the health of college students for the Year 2000 National Health Objectives, the Division of Adolescent and School Health, Centers for Disease Control and Prevention, developed the National College Health Risk Behavior Survey in 1995, using input from experts in higher education, ACHA, and other federal agencies and national organizations. This instrument and its accompanying data collection system provided validity, reliability, and comparability with which to track health risk behaviors of college students and to contribute to a national database that could lead to a fuller understanding of the health of college students. It also strengthened the capacity for data-driven decision-making and the collection of outcome evaluation.

However, use of the National College Health Risk Behavior Survey brought awareness of a second and equally pressing need—to create a database to further assess health factors that impact academic performance, retention, and quality of campus life. These factors include not only the incidence and prevalence of key risk behaviors, but also protective behaviors, health status, health outcomes, perceived norms, and access to health information. Data was also needed on safety and violence; alcohol, tobacco, and other drug use; depression; suicide; sexual behavior; body weight; nutrition; and physical activity consistent with measurement of progress on the year 2010 health objectives. This data was needed to assist institutions of higher education with priority setting, campus-wide program planning, and resource allocation.

Recognizing the need for a national effort to develop a more comprehensive data collection approach, the American College Health Association created a workgroup in 1997 to develop the American College Health Association National College Health Assessment Survey (ACHA-NCHA).[46] This workgroup used a number of validated surveys in the development of their own instrument, including the National College Health Risk Behavior Survey, the Student Health Survey from the University of Minnesota Boynton Health Services, the Core Alcohol and Drug Survey,[47] the College Alcohol Study,[48] the Student Health Behavior Assessment from Northern Illinois University, and the Monitoring the Future questionnaire.[49]

The National College Health Assessment Survey has been piloted and implemented in institutions of higher education throughout the country, filling a gap in data-driven needs assessment that will allow college health professionals and health promotion planners to more fully understand the status of student health and its influence on retention, learning, and quality of campus life as well as tracking higher education's progress on meeting the year 2010 national health objectives for college students.

THE FUTURE

Looking toward the twenty-first century, the future is filled with challenges and opportunities. Eroding public confidence in higher education, demands for accountability, and demographic shifts in student populations require the application of the highest science and creativity to individual, community, and social issues that profoundly impact health, learning, and productivity on college campuses. New paradigms of college health will require an increased commitment of human and fiscal resources targeted to specific environmental and public health concerns as well as to the physical and emotional aspects of health on which health care has traditionally focused.

A research agenda will need to be created to better understand variables that affect successful academic performance and quality of campus life. The integration and creative synthesis of both behavioral and social sciences will be required for deepening our understanding of risk and protective factors related to health priorities, including injury prevention, the harmful use of alcohol and other mood-altering substances, depression, and suicide, and responding to those concerns with the most appropriate and effective health education and health promotion strategies.

The future will require creative partnerships with a spectrum of campus and community members. Active collaboration with public health departments and community-based organizations will be needed to address issues of social injustice, interpersonal violence, and an array of socioeconomic variables that have profound effects on living-learning environments, the campus community, and the communities that border or surround our colleges and universities. Formal health management networks led by experienced health promotion planners will be needed. They will be charged with integrating fragmented health resources across an institution with the creation of a common mission and strategic plan. This will necessitate quantitative and qualitative assessment of student and employee health to establish priorities, as well as community resource mapping that will focus on gaps and deficiencies in institutional processes, services, and systems that support health and learning.

More effective partnerships will need to be established with faculty members to participate in building curriculum infusion paradigms that validate individual and community health as essential components of social responsibility, and to partner in research initiatives that can deepen the impact of our work. Improving the ability of faculty, staff, and academic advisors to support early identification, intervention, and referral of students with health and learning issues will also strengthen a systems approach to campus-wide health and learning.

Clinical preventive services and patient education systems will also need to focus on methods for integrating prevention education into the clinical visit in order to improve patient outcomes. New strategies for optimal teaching/learning outcomes will be employed. Clinical teams will need to build skills through which education for prevention, early intervention, referral, and follow-up for improved health outcomes will occur in a systematic, interdisciplinary process. The development of clinical and community health networks based on an interdisciplinary systems approach to health and disease management will maximize available resources for prevention, early intervention, assessment, and treatment of health issues that interfere with personal health and academic performance. With this new approach, advocacy for third-party reimbursement for clinical preventive services will be essential.

Unlike local public health providers, whose funding focuses on the improvement of community health status, campus health service funding currently focuses on the delivery of clinical services. The future will require a commitment to funding for health promotion staffing levels that will allow targeted as well as campus-wide interventions for health protection and risk reduction. Building the capacity for best-practice health education and promotion planning, implementation, and evaluation within institutions that have not previously invested in health promotion or public health expertise will be necessary and may require a paradigm shift, particularly in smaller institutions.

Two important questions remain. First, does the health of college students decline or increase as a result of their college experience, and second, how does maintaining and improving the health of students enhance lerning, retention, and academic success? The challenge of the future will be to create environments and services that advance and protect the health of higher education communities and link the mission of higher education with national health priorities.

GLOSSARY

Definition of Terms

Health Promotion
Any planned combination of educational, political, regulatory, and organizational supports for actions and conditions of living conducive to the health of individuals, groups, or communities.

Health Education
Any combination of learning experiences designed to facilitate voluntary actions conducive to health.

• Combination—emphasizes the importance of matching the multiple determinants of behavior with multiple learning experiences or educational interventions.
• Designed—distinguishes health education from incidental learning experiences as a systematically planned activity.
• Facilitate—means predispose, enable and reinforce.

- Voluntary—means without coercion and with full understanding and acceptance of the purposes of the action.
- Actions— means behavioral steps taken by an individual, group, or community to achieve the intended health effect or to build their capacity for health.[1]

Prevention
In the health field, prevention is the process whereby specific action is taken to prevent or reduce the possibility of a health problem or condition developing and to minimize any damage that may have resulted from a previous condition.[2]

In public health, it can include primary prevention (stop a process before an undesirable health condition arises), secondary prevention (early intervention into illness episode or undesirable behavioral sequence), and tertiary prevention (interruption of chronic disease process or rehabilitation).[3]

1. Green, L., Kreuter, M., Health Promotion Planning: An educational and ecological approach. Third Ed. Mountain View, Mayfield Publishing, 1999.
2. Modesto, N. Dictionary of Public Health and Education Terms and Concepts. Thousand Oaks. Sage Publications, 1996.
3. Standards Revision Work Group. Guidelines for a College Health Program. Baltimore Maryland, American College Health Association, 1999.

REFERENCES

1. *Healthy People 2000—National Health Promotion and Disease Prevention Objectives.* DHHS (PHS) 91–51212, Washington, D.C., 1991.
2. U.S. Department of Health and Human Services. *Healthy People 2010* (Conference Edition, in Two Volumes). Washington, D.C.: January 2000.
3. DeArmond, M. The future of college health. *J Am Coll Health.* May 1995: 43(6): 258–261.
4. Levine, A., Cureton, J. *When hope and fear collide: A portrait of today's college student.* San Francisco, Jossey-Bass: 1998.
5. Patrick, K. Medical care within institutions of higher education. *JAMA,* 1988:260:3301–3305.
6. Means, R. *A history of health education in the U.S.* Philadelphia, PA: Lea-Febiger: 1962.
7. Boynton, R. Historical development of health services. *Student Medicine.* 1962: 10:294–305.
8. Lockhart, A., Spears, B. *Chronicle of American Physical Education: Selective readings, 1855–1930.* Dubuque, IA: WC Brown Co: 1972: 66.
9. Raycoft, J. History and development of student health programs in colleges and universities. *Proceedings of the twenty-first annual meeting of the American School Health Association.* Ann Arbor, Mich. 1940:37–43.
10. Christmas, W. The evolution of medical services for students at colleges and universities in the United States. *J Am Coll Health.* May 1995:43: 6: 241.
11. Hitchcock, E. *An anthropomorphic manual giving the average and mean physical measurements and tests of male college students and methods of securing them.* Amherst, Mass.: JE Williams: 1889.
12. Canuteson, R. Looking ahead in college health. In: *Proceedings of the twenty-fourth annual meeting of the American School Health Association.* Minneapolis, 1946: 7.
13. Conant-Sloane, B., Zimmer, C. Health education and health promotion on campus. *Principles and Practices of Student Health.* Oakland, Calif., Third Party Publishing Co., 1992, 540–541. Ed. Wallace, H., Patrick, K., Parcel G., and Igoe, J.
14. Sloane, D., Conant-Sloane, B. Changing opportunities: An overview of the history of college health education. *J Am Coll Health.* 1986: 271–273.

15. Boynton, RB. Historical development of college health services. *Student Medicine.* 1962.10: 298.

16. Davenport, J. Thomas Denison Wood: Physical education and father of health education. *JOPERD.* Oct. 1984, 63–68.

17. Mitchell OWH: Health services in colleges and universities of New York state. *NYSJ of Medicine.* Nov. 1930: 1:30(20): 1283–1286.

18. Christmas, WA. The history of sections in the American College Health Association. *J Am Coll Health.* 1992: 121–126.

19. Zimmer, C. The health education section: 38 years of growth. *J Am Coll Health.* May 1995: 43: 6: 276–278.

20. Richmond, J. *The surgeon general's report on health promotion and disease prevention.* USDHEW/ USPHS Pub 79–55071. Washington, D.C.: 1979.

21. *Promoting health/preventing disease—objectives for the nation.* DHHS/USPHS/CDC. Atlanta: 1980.

22. Chervin, DD., Conant-Sloane, B., Gordon, K., Gold, RS. Achieving the health objectives for the nation in higher education. Report of the Task Force on Achieving the Health Objectives for the Nation in Higher Education. *J Am Coll Health.* 1986: 35: 15–20.

23. Gordon, K. College health in the national blueprint for a healthy campus 2000. *J Am Coll Health.* May 1995:43:6: 273–275.

24. Guyton, R., Corbin, S., Zimmer, C. et al. College students and national health objectives for the year 2000: A summary report. *J Am Coll Health.* 1989; 38:1: 9–14.

25. Task Force on the National Health Objectives in Higher Education. *Healthy campus 2000: Making it happen.* Baltimore, Md., American College Health Association, 1995.

26. National Commission for Health Education Credentialing, Inc. *Self-assessment for health educators.* New York, NCHEC, Professional Examination Service, 1990.

27. Glanz, K, Lewis, F., Rimer, B., ed. *Health behaviors and health education: Theory, reseach and practice.* 2nd ed. San Francisco, Jossey-Bass, 1997.

28. Green, L., Kreuter, M. *Health promotion planning: An educational and environmental approach.* 3rd ed. Mountain View, Calif., Mayfield, 1991.

29. Gielen, A., McDonald, E. The Precede-Proceed planning model, in *Health behaviors and health education: Theory, research and practice,* Ed. Glanz, K., Lewis, F., Rimer, B. 2nd ed., San Francisco, Jossey-Bass, 1997, 359–384.

30. Prochaska, J., Redding, C., Evers, K. The Transtheoretical model and stages of change in *Health behaviors and health education: Theory, research and practice,* Ed. Glanz, K., Lewis, F., Rimer, B. 2nd ed., San Francisco, Jossey-Bass, 1997, 60–84.

31. Miller, RM., Rollnick, S. *Motivational interviewing: Preparing people to change addictive behavior.* New York, Guilford Press, 1991.

32. Prochaska, JO., DiClemente, CC. Stages and processes of self-change of smoking: Toward an integrated model for change. *Journal of Consulting and Clinical Psychology.* 1983; 51: 390–395.

33. Oldenburg, B., Hardcastle, D., Kok, G. Diffusion of innovations in *Health behaviors and health education: Theory, research and practice,* Ed. Glanz, K., Lewis, F., Rimer, B. 2nd ed., San Francisco, Jossey-Bass, 1997, 270–286.

34. Basch, C. Research on disseminating and implementing health education programs in schools. *J Sch Health* 1984; 54: 57–66.

35. Basch, C., Eveland, JD., Portnoy, B. Diffusion systems for education and learning about health. *Fam and Comm Health* 1986; 9: 1–26.

36. Andreasen, AR. *Marketing social change: Changing behavior to promote health, social development and the environment.* San Francisco, Jossey-Bass, 1995.

37. Berkowitz, AD. From reactive to proactive prevention: Promoting an ecology of health on campus. Chapter 6 in *Substance abuse on campus: A handbook for college and university personnel.* Ed. Rivers, P., Shore, E. Westport, Conn., Greenwood Press, 1997.

38. Haines, M. *Community-generated protective norms reduce risk and protect health.* April/May/June 1998. *Action.* American College Health Association, 37:4: 1–3.

39. Zimmer, C., et al. Proposal to create and fund a tast force on health promotion in higher education. In *Standards of Practice for Health Promotion in Higher Education,* American College Health Association, Baltimore, 2001, 15–19.

40. Task Force on Health Promotion in Higher Education. Survey on health promotion and education in institutions of higher education. In *Standards of Practice for Health Promotion in Higher Education*, American College Health Association, Baltimore, 2001, 21–30.

41. Task Force on Health Promotion in Higher Education. Background development of the standards. In *Standards of Practice for Health Promotion in Higher Education*, American College Health Association, Baltimore, 2001, 2–3.

42. Modesto, N. *Dictionary of Public Health and Education Terms and Concepts*. Thousand Oaks, Sage Publications, 1996.

43. Task Force on Health Promotion in Higher Education. Survey on health promotion and education in higher education: Preliminary findings. In *Standards of Practice for Health Promotion in Higher Education*, American College Health Association, Baltimore, 2001, 31–45.

44. Task Force on Health Promotion in Higher Education. Standards of practice for helath promtion in higher education. In *Standards of Practice for Health Promotion in Higher Education,* American College Health Association, Baltimore, 2001, 4–8.

45. Task Force on Health Promotion in Higher Education. Program self-assessment tool. In *Standards of Practice for Health Promotion in Higher Education*, American College Health Association, 2001, 9–13.

46. American College Health Association. *National college health assessment 2000 user's manual.* Spring 2000, Baltimore, Md., American College Health Association.

47. Presley, C. *Core alcohol and drug survey: Long form.* Core Institute, Carbondale, Southern Illinois University at Carbondale. 1994.

48. Wechsler, H. *College alcohol study.* Boston, Harvard School of Public Health, 1997.

49. Johnston, L., O'Malley, P., Bachman, J. National survey results on drug use from the Monitoring the Future Study, 1975–1995: Vol II. College students and young adults. Rockville, Md.: US Dept of Health and Human Services, National Institute on Drug Abuse. 1997: Public Health Service, National Institutes of Health 98–4140.

CHAPTER 17

STUDENT HEALTH INSURANCE

Stephen C. Caulfield, MSW

INTRODUCTION

Student health insurance has an important component role as it relates to the economics of student health programs, and to the shaping of the direction and content of student health services.

Health insurance for students is strongly influenced by the larger context of employer-sponsored health insurance programs. In that context, the health insurance industry in the United States has undergone three significant changes in the past decade. The first is consolidation. In 1990, health insurance was provided by Travelers, Metropolitan, Prudential, Mass Mutual, Hancock, or a variety of state-based Blue Cross plans. Today, many of these insurers have been acquired by, or merged into, Aetna, CIGNA, United, Wellpoint, and Anthem. And the consolidation has not stopped.

A second important change has been the conversion of the health insurance industry into the managed care industry. "No longer is there a clear separation between the companies organizing populations into risk pools and the people managing the delivery system. Managed care organizations have the responsibility to do both. As a result, both payer and provider are now thrown together to face financing, marketing, capital formation, and systems issues."[1]

A third change is the health insurance "product" itself. Health insurance is not intended to be primarily economic protection from an unanticipated, significant, and expensive medical event—an insurance product which for decades was called "major medical and hospitalization insurance." Now the consumer has demanded, and the industry has provided, a prepaid program of benefits covering routine dental care, physician office visits, prescriptions, and nearly every imaginable variety of diagnostic testing and imaging. In pure economic terms, this is no longer "insurance," whereby a large number of people pay a small premium for protection against those economic costs for events that are known to occur to only a few. Now "health insurance" means a program which will pay most of the costs for routine care that virtually everyone will access in their foreseeable futures. Of course, health insurance continues to have an "insurance" component (e.g., protection from the significant or catastrophic event), but it also has a large number of "prepayment" features. Inevitably, this dramatic change has led to increasing costs and increasing premiums. From the consumers' point of view, these expansions of benefits are quite attractive, since their employer usually pays the majority of these costs with pre-tax corporate dollars. Thus, a tax-advantaged benefit is provided to the employee at a relatively low cost. And, although employees' shares of premium are now steadily rising,[2] most still view the employer-based health benefit as an important part of their compensation.

In addition to these three major trends in health insurance, other significant changes have occurred, particularly in the mix of health care services utilized. The use of inpatient care has declined, while outpatient care, particularly for ambulatory surgery, has escalated. Today, three out of every four surgical procedures are done on an outpatient basis.[3] New technology has dramatically improved both diagnostic and procedurally based medicine. The use and cost of prescription drugs have exploded.[4]

Two other significant changes are unfolding. First, expanding knowledge of genetics is creating new screening tools and new pharmacology. Second, the increased use of the Internet for patient information and as a platform on which patients and caregivers can interact is creating both opportunities and concerns.

In this swirl of change, certain features of the health care system in the U.S. have remained quite constant. Despite some fluctuations in the trends of component costs, at the beginning of the 21st Century, the United States still spends about 13.5% of its GDP on health care, up just slightly over the past decade.[5] Despite this high level of expenditures, more than 44 million Americans are uninsured.[6] Further, belying their top rank in expenditures, Americans have made relatively little progress in infant mortality and other population-based measures of health status, and also appear to be losing ground in youth smoking, nutrition, and fitness.[7]

Against this background of national trends in both health care and health insurance, student health insurance is undergoing less dramatic, but still significant changes.

First, colleges and universities are increasingly concerned that all students have adequate health insurance; thus a trend seems to be emerging towards hard-waiver or mandatory programs.

Second, as employer-sponsored parental plans impose limits on age, out-of-area non-urgent care, and non-network providers, these plans may provide less than adequate coverage for students, if they provide any coverage at all. "Shortly after the failure of the Clinton Health Reform effort, employers began (the) gradual withdrawal from the provision of health benefits. This has taken the form of limitations on coverage provided to retirees, dependents and most powerfully, the limits on the costs of employee (health) benefits."[8] A recent study at the University of California at Davis, found that over three-quarters of claims submitted to parental plans by Student Health Services were totally denied either because deductibles were not met or because non-urgent out-of-area care was rendered.[9]

Third, as the counterbalancing pressures to have both broad coverage and affordable premiums are imposed on student health-insurance plan designs, some insurers have introduced exclusions and/or plan limits, exposing some seriously ill or injured students and their families to significant economic liability. (Uninsured health care costs are the leading cause of personal bankruptcy in the U.S. today.)[10]

Finally, as colleges and universities struggle with affordability and access for a diverse but qualified group of students, university support for campus-based student health services has become increasingly constrained. This raises a complex set of questions about the role of student health insurance in financing student health services.

THE NEED FOR STUDENT HEALTH INSURANCE PLANS

For a number of years, the American College Health Association (ACHA) has recommended that "colleges require students to demonstrate adequate health insurance coverage or adequate financial resources to pay for expected and unexpected medical conditions as a condition of enrollment."[11] More recently, ACHA has adopted new guidelines, which are somewhat stronger in their recommendation. "Students are required to provide evidence that they have health insurance coverage as a condition of enrollment."[12] And these guidelines go further, describing "an appropriate scope of coverage."[13]

The rationale for these recommendations is quite straightforward: the college-aged population is among the largest group of uninsureds, with the 19–21 year old cohort representing 30% of the 44 million Americans without health insurance.[14] These data are more impressive when one considers that the student population is aging or, more correctly, that there is a growing group of 25–30-year-olds. Further, the female enrollment is rising both proportionally and in absolute terms, and women are more frequent users of health care in every age group.[15]

Certain important characteristics of the older group are that they tend to be enrolled in public institutions, they tend to be married with children, and some member of the family is employed. This employed cohort, however, is at higher risk to be uninsured because of frequent employment in lower-wage service industries and part-time or seasonal employment.[16] This results in a group of students with higher morbidity than more traditional college-aged students, more expenditures, no access to parental insurance, lower probability of employer-sponsored health insurance, and limited disposable income. Kronick and Gilmer have observed, in their comprehensive analysis of the decline in insurance coverage, ". . . persons with assets to protect will see an increased financial risk from being uninsured, and many will find higher premiums worthwhile. However, persons with few assets to protect will get no greater benefits from insurance when health care prices are higher."[17] Left to their own choices, many students without access to parental plans will elect to "go bare," and many will even misrepresent coverage availability on waiver enrollment.[18]

Further, access to parental coverage is declining. Most family plans have dependent age limits of 21 to 23, although some plans drop coverage at age 18. Also, as previously noted, managed-care plan rules and plan designs have further limited coverage, particularly for non-urgent, out-of-area care. For example, it is virtually impossible to find managed care coverage for remedial orthopedic procedures to treat sports injuries proximate to the campus. Faced with the choice of interrupting their course of studies or relying on the school's sports insurance, the choice is almost always the latter. This cost-shifting then burdens the loss ratios of the athletic coverage, which is usually paid for in full by the institutions.

For graduate students, the availability of parental insurance is dramatically lower than for undergraduates, as most graduate students, whether in arts and sciences or in professional schools, will "age out" of eligibility before they earn their terminal degrees.

Thus, if a university wishes to ensure compliance with ACHA guidelines, it is likely it will have to adopt a "hard-waiver" plan, where the student affirmatively demonstrates having coverage, or otherwise is required to purchase the college's offered plan.

In 1989, The Commonwealth of Massachusetts enacted legislation requiring college and university students to have student health insurance as a condition of enrollment. The Qualified Student Health Insurance Program, QSHIP, requires that every full-time and part-time student enrolled in a public or private institution of higher education participate in a qualifying student health insurance program. (Part-time is defined as 75% of the full-time curriculum.) Students who do not demonstrate enrollment in a similar plan are required to purchase the insurance plan sponsored by the specific institution.

To ensure at least minimal protection against sickness or injury, QSHIP mandates the following minimum benefit levels:*

- Aggregate Maximum—no less than $25,000*
- Inpatient Hospitalization—80%
- Outpatient Services—80% to $1,500
- Surgeon Fees—80% to $5,000
- Maternity—(treated as any other condition)

It is important to note that the QSHIP law is based on the "per condition" concept. Therefore, all of the benefit limits noted above are on a per-condition, per-year basis.

For policy year 1998–99, 31.6% of the students matriculating in Massachusetts colleges and universities were required to purchase the institution-sponsored insurance program, according to a report produced by the Massachusetts Division of Health Care Finance and Policy.[19] Currently, Massachusetts is the only state with a mandatory student health insurance statute. Massachusetts is the eighth-lowest state in terms of uninsureds and one of only six states where the number of uninsureds is declining.

The author's experience with a broad range of institutions across the country is that Massachusetts's experience is representative of the general exposure of students with inadequate or no health insurance. Applying the 31.6% enrollment statistic to the 14.5 million students enrolled in colleges and universities across the U.S. suggests that as many as 4.3 million students may not be covered by an adequate student health insurance program.

ACHA, at its annual meeting in Toronto in 2000, adopted a resolution supporting the adoption of legislation similar to QSHIP in other states.

---

* Many institutions select enhanced benefit plan.

But even a hard-waiver program may not ensure adequate student coverage. A recent audit at a large university found that 8% of undergraduates had no insurance and 32% had inadequate coverage. Among international students, 12% were uninsured and 74% were underinsured. These numbers may actually understate the problem, because a number of the insurance companies noted on waiver forms were unreachable, even after repeated telephone calls.[20]

Underscoring these observations, in September 2000, the University of California Board of Regents authorized mandatory health insurance as a non-academic condition of enrollment for undergraduates. The press release announcing this decision noted "Responding to growing concern about the estimated 40 percent of UC undergraduates without adequate health insurance and alarming medical-related student drop out rates . . ."[21]

Adequate student health insurance is an essential element of the multiple components of student health care, including the campus-based student health service, access to community-based providers, global access, medical evacuation and repatriation (because of frequent student travel), and adequate financial protection.

Until the 1950s, many employers ran employee health services, but only a few remain today. As a result, many employer-sponsored plans and most insurers who deal mostly with employer plans have little experience in providing insurance where the student health service (SHS) is the centerpiece of the student health delivery system. This lack of experience is seen in plan design, premium, administrative flexibility, and particularly, their general unwillingness to reimburse student health services for covered benefits. The intimate financial linkages among health insurance, the campus-based student health service, and referral relationships with providers in the community and elsewhere have few comparable models in employment-based insurance plans.

Further, many would argue that the college health model is superior to most managed care organizations because it incorporates both the best of the "staff model" HMO features and current best practices in public health for primary and secondary prevention for a known population at risk. When the college or university integrates the SHS and public health approaches into specifications for a student insurance plan, with particular emphasis on making care in the community a fully integrated part of the SHS program, students and parents are offered an alternative to employer-sponsored plans that truly fits students, their health care needs, and the student health service, usually at a reasonable premium.

DECIDING ON A STUDENT HEALTH INSURANCE PROGRAM

Typically, student health insurance decisions are made by a committee that almost always includes the director of the student health service and student representatives. The administration is also usually represented by someone from student affairs, finance, or both. Technical expertise in insurance matters from the risk management function is involved in only about 20–25% of the committees.[22] The use of risk management expertise, either internally or through consultants, should be the rule, rather than the exception. Many schools, particularly public institutions, use the purchasing office to run the process. While a disciplined process is desirable, care must be exercised to ensure that function prevails over form.

Whatever the historic process, the leadership role in the student health insurance decision should be held by the student health service director. While the student health service director is typically a health care professional and often a physician (and thus, by education and training, not an insurance expert), it is critical that the financial access to care, represented in part by adequate health insurance, be seen as a key responsibility of the student health service director. While the leadership function should lie with the SHS director, expertise on the various components of a well-performing student health insurance program can reside within the committee or be brought to the decision-making process from elsewhere in the university, for example, from consultants or from brokers.

There are additional concerns about "process." Academic institutions are sometimes slower to make decisions than other organizations, "chewing more than they bit off," as one cynic has commented. To avoid this trap, two separate strategies may be used: the use of outside experts, either consultants or peers from other colleges and universities (or both); and establishing a multiple-year insurance program, with an annual review and evaluation mechanism, while limiting rebidding to three- to five-year cycles. The former moves the process along by adding data and information on best practices; the latter amortizes the decision process over multiple years.

KEY DECISIONS WHICH MUST BE MADE TO ENSURE A STRONG STUDENT HEALTH INSURANCE PROGRAM

As noted above, *who is to be covered* is the first decision, with "best practice" being to provide coverage for *all* students through either parental or spousal coverage, or through the university-endorsed plan.

The determination of "adequacy" forces the second decision, which is *plan design*. Plan design will determine which benefits are covered, at what level of payment (including co-payments, deductibles, and other plan limits), and through which providers. For college health, broad geographic coverage is particularly critical, both in the campus environs and worldwide, because of high student mobility.

Plan design drives a third critical decision, which is *affordability*. Those making the insurance decision, whether a committee or an individual, should know, going into the process, what range of premiums will be acceptable. Obviously, premium will be variable, influenced primarily by plan design, so these two decisions, plan design and affordability, should be made in tandem.

A fourth decision will be how the student health insurance program will work together with *the student health service*. If basic primary care services are available at little or no cost to the student, the premiums are likely to be lower. Another financial consideration that will affect the plan (and the premium) is whether to require referral management by the health service.

With eligibility, plan design, affordability, and partnership decisions at least sketched out, the college or university must then decide whether to select an insurer or to manage the program on a self-insured or self-funded basis. These terms are used here synonymously, although there are technical differences.[23] (This is a complex decision, so a separate section is included in this chapter on how to manage self-funding.)

Because so many of the elements of a high-performing student health insurance program are the same, without regard to who bears the ultimate financial risk, the characteristics of best practices are described first.

Most institutions are required to release a Request for Proposal (RFP) or go out "to bid." The RFP process is preferable to the bid process in most instances, because it allows the institution the flexibility to evaluate responses on several criteria, as opposed to a bid, which focuses predominantly on costs. The RFP process has five critical steps:

1. Preparation of bid/RFP specifications
2. Selection of qualified bidders
3. Bidders' conference
4. Finalist selection and negotiation
5. Selection and contracting

If the university has decided to self-insure, it is likely it they will bid out at least the claims payment function to a third party administrator (TPA), so these same steps will need to be followed.

There are 12 attributes of a high-performance student health insurance program, as shown in Figure 1. The discussion below on eligibility, plan design, and premium should guide both the preparation of bid specifications and the development of selection criteria. Broadly speaking, the twelve criteria may be grouped into insurance issues, service issues, and SHS partnership issues. While each institution will develop its own weighting system, the author suggests weighting the insurance factors at 45–55%, the service issues at 25–35% and the partnership issues at 20–30%.

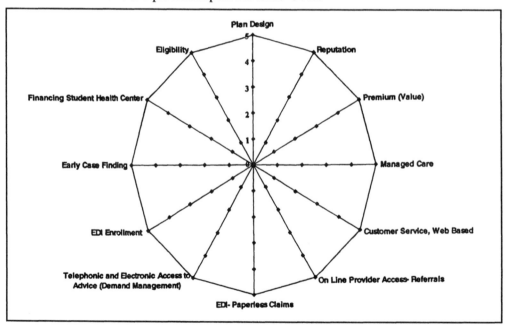

ELIGIBILITY—COVERAGE BY THE STUDENT HEALTH INSURANCE PROGRAM

As noted earlier, evidence is mounting that students are increasingly not covered by parental insurance because of lower age limits or because employers are charging employees substantially more for dependent coverage. Further, underinsurance is a growing problem because many family insurance policies do not cover out-of-area, non-urgent care or care rendered by non-network providers, and because plans are imposing higher deductibles. Students without insurance or with inadequate insurance represent 25–40% of the student population (both undergraduate and graduate students).

Immigration laws require international students to have a minimum level of insurance, although many institutions have raised the requirements to levels of coverage higher than those required by law.

The insurance plan should be available to all students, undergraduate, graduate, and professionals. A single premium rate for all undergraduate students, regardless of age, is strongly recommended, as "age-rated" programs (programs that charge different premium rates based upon different ages of students) often become unaffordable to older students. Coverage for graduate students may or may not be priced differently, at the discretion of the school. Increasingly, graduate students are receiving support from the university for some or all of their health insurance premium. Inclusion of graduate students, regardless of the source of premium payment, with the undergraduate population raises the undergraduate premium. It is also important for institutions to make available coverage for spouses and dependents. This family coverage is usually significantly more expensive than the coverage for the individual student, as the number of insureds is typically smaller, and the adverse selection much greater. Institutions need to make a conscious decision as to whether or not to allow "cross subsidies" by the larger student group of insureds to help lower the premium for spouses or children.

There are four basic types of enrollment by students into university-sponsored insurance plans; voluntary, soft waiver, hard waiver, and mandatory programs. Voluntary enrollment means that all individuals in a defined class, such as "all students," will have the option to enroll in an institutionally sponsored insurance plan.

A soft-waiver plan is a process whereby students are expected to have insurance and are billed for it on their bill from the university. They are instructed to delete the charge if they have insurance. However, no proof of insurance is required.

Hard-waiver insurance programs are designed around the concept that all students will be automatically enrolled in, and billed for, along with all other student fees, the university-selected and approved insurance plan; students who have other comparable insurance must submit proof to the university to have the charge removed.

Finally, for mandatory programs, all enrolled students of a college or university are automatically considered covered by the university-sponsored insurance plan; charges for these plans are included on the student's bill for tuition and fees and must be paid, without exception, by all students.

In addition to ensuring coverage, hard-waiver or mandatory programs reduce a process known as adverse risk selection. In a voluntary plan, solely at the election of the student, two things happen. First, many fewer students sign up. Second, most of those who do, do so because they have a chronic or recurring illness or condition which will result in claims greater than the premium, or because they want access to care without the limitations parental plans may impose. This combination of a smaller population across which to spread risk and a higher-than-anticipated level of claims may result in loss ratios far above 100%; i.e., expenses will exceed premiums—the result of adverse risk selection. If adverse risk selection is allowed to continue over time, premiums increase to the point that only the very sickest of the population enroll. This phenomenon, called a "death spiral," effectively kills the plan. In employer-sponsored plans, COBRA coverage has become a classic case of adverse selection. By extension, student continuation plans usually have similar characteristics.

GOOD PLAN DESIGN

College health insurance plan designs tend to mimic those benefits offered by employers, even though the needs of the student population are significantly different. The trend in employer-sponsored health insurance has been to add benefits that are frequently used by most of those insured, such as prescription drugs, dental care, and vision benefits. Although the unit costs of these services are not prohibitive, the high utilization rates of these types of benefits add significantly to premium costs. When someone else pays the premium (e.g., an employer), the demand for these benefits is high. With college health insurance, however, the premium is usually paid by students themselves or parents (or, increasingly, by the institution as a benefit for certain categories of graduate students), making price critical. This requires that the costs of these popular types of coverages be offset in other ways, such as deductibles, coinsurances (or co-payments), and plan limits.

A well-designed plan must first and foremost have adequate protection against significant economic costs because of a major illness or injury, not just the "popular coverage" for benefits like prescription drugs. Two strategies are often used to resolve the inherent tension between cost-sharing and economic protection. The first is the out-of-pocket maximum (OOPM), meaning when the combination of deductibles, co-payments, or plan maxima reach a threshold, the insurer pays 100% thereafter, protecting students and families from unduly high bills. Similar to automobile or homeowners' insurance deductibles, the higher the OOPM, the lower the premium.

The second strategy is to simply avoid plan limits and/or exclusions that can lead to significant financial burdens for the seriously ill or injured student. Unfortunately, it is common to see low limits on surgery (particularly outpatient) and prescription drug benefits. It is also common to see exclusions for alcohol-related injury or treatment resulting from an attempted suicide or other self-inflicted injury. Because these are not uncommon claims in student populations, significant plan limits in these areas of coverage can leave some students and their families with very significant uncovered costs. Some exclusions, however, are appropriate and consistent with either common practice and/or university policy. An example of the former is elective cosmetic surgery; an example of the latter is an injury incurred during a riot.

Insurers will, of course, write plans to the specifications suggested or requested by each school. Some insurers, however, may use narrow internal plan limits, such as indi-

RECOMMENDED RX PLAN DESIGN

The recommended attributes for a successful pharmacy benefit component in a student insurance plan are as follows:

- **Pharmacy Management Service Contract**—the use of an outside agency ensures ease of use for insureds and greatest access to discounts for long term cost control for the plan as well as avoiding the "shoe box effect".
- **Cost Sharing**—to promote consumerism, some level of cost should be shouldered by the insured. Most often this component also includes a steerage mechanism aimed at encouraging the use of less costly medications. Typical examples include co-payments of $5 for generic drug and $10 for brand name drug or $10 for generic and $20 for brand name.
- **Low Annual Maximum**—In order to control the overall impact on the insurance plan, it is important to limit the negative effect that prescription drugs can have on the total plan losses. Commonly, the annual maximum for prescription drugs in a student plan is$500–$1,000 per policy year (at the time of publication).
- **Exclusion of certain drug types and classification**—Generally, plans exclude medications such as oral contraceptives, allergy sera, non-self injectables, and acne medications. Since the general intent of student insurance plans is to cover medically necessary incidents that arise during the course of one's education, it follows logically that elective medications would not be covered. However, since all of the above noted medications are also used to treat medically necessary conditions, most plans will include a mechanism to approve coverage on an ad hoc basis as necessary. These drug classifications can also be said to be knowable and predictable in their usage, so that should a plan choose to include them for coverage, an appropriate premium increase may be budgeted to offset the expected utilization.

SUGGESTED MEDICAL BENEFIT DESIGN

The recommended attributes for a successful student insurance plan include the following components:

- **Plan Maximum**—250,000–500,000 lifetime
- **Annual Deductible**—$100–$150 per occurrence but waived if treated or referred by the Student Health Center.
- **Managed Care Elements**—Should include pre-certification, use of a gatekeeper & PPO networks
- **Coinsurance**—90% in network / 70% out of network
- **Co-payments**—Additional $25–$50 co-payment for emergency room usage, which would be waived if admitted. $10–$15 co-payments for office visits
- **Internal Benefit limits**—Certain highly utilized benefit types should be capped to protect plan performance while still protecting insureds. Generally, internal limits are placed on physical therapy, chiropractic care, and outpatient mental health. Benefit limits may be expressed as dollar amounts, as limits on the number of visits per policy year, in co-insurance percentages that are lower than the general plan design, or in varying combinations of these three.
- **Out-of-Pocket-Maximum**—To control annual premium for student, many plans utilize an OOPM of $1,500 in network, $4,500 out of network. As noted in the chapter, the higher the OOPM, the lower the annual premium.

vidual condition limits of $10,000, or hospital room and board limits of $300/day, to lower premiums. These should be avoided, because they place the insured at significant economic risk. Where possible, the university should try to balance coverage of high-frequency care (e.g., office visits, Rx's, etc.) with deductibles and co-payments.

While there is no ideal plan design for student health insurance, the better plan designs meet five tests:

- Coverage will offer solid economic protection against significant unanticipated medical costs.
- Coverage for anticipated medical costs (Rx, routine office visits, labs, etc.) will provide good value for premium.
- Coverage will follow the student as they leave school on holidays, breaks, and travel and provide medical evacuation and repatriation coverage.
- Coverage will fit hand-in-glove with the programs of the SHS.
- Provider contracts will allow broad geographic access with minimal balance billing.

AFFORDABILITY, PREMIUM, TOTAL COST, AND VALUE

Decisions on plan design and affordability must go hand-in-hand. While premium is primarily a function of plan design, historic claims experience and provider network arrangements are also critical. Plan design provides information on what is covered and, importantly, what levels of cost-sharing exist. Historic claims experience reflects the specific demographics of the insured population (male vs. female, undergraduate vs. graduate, domestic vs. international), the medical costs in that specific geographic area, and historic patterns of utilization (which may be modestly altered by cost-sharing). Broad provider networks allow both the plan and the health center the freedom to direct care to selected providers within the network and, thus, to manage both utilization and cost. Three additional factors can also influence affordability and are very important in evaluating premium: annual trend—the anticipated change in costs and utilization; pooling with other policies or other institutions; reinsurance levels with other carriers, particularly for very high claims; and the target loss ratio (TLR) the insurer wishes to achieve. TLR is defined, simply, as the ratio of dollars expended to pay benefits with dollars paid in premiums.

If one assumes actuarial science and underwriting methodologies are based on well-established practices and broadly accepted assumption principles, then it is likely that multiple insurers quoting on the same plan design, with the same historical claims experience data and comparable provider networks, will price the case to the same, or very similar, premiums. Indeed, this frequently happens, often within a few dollars. Where premiums differ more substantially, the insurer with the lower premium may have discounted recent large claims, hoping they will not reoccur (an actuarial sin!), may make lower trend assumptions, may have more favorable provider arrangements, or may be willing to assume a higher loss ratio. In some cases insurers deliberately try to "buy" the business with unrealistically low premiums, expecting substantial premium increases in future years to cover early year losses.

Realistic premiums accurately reflect the anticipated costs of specified plan design according to accepted underwriting practices, which combine historic utilization with future price expectations or trend. The "trend" assumption will incorporate all the guess-work of how the future will play out relative to the historical experience; it is, at best, an extrapolation of everything known to date. The trend assumption, thus, is a judgment call (others might say an educated guess), but can be checked against a variety of cred-ible surveys which should provide a confluence of values. Trend assumptions that are outliers on either side of the average should be questioned.

Among all the pricing variables, it is the provider arrangements which require the most careful analysis. An insurer paying a percentage of usual, customary, and reason-able charges (UCR) is a risky proposition for two reasons. First, "charges" are deter-mined only by the provider, without any negotiation with the insurer or managed care organization. Charges can be whatever the provider says they are. Thus, the difference between charges and an individual provider's UCR can change at any time and may often become significant. Worse, this difference may be billed directly to the student. This practice is called "balance billing," and represents a direct cost to students and/or their families. A more significant risk, however, is that the provider may not accept the insurance at all because the UCR percentage is too low, requiring the student to pay the entire bill directly and then seek reimbursement from the insurer. Although this process of paying first and then submitting bills to the insurer is both costly and inconvenient to the student, many insurers deliberately design plans to encourage direct patient payment for some benefits, particularly benefits like prescription drugs, where costs are rising rapidly. This direct patient payment theoretically focuses the student on price at the time of purchase, with the stated intent of imposing some consumer discipline. But it is also known that many students fail to file for reimbursement by losing bills, through neglect, or for other reasons. This "shoe box effect," as it is called, can save the insurer signifi-cant numbers of claims that are relatively expensive to process and cost even more in dollars.

Far preferable to UCR contracts are provider arrangements where the provider and insurer agree contractually to a payment program with no balance billing and guaranteed open access for the insured. And despite the cost-saving attractions of the "shoe box effect," the author does not favor direct patient billing other than for co-payments, coin-surance, or deductibles.

In the end, "value" is determined by, first, adding to the premium the expected out-of-pocket costs for deductibles, co-pays, and plan limits and any balance billing, the sum of which might be called the "full price." What is purchased for this full price is plan design, geographic access, the ratings and reputation of the company(ies), and the qual-ity of service for students, providers, and the university. The lowest premium is often *not* the best value, because it may have hidden, higher out-of-pocket expenses to the student, limited access to preferred specialists, disjointed service, and higher than average pre-mium rate adjustments in the future. Self-insured plans should be subject to the same value calculation to ensure that premiums and co-payment features do not unduly bur-den the ill or injured student.

CROSS-SUBSIDIES ACROSS PREMIUMS AND AMONG DIFFERENT RISK GROUPS

Within student populations different subpopulations will exhibit different patterns of utilization and cost. Some of these differences can be both stable over time and significant. For example, graduate students typically access health care more than undergraduates, attributable to age, planned pregnancies, and the number of eligible dependents.[24] If a university decides to have a single premium for both undergraduate and graduate students, then the undergraduate group is most likely subsidizing the graduate population. There is nothing inherently wrong with this type of cross-subsidy. Indeed, one could argue that all insurance involves the non-user or low user subsidizing the higher user. Those making student health insurance decisions should, however, be aware of all significant cross-subsidies and consciously make the pricing policy decision about the degree to which they should continue.

These decisions can become complicated when groups of students have different mechanisms for purchasing insurance, for example, when graduate students are self-pay (as in most professional schools) rather than receiving university funds through grants, fellowships, or financial aid to subsidize their student insurance premium.

In any program some level of cross-subsidies is likely to exist. At the minimum, those making plan decisions should be fully aware of what is occurring, and be prepared to defend these practices to student groups. As noted, the larger the pool of insureds, the lower risk selection becomes. Risk selection can dramatically distort cross-subsidies. This is another argument for hard-waiver programs or, for graduate students, even mandatory coverage.

INCLUSION OF INSURERS ON RFP/BID LISTS AND EVALUATION OF FINALISTS

Obviously, the criteria for inclusion on the initial RFP/ bid list are less stringent than those for the final selection process. For initial inclusion, a minimum screen should be those insurers who have provided credible service and coverage to colleges and universities in the past and have the requisite licenses and plan filings in one's state. A slightly more rigorous process involves a verbal reference check with other colleges and universities. A check of current ratings with AM Best, Moody's, Duff & Phelps, and other publicly available rating groups is also appropriate *prior* to developing the bid list, since this is useful information which is readily available through the Internet.

Another criterion, which may be used to determine an RFP/bid list is the degree to which the college or university is prepared to consider proposals for "unbundled" services. Student health insurance has several component parts:

- The relationship with the college or university
- The relationship with students and families
- The paying of claims (often called the TPA or third party administration function)
- The assumption of risk and the adequacy of compliance with insurance regulations
- The relationship with providers, including the complex task of negotiation and maintaining favorable contracts.

Different groups are qualified to provide these functions and are often discrete corporate entities that have partnered only to serve a specific school. In the most disaggregated model, a broker, a TPA, an insurer, and a network manager are four separate entities servicing a single school's student health insurance program. Additionally, to cover student travel, multiple network managers may also be involved in various locations. Among these entities, only the insurer has publicly available business ratings as described above. Brokers and TPAs are usually licensed and regulated by the states in which they do business. Provider contracting companies, sometimes called managed care organizations (MCOs), are generally not licensed, although the divisions of insurance in several states, for example, California and New Jersey, now oversee providers and MCOs which take "downstream insurance risk" (e.g., risk capitation).

In deciding whether to select proposals from "unbundled" components, two issues should be considered: responsibility and accountability. The author's prejudice is toward a fully integrated, single corporate entity, although disaggregated models have been effective for some. However, if one entity controls the entire service and insurance function, the focus of responsibility and accountability is the highest. Conversely, the adage, "what's two people's responsibility is nobody's responsibility" would not be an adage if it weren't true.

Once an RFP/bid list is established, all vendors should receive the same information and have the same access to the college or university for supplemental data and information. Care must be taken to ensure that the incumbent carrier provides to the university complete, accurate, and current claims experience data in the format specified by the institution. These data, in turn, are made available to each bidder.

As bids are examined, it is imperative that the quality and the reputation of the insurer, TPA, and broker be carefully evaluated. Reputation is discoverable at three levels—publicly available ratings, retention of clients, and written or oral references. All three should be evaluated with care. Human nature is such that if the premium is competitive, if claims get paid, and if reference customers are happy, the soundness of the insurer is rarely questioned. Recent failures of managed care organizations and insurers in several states, and receivership and government oversight of plans in other jurisdictions, have made a close examination of the financial health of insurers a critical and necessary part of every student health insurance program. The line from Gilbert and Sullivan is apt: "All is not what it seems when the milk masquerades as cream." And worse, sometimes the milk sours. To effectively probe references it is often useful to ask bidders to list at least two schools they have lost as customers in the past year. Talking to those schools may be quite helpful. Losing a customer on price when service has been excellent is less concerning than a situation where service has deteriorated.

The evaluation of the soundness and reputation of the insurer may benefit from the participation of the college's or university's risk manager or a consultant. Critical ratios established by the National Association of Insurance Commissioners should be reviewed, as well as reserves, debt ratings, and interdependent corporate financial structures. Failures in non-insurance subsidiaries have been known to draw essential assets away from the insurance company. Publicly traded companies may be reviewed in depth through the Internet and publicly available documents. At a minimum, the most recent 10K and

10Q filings with the Securities and Exchange Commission should be reviewed for publicly traded companies.

Beyond the careful analysis of the financial stability of the insurer, references from other colleges and universities should be weighted heavily. Although plan design and premium may vary considerably from one school to another, service needs and partnership issues should not.

CRITICAL SERVICE CONCERNS AND ENROLLMENT AND ELIGIBILITY BEST PRACTICES

There are five critical service concerns common to most programs.

- Enrollment and maintenance of accurate eligibility files
- Paperless claims, high quality, and timely claims adjudication
- Customer service (telephone, Internet, and email)
- Provider access and "hassle-free" referrals
- Telephone and Internet medical information

With most plans today, many of which include pharmaceutical coverage, the need for correct and timely enrollment data is critical. In the past, enrollment data were submitted as registration periods came to a close and the designated office on campus could be sure the list or roster was accurate, usually sometime late in October or early in November. For the most part, this late submission pattern was based on hard-waiver schools wanting to make sure that everyone who wanted to waive the plan would not be charged. Although administratively effective, this process did not provide timely coverage for those who needed it between the inception date of the insurance coverage, usually mid-August, and the actual submission of eligibility. Claims incurred during this gap period would usually be denied, leading to exasperated students and angry parents who felt they had enrolled in the university plans in a timely manner.

In an effort to link enrollment more closely to plan inception, and to provide high levels of customer service to students and dependents who want the insurance plan, several strategies have recently been implemented on many campuses.

- Use of an enrollment/waiver card. This allows students to indicate their coverage choice as early as possible, not leaving those who wish to enroll in the plan to be enrolled by default when the institution is sure that the waiver process is complete.
- Waiver deadlines and clear administrative policies.
- Incremental submission of positive enrollment. Institutions submit "rolling" lists of students actively electing insurance coverage as early as mid-July. These students can then be enrolled in the plan, be issued ID cards, and obtain pharmacy and all other benefits as soon as the coverage begins, usually mid-August.
- Multiple electronic file submissions. Most eligibility is now submitted using Internet FTP protocol or email between five and ten times during the plan year. Each file is a complete replacement, thereby forcing the system into reconciliation with each update.

- Decoupling premium billing between the carrier and institution. In the past, it was common practice for payment checks to be sent to a carrier or administrator along with the initial enrollment roster, often delaying submission of that roster. With a pre-negotiated payment and reconciliation schedule, there is no need to delay roster submission for payments.

These five strategies, as well as individual institutional initiatives, have served to increase student satisfaction with insurance programs while reducing the level of stress placed on the administrator of the plan. As all institutions have unique needs and capabilities, each must work closely with the claims administrator to develop a customized plan that will best serve its specific program.

Enrollment involves not only determining and maintaining eligibility, and issuing ID cards, but also involves preparing and distributing brochures. Increasingly, it is important to provide brochures on line so that students may quickly find a clear description of covered benefits and how to take advantage of them. The development of high quality brochures requires "serving three masters" who often have only marginally aligned interests. First and foremost is the student who needs to know, in plain English, what is covered and how to access care. Second, the university, particularly the student health service, wants the brochure both to accurately describe the relationship between the SHS and the insurance program and to encourage the appropriate use of the SHS. Finally, the insurer and TPA have two critical requirements: language that is legally compliant with the Division of Insurance regulations, and clarity and specificity to ensure a well-informed customer. Brochures that are clear, concise, readable, and compliant require hard work and cooperation. Sadly, many are "pasted" together on a word processor and are often more obscuring than illuminating. To the degree a university selects "unbundled" vendors, separate brokers, TPAs, and insurers, brochures can become even more unintelligible. By contrast, a well-thought-out brochure and a well-designed web site can improve a program's value greatly and result in high consumer satisfaction and administrative efficiency.

PROVIDER ACCESS AND IMPROVING THE REFERRAL PROCESS

Most student insurance plans recommend or require a student to initiate treatment at the college health center before seeing an off-campus provider. When referrals are necessary, this referral information must be accurately communicated to the plan administrator in order to properly process a student's benefit. Historically, insurers and college health centers have used a manual process of matching the health center referral with the physician's itemized bill. The challenge has always been in the timing and location of the two separate mailings.

When a student receives specialty care, it is now possible, with the use of the Internet, for the provider to fulfill the plans referral administrative requirements electronically. Best practice also allows college health centers to transmit important patient referral information through a password-protected web site. Insurers partnering with the student health services on these provider referral programs create a win-win situation for everyone. College health centers benefit by no more batching, mailing, or faxing referrals, and by access to real-time patient status. SHSs can add or delete a referral, providing better customer service for students, reducing the number of student follow-up calls, and limiting confusion from duplicate paperwork.

Students benefit by receiving immediate feedback from the insurer or the SHS on their referral status. This "real-time status" tool provides a comfort to the student in knowing he or she has properly fulfilled his or her referral requirement before seeking outside medical care. The insurer benefits by reduced patient documentation turnaround time, increased responsiveness to student inquiries, and less manual entry of mailed or faxed referrals.

Other service components of claims processing, customer service, and provision of medical information are also dramatically improved by applications of information technology. In the end, of course, it is the people and the service orientation of the insurer and TPA that differentiate good service from bad. While reference checks are of great value, site visits may also be a useful tool in evaluating service performance and commitment.

CASE MANAGEMENT/PARTNERSHIP ISSUES

It is important to emphasize again a key distinction between student health insurance and employer-sponsored plans. That difference is that virtually all student plans are centered around a campus-based student health center, which offers a number of health education and screening programs, as well as primary care and some specialty care. Employees and clinical staff of the SHS are typically salaried or paid fee-for-time (sessions) and thus function very much like a staff model HMO. Unlike the situation in college health, employer-based clinics do not exist, except in a very few companies. Thus, family plans, which are almost always employer-based, do not have any predisposition to work with the student health centers, and often reject SHS insurance claims as non-network providers. The implication of this difference is that insurers who work primarily with employee groups may not have experience in collaborating with typical SHS programs.

The critical components of the partnership between student health insurance programs and student health centers are fourfold: first, early case finding, health education, and prevention programs; second, contributing to the financing of the SHS; third, managed care strategies, including demand management and disease management; and fourth, a shared commitment to information technology.

The Importance of Early Case Finding, Health Education, and Prevention Programs

Insurers have historically been somewhat reluctant to pay for these kinds of "soft" services for several reasons, including the difficulty in projecting costs and, more importantly, the inability to measure their benefit in any reasonable (by insurance standards) time period. Over the past several years, as employers have pushed for plans to provide pediatric immunizations, Pap smears, mammography, and other proven case-finding and screening mechanisms, (for example, HEDIS—Health Plan Employer Data Information Set), insurers are now covering a broader range of these preventive and early diagnostic procedures.

For students, however, beyond vaccine-preventable disease and Pap smears, much of the early screening and case finding focuses on lifestyle risk behaviors, such as alcohol and other substance abuse, tobacco use, eating disorders, unprotected sex, lack of physical activity, and aggressive behaviors.[25] These risk factors do not lend themselves to simple clinical procedures or lab tests, but involve carefully designed, multidisciplinary human interventions. (Surveys have utility in defining the population at risk, but are limited in helping individuals or groups modify behaviors.) It is typical for student health centers to fund these early case-finding programs through student health service fees, university funds, or special grants. It is difficult to build support for these kinds of programs into student health insurance premiums; nonetheless, it should be expected that student insurers actively support any direct clinical interventions that flow from early case finding. Further, if the student health insurance enrollment is large enough to represent a significant subset of the total population, say 40% or greater, and the university is willing to build these costs into the premium, the insured and the insurer should consider supporting these activities on a capitated basis financed through the premium.

The insurer's role in financing student health centers

Student health centers are increasingly limited in their ability to raise student fees or increase their support from university funds. The student health service as the primary care center for the campus is uniquely positioned to help keep costs down for the university student insurance plan by the care they render and by managing and coordinating, to the extent possible, that care which is delivered in the surrounding community, including consultations and hospitalizations. Given this important role in both care and cost management, logic would suggest that a student insurer's self-interest would be to partner with an adequately funded student health center. The reality, however, is different. Asking (or expecting through contract negotiations) the student insurance carrier to provide general financial support for the SHS by virtue of a higher premium places an unfair burden upon those who use the university-sponsored plan as primary insurance. Since many (or, with HMOs, most) family insurance plans will not reimburse an SHS for medical services, general fund support from the student carrier to support the SHS amounts to an indirect subsidy of other plans which won't pay for these services.

One solution is for the student health insurance program to work closely with the student health center to pay for all covered benefits provided by the SHS which are not covered by the student fee. This cooperative reimbursement philosophy will, in turn, encourage the SHS to add capacity by moving some specialist care from the fee-for-service community to the student health service. The two keys to this successful partnership are flexibility and data. Best practice is to know what care which could be rendered in the SHS is actually finding its way into the community (this can be facilitated by a web-based referral system as discussed above) and then creating a financial partnership to bring that care back to the student health service. Payments from the student health insurance program to the student health center may take several forms: capitation, periodic interim payment (PIP) with register billing, fee-for-time (sessions reimbursement), or fee for service.

Best practices for managed care strategies for student health insurance

The core of managed care is "evidence-based medicine," or following the most effective and efficient known course of treatment. Unfortunately, much of what is called managed care is actually "managed fee" medicine. Examples of current best practices in evidence-based medicine are in the management of certain high-frequency, high-cost diseases such as asthma, diabetes, hypertension, and congestive heart failure. Most of these conditions, however, have a low prevalence among college students. However, students typically have three areas of high utilization, which may be amenable to "evidence-based medicine" managed care interventions: prescription drugs, ambulatory surgery, and behavioral health.

Best practice in bringing evidence-based medicine to these three areas involves a close working relationship between the student health center and practitioners who treat students appropriately, achieve good outcomes, and conserve resources. The role of the insurer is twofold: first, to provide a broad network of providers who have agreed to economically fair provider contracts; and, second, to identify for the student health service directors those significant practice pattern variations among network physicians which persist over time. It is *not* the insurer's role to tightly restrict a network; rather, the SHS should have the information to develop its own preferred providers. The concept is "a network within a network," which is facilitated by information.

Insurers should also furnish to each insured school current information on best practices in plan design, which also can support managed care by creating economic incentives through different levels of co-payment or co-insurance for the student to use preferred providers.

In summary, best practices in student health insurance yield *real economic protection*, to *all students without other adequate health insurance*, through *a broad network of providers* at a *competitive and stable price*. This insurance program should be a *close working partner* with the student health service to *support early case finding*, to provide *appropriate financial support* and to identify best practices in *evidence-based medicine*.

The challenge to colleges and universities is to work with insurers to create these kinds of high-quality/high-value programs.

SELF-INSURANCE OR SELF-FUNDING IN COLLEGE HEALTH

Self-Insurance in its simplest definition is the assumption by a college or university of the economic risk of an insurance program, a risk normally assumed by an insurance company. Assumption of this risk requires that the institution recognize the full responsibilities of risk management, i.e., funding all claims and maintaining adequate financial reserves for all outstanding liabilities and making provisions for potentially adverse and unanticipated claims loss experience.

Self-insurance found its way gradually into the employer-sponsored health benefits world in the mid-1960s, as insurers developed innovative financing arrangements, including minimum premium plans and Administrative Services Only (ASO) contracts. The concept was to reduce risk to the insurer and attempt to minimize premium increases by shifting a portion of the risk to the policy holder (the employer, not the individual), thus reducing both the state premium taxes and the reserves being held by the insurer, and thereby "recapturing" for the plan sponsor both cash flow and its concomitant investment income.

The trend among large employers to move to self-insurance accelerated in the mid-1970s as group benefits consultants promoted the idea and provided the actuarial and underwriting services to set premiums and establish reserve levels. The federal Employee Retirement Income Security Act of 1974, as amended (ERISA), exempted these group plans from state insurance regulations, including those related to mandated benefits, adding the legitimacy of the federal government to the self-insurance trend. (ERISA does not, however, preempt self-insured student health plans.)

Another significant factor in the self-insurance movement of the 1970s was a desire by large employers to become more involved in the direct management of health costs, believing that self-insuring would provide access to key utilization management information which insurers were either not collecting or not using. Furthermore, it put employers in a position to negotiate directly with providers for favorable reimbursement arrangements, eliminating the insurance "middle man."

The ability of self-insured plans to effectively manage the medical loss ratio has, over time, differentiated the various self-insured programs. In an important text on self-insurance, published in 1979, at the height of the self-insured trend, Egdahl and Walsh quote expert after expert that the majority of insurers are managing "retention" (administrative costs) efficiently and providing value for those few cents on each premium dollar.[26]

> The two components of the premium—the monies allocated for administration and those dedicated to paying claims—are inseparable. Trade-offs make it impossible to look at one in isolation and then move on to the other. I would especially caution against overlooking the dimensions of administration . . . quality assurance, utilization review, data evaluation, consumer education, and things of that kind.[27]

Currently, successful self-insured programs in both college health and employer-sponsored plans embrace the concept that management of the medical loss ratio is part and parcel of an effective self-insurance program.

> There is no magic formula nor anything approaching unanimity on how to estimate the cost-saving potential of bringing the reserves and the risk in-house. Even the most optimistic concede this essential caveat: Shaving percentage points off the fifteen to ten percent constituting administrative expense will be the height of folly if the exercise obscures the employer's (university's) sight of the other eighty-five or ninety percent of the premium.[28]

For the college or university, self-insurance requires one of two strategies: either enter the insurance and managed care business "with both feet," or contract with a vendor for some or all of the components of actuarial and underwriting expertise, claims payment, provider contracting, investment management, and customer service. If the contracting approach is taken, the vendors are likely to be benefits consultants, third party administrators (TPAs), network managers (often managed care organizations— MCOs), or insurers. With the contracting approach, the one piece the university *must* retain to be self-insured is the economic risk (although even a portion of that can be insured through stop-loss or reinsurance).

Further, before considering self-funding, a college or university must examine the relevant statutory legalities for self-insurance or self-funding. Most states establish statutory definitions of what constitutes being engaged in the business of insurance and therefore subject to licensure and other requirements of the division of insurance. In some jurisdictions, self-funding student health insurance is currently prohibited. Further, some jurisdictions now regulate those entities assuming "downstream risk" in the form of capitation or other risk-bearing financial arrangements. These restrictions could potentially apply to student health centers.

The election of self-insurance by a college or university requires a three-part commitment: economic risk, health cost management, and beneficiary and provider services. Few institutes have the expertise to do all three well.

The following ten points represent the minimum requirements for running a successful self-insured college health program:

1. An insured population large enough to provide a credible and stable risk pool. (Experts vary widely on this subject, and variables include the homogeneity of the group, plan design, and underwriting selection.)
2. Adequate premiums.
3. Adequate reserves. (Accounting firms now routinely require actuarial certification of reserves.)[29]
4. Professional investment management.
5. Appropriate stop loss coverage.
6. Independent actuarial and underwriting support to set premiums, reserves, and to advise on stop loss.
7. Solid provider networks, both locally and across the country.
8. Efficient and timely claims adjudication. Two "tests" must be applied: Does the TPA have both the incentive and the rigor to adjudicate all claims accurately?; will the self-insured school take the "heat" for appropriately denied claims?
9. Customer service to both insured students and their families and providers.
10. An administration committed to protecting the program with a full appreciation for the elements of risk protection, particularly reserves, and the requirement for adequate premium. (Starting a self-insured program presents the additional challenge of creating adequate reserves from the outset.)

Further, self-insurance plans, like traditional insurance programs, should coordinate with the student health center on plan design, referral requirements, and payment mechanisms.

Considering self-insurance from an objective "make" or "buy" decision matrix requires demonstrating the college or university can outperform the specialists in the field, and continue to do so over time. Self-insured plans may be exempt from state premium tax (whereas insurers are not), representing an advantage which is variable state by state. On average, state premium tax will be in the range of 1.5 to 2.5% of the premium, thereby "saving" the plan that amount. That advantage, however, may be more than offset by a third party administrator who is "writing checks" on the university's checkbook without an aligned interest in paying only contractually agreed-upon rates for covered benefits or for eligible beneficiaries.

Another quote from Egdahl and Walsh's text on self-insurance is instructive:

> Let's look at the retention battle as if we haven't reached the saturation point and reduce the three percent to one percent. Isn't it fair to assume that if the caretakers of the funds were paid next to nothing, they would do next to nothing? Solid cost containment and administration has a price. The lowest bidder is not always the best—I would not go to the moon on a rocket built by the lowest bidder.[30]

The few programs in college health that have continued to be self-insured tend to be large, private schools with relatively high tuition, large endowments, a close collaborative relationship with the local provider community (often their own academic medical center), and a student health service director and supporting staff of exceptional talent and experience in the self-insurance field. The leadership typically enjoys a high standing with the administration. Further, colleges and universities with successful self-insured programs will likely not have embraced outsourcing of other services. They can tolerate (indeed they may support) business ventures outside their institutions' core mission of higher education.

Some colleges and universities have been self-insured for several years and then have reverted to the more traditional insurance product. Some have experienced higher than anticipated losses and felt it prudent to divest themselves of the economic risk. Almost all, however, have experienced "fatigue" from trying to maintain a well-run insurance company within a university. Many cite a relentless attack on their reserves by other parts of the university community. Some cite frustrations in dealing with multiple and non-aligned vendors; some have concerns about the ethical problems of a natural underwriting or risk cycle which runs beyond the average tenure of a four-year undergraduate, requiring future students to fund historic adverse experience, or the reverse.

While self-funding is quite uncommon in college health, it still is used by some large group employers. More typically, employers now offer the choice of several plans, including HMOs, limiting the pool of employees available for self-insured plans. But the risk of self-funding has changed even for these employers. Increasingly, employers are moving toward defined contribution plans, where the incremental risk of premium increases is largely born by the employee.[31]

In short, while self-insurance can be a preferred option for a few colleges and universities, for most, an insured product, professionally administered, will be the choice after a careful "make or buy" analysis.

REGULATORY ENVIRONMENT FOR STUDENT HEALTH INSURANCE

The legal and regulatory environment for student health insurance generally follows group health insurance in that the primary level of regulation is by the state insurance division, with federal law preempting state jurisdiction only occasionally.

Regulatory requirements are determined by how a student health insurance plan is filed in each jurisdiction. Most student health insurance plans are filed as "blanket" plans with time limited coverage, as opposed to group plans, the more typical product filing for employer-sponsored plans. Further, unlike employer plans, which are governed by ERISA, there is no federal preemption for student insurance plans, even if they are self-funded. As a result, all student plans are subject to the regulatory environment of their respective states. Thus, the first rule of compliance is to know one's plan filing status.

The state's jurisdiction typically covers licensure, filing, reporting, solvency, and mandated coverage. Federal law covers issues such as nondiscrimination, civil rights, compliance with the Americans with Disabilities Act, coverage provided under Medicare and Medicaid, and benefits for international students on J1 and J2 visas. Other applicable federal laws can be grouped broadly under mandates and patients' rights, including, for example, the Mental Health Parity Act of 1996, and the Newborns' and Mothers' Health Protection Act of 1996. (Of interest is that both of these federal laws apply to group plans and are not, therefore, applicable to student health insurance plans filed as blanket plans.)

Currently, insurers, TPAs, and student health services are developing plans to comply with regulations supporting the Health Insurance Portability and Accountability Act of 1996 (HIPAA). Under these regulations, standards will be established for electronic transactions in a variety of areas, including claims, enrollment, eligibility, payments for services, premium payments, referrals, coordination of benefits, and coding (ICD-9-CM, CPT-4, HCPCS, CDT-2, and NOC).[32] Of particular note regarding HIPAA is that the federal regulation establishes a floor upon which the states may establish further requirements.

Colleges and universities, in contrast to many businesses, have the advantage of conducting business in only one state's jurisdiction. This is helpful when ensuring compliance for both the student health service and the student health insurance program. However, certain federal laws do apply to colleges and universities by virtue of grants and/or contracts which include federal funds. Colleges and universities should understand that these requirements may not apply directly to the insurer, or be known or understood by the insurer, and are the unique responsibility of the institution. Thus, as a general rule, colleges and universities must ensure that their student health insurance program is in compliance in all areas of legislation or regulation.

This can be a daunting task, particularly since legislation and regulations are constantly changing and the distinctions between blanket and group-filed plans are becoming more difficult to discern. This rate of change may accelerate because the current political environment has placed managed care, patients' rights, prescription drug benefits, and access to insurance high on the public policy agenda. Over the next several years it is likely that both federal and state initiatives will create a highly dynamic regulatory insurance environment.

Since this chapter is being written at a specific point in time (Autumn 2000), it would be imprudent to attempt to specify the myriad of laws (or case law) and regulations in each state which currently govern student health insurance. In the alternative, the following suggestions may help institutions with both compliance and advocacy, to ensure compliance is reasonable and equitable.

The guiding principle is to place the burden of compliance on the regulated entity. The three groups subject to regulation include the broker, the TPA, the insurer; the health care providers (student health service); and the college or university. Not only should all contractual relationships indemnify the institution for compliance, but the college or university should require the vendor to disclose its internal compliance mechanisms. For example, every insurer and/or TPA should have a standing policy council or regulatory compliance group which meets regularly to review all applicable new legislation and regulation for all states and the federal government. This group should issue periodic directives to its claims unit, customer service departments, and online brochure group to ensure timely compliance. When preparing an RFP or bid for insurance, the college or university should ask for recent minutes and/or policy directives from these groups to ensure the mechanisms for compliance are in place and functional.

Most regulations are issued in draft form with provisions for comments. Institutions may want to ask vendors (brokers, TPAs, insurers) to keep them abreast of comments being offered or, at the very least, ask for notice on issues of direct relevance to the university or the student health service.

Universities also should work with the American College Health Association to support a fair and reasonable regulatory environment. The ACHA can be an important resource for timely publications and directives on compliance.

Finally, student health insurance and student health programs are subject to general liability. The standards for general liability are broad and include failure to act in the best interests of the covered population, self-dealing, arbitrary and/or capricious exclusions, and knowingly engaging in illegal practices such as "rebating" or acceptance of gifts to influence the purchase of an insurance product. Perhaps the most common exposures to general liability for a college or university are an insurer's exclusions or plan limitations which could be judged to be arbitrary and capricious. These might include illnesses or injuries which are self-inflicted, resulting from consumption of alcohol or other substances, or other behaviors judged to constitute unnecessary or inappropriate risk. General liability can also include contingent medical malpractice liability associated with the student health service and provider contracting into which it may enter.

To ensure compliance in student health insurance and student health programs, most universities find it useful to designate a compliance officer. This individual typically works closely with both the university counsel and the risk manager to represent the unique needs of the student health program.

In summary, a student health insurance program must comply with a variety of federal and state laws and regulations. Properly administered plans, however, should not be unduly burdened by compliance. Insurers, brokers, and TPAs are engaged in regulated industries; compliance should be efficiently embedded in their day-to-day activities. The challenges are twofold. First, every institution must affirmatively review its vendors' compliance activities and obtain the appropriate indemnification. Second, because of the unique nature of the intersecting enterprises of higher education, health care delivery, and health insurance, each college or university should have a multidisciplinary compliance team in place, probably under the oversight of the general counsel, with a single designated compliance officer for student health.

FUTURE TRENDS IN COLLEGE HEALTH INSURANCE

As discussed from the beginning of this chapter, it is predicted that more undergraduate students will be without any, or adequate, parental or other family coverage in the future. Simultaneously, leaders in higher education will continue to be concerned about retention and successful academic experiences and may thus move toward hard-waiver or even mandatory insurance programs to ensure that all students have economic barriers to health care removed.

Among employer plans there will be a trend toward a greater employee contribution towards premium rather than the defined benefit approach which has existed since World War II, where employers paid for most of the health insurance premium.[33] This shift will lead to plans with very high deductibles which, in turn, may be covered by equivalent medical spending accounts. This will bring a new consumerism to American health care as families make "point-of-purchase" decisions with their own money. This "new consumerism" will have its largest impact on those medical expenses which can be deferred or where there is significant price differential, with the two leading categories, being respectively, primary care (for self-limiting disease) and prescription drugs.

If student health insurance follows this pattern of higher deductibles, both the insurers' ability to use student health insurance to help finance student health services and students' willingness to use student health centers if fees are involved, may be reduced. Either result would be unfortunate. On the other hand, high-deductible plans can serve as popular "bridge" plans, providing good insurance coverage without the limitations of employer-sponsored plans. Whatever the plan design, it is likely that the popularity of bridge plans will grow.

Graduate student health insurance may be separated from undergraduate plans because of the differences in need, coverage, and financing.[34] Student health insurance programs will continue to invest heavily in technology. As a result, enrollment, eligibility, and information on coverage will be readily available.

As regards public policy and student health insurance, with the possible exception of other states following Massachusetts' thirteen-year-old model of mandatory student health insurance, relatively little change is expected. State legislatures and the federal government are more focused on expanding Medicaid for the near-poor, dealing with the coming crisis in long-term care, and solving the problem of prescription drug costs for seniors.

Public opinion on higher education (which will influence public policy) will continue to focus on affordability, diversity, and quality. Health care and health insurance will not likely be a priority for chancellors, presidents, regents, and trustees of universities, except in certain areas of high-risk behavior such as alcohol abuse.

Anticipating the future is always a risky proposition. But to not anticipate the future is more risky. The watchword in student health insurance will be adaptability. We do know this: student health insurance and student health services have been far more successful in trying to address the public health and lifestyle risk factors than have employer-sponsored plans. This is a significant achievement and one in which all colleges and universities should take pride. Although much more can be done, this tradition of college health services and student health insurance committing to prevention, as well as to clinical care, should be continued. One important measure of success will be economic access to good health care, including health education and prevention, for all students within a system that is the prudent steward of limited resources.

GLOSSARY

Aggregate maximum—The maximum benefit that will be paid under the policy for all covered medical expenses incurred by a covered person that accumulate from one year to the next.

AM Best—An insurance industry standard rating service that provides information on the financial stability of insurance carriers.

American College Health Association (ACHA)—The professional organization comprised of and representing College and University Health Centers and professionals.

Bridge plans—Health plans intended to fill a gap in coverage created by an insured's existing plan. Modest in terms of maximum benefits, bridge plans can be used to offset an existing plan's deductible by providing first-dollar coverage or to supplement an HMO plan by providing non-emergency, out-of-area coverage.

COBRA coverage—Under the Consolidated Omnibus Budget Reconciliation Act of 1985 a provision was made for employers with 20 or more employees to continue to offer coverage in their group health plan for certain former employees, retirees, spouses, and dependent children.

Co-insurance—A variable dollar amount expressed as a percentage of the covered benefit. If the covered benefit is UCR for office visits and the co-insurance is 10%, the plan will pay 90% of UCR. If the provider charges more than UCR, the insured may be billed for the full difference between plan payment and the bill.

Co-Pay—A fixed dollar, out-of-pocket expense applicable to certain benefits (e.g., office visits, prescription drugs) and collected by the provider at the time of service.

Defined benefit—An employee benefit plan under which benefits are specified when a participant first becomes eligible. Under defined benefit plans the benefit remains constant, while the premium is adjusted to reflect current costs.

Defined contribution—An employee benefit plan under which each participant's benefits are based solely on the contributions made to the participant's account. Income or gains are credited to the account and expenses; losses or forfeitures assigned to the participant's account are deducted. Here the employer's contribution is the constant feature.

Distance learning—Course work facilitated via the Internet. These students may never actually set foot on a college campus.

D.R.G.'s—Diagnostic related groups are an industry standard coding convention which groups all diagnostic codes (ICD-9–CM—International Classification of Diseases, 9th revision, Clinical Modification) into 511 groups. DRGs are often used for defining payments.

Duff & Phelps—Industry standard rating service. Duff & Phelps Credit Rating Company is based in Chicago.

Evidence-based medicine—The use of empirical data to shape clinical judgment and to reduce practice pattern variation.

Gatekeeper—Typically a primary care physician who is responsible for managing the health care needs of the covered member. Maximum reimbursement is available only for services rendered by the gatekeeper or upon referral to a specialist by the gatekeeper.

Hard-waiver Eligibility—All students must meet pre-specified registration criteria for adequacy of health insurance and must affirmatively declare they meet these criteria (thus, "hard") to waive the university-sponsored student health insurance program.

Hard-waiver programs—Insurance programs designed around the concept that all students who cannot furnish proof of other comparable insurance coverage will be automatically enrolled in and billed via their bursar bill for a university-selected and approved insurance plan.

HEDIS—Health Plan Employer Data Information Set—A set of standardized performance measures designed to ensure that purchasers and consumers have the information they need to reliably compare the performance of managed health care plans. The performance measures in HEDIS are related to many significant public health issues, such as cancer, heart disease, smoking, asthma, and diabetes. It is sponsored, supported, and maintained by the National Committee for Quality Assurance (NCQA).

HIPAA—Health Insurance Portability and Accountability Act.

Individual condition limits—The maximum amount that will be paid for a service or event based on a specifically defined illness or injury. Individual conditions are usually signified by specific related ICD-9 codes.

Internet FTP (Internet File Transfer Protocol)—Standard process for transferring electronic files via the Internet.

Mandatory eligibility—All individuals in a defined class, such as "all graduate students," will be required to enroll in the insurance plan. The covered class may be specifically defined to meet the needs of the institution or benefit plan.

Mandatory programs—All enrolled students of a college or university will be automatically considered covered by the university sponsored insurance plan. Charges for such plans are included on the bursar/tuition bill and must be paid without exception by students.

MCOs—Managed care organizations

Moody's—A credit and debt rating company, which provides information on the financial soundness of the insurance industry.

National Association of Insurance Commissioners—This organization, originally created in 1871, is responsible for the coordination and regulation of multi-state insurers and industry standard forms and practices. The organization is comprised of the insurance commissioners of all 50 states, the District of Columbia, and the 4 U.S. territories, and is headquarted in Washington D.C.

Negotiated rates—Contractual arrangement with providers for reimbursement of services rendered using a specific methodology or table of rates. Negotiated rates are customarily in the form of discounts off published charges, per diem charges, DRG's, flat fees, case fees, or fee schedules based on CPTs (Current Procedural Terminology).

Non-network provider—A health care provider that has not contracted to furnish services or supplies at a negotiated charge.

Non-urgent care—Care or treatment which could be provided by a physician or other primary care provider at some future time.

Out-of-area providers—Hospitals, physicians, and other medical services providers who are not in the geographic area covered by the plan or proximal to the institution.

Out-of-pocket maximum (OOPM)—The maximum amount that an insured will be required to pay for services rendered within any given policy year. The calculation for OOPM includes all applicable deductible, co-payment, and coinsurance amounts. It does not include amounts in excess of URC or non-covered services or amounts.

Password-protected web site—A home page or site on the World Wide Web that may be accessed only by using a user-specific log-on ID and password. Sites of this type are created to protect both the security of the site and the user's data input.

Periodic interim payment (PIP)—The practice of an insurer or other payer providing regular scheduled payments to providers which are adjusted, up or down, periodically, to reflect the number and value of services actually rendered.

Risk Management—The process of reducing adverse effects of harm or loss at the lowest possible cost, by identifying, measuring, and controlling underlying risks.

Risk selection—An underwriting process that allows for the average morbidity/mortality of an individual or group of individuals to be assessed and maintained. The typical process may or may not include such screening or selection techniques as health statements or physical examinations, specific eligibility criteria, and conditions and exclusions (e.g., preexisting condition limitations) in the benefit plan. Plan design features such as excluding prescription drugs while including rebates for health club memberships can be used to attract more favorable risks.

Self-insured (or self-funded) option—A benefit plan funded through financial vehicles other than insurance contracts. The institution assumes the risk of paying all claims costs incurred by the covered members.

"Shoe box effect"—The practice of putting receipts for paid services aside for submission to the insurance company at a later date. In general, the set-aside bills are rarely submitted for reimbursement.

Soft-waiver plan—The process whereby students are asked to provide proof of insurance coverage to their college or university, but are not automatically billed or barred from class registration if they do not submit the information. In this model all students wishing to participate in the school-sponsored plan must fill out an individual application and remit premium either to the school or directly to the carrier.

"Staff model" HMO—An organization which retains employed physicians on salary. The physician group is controlled by the HMO unit. The two other models are group, where a physicians group practice assumes economic risk for a population, and IPA or independent practice association, where many unrelated practices contract with the HMO to provide care.

Standard & Poor's—Standard & Poor's is a New York-based division of The McGraw-Hill Companies that independently rates the financial security of companies, including insurance carriers.

Target loss ratio (TLR)—In the prospective rating of a group or specific book of business for a defined period, the TLR is the expected incurred claims for that period divided by the expected premium to be generated for that period, expressed as a percentage.

10K filings with the SEC—An annual report disclosing a variety of information, including audited financial reports, material business events, executive and board compensation, pending litigation, contracts and agreement with parties at interest, and other matters that may materially affect the performance of the company.

10Q filings with the SEC—Quarterly updates to the 10K (see above).

Usual, customary, and reasonable charges (UCR) – The charge which is the smallest of: (a) the actual charge, (b) the charge usually made for a covered service by the provider that furnishes it, and (c) the prevailing charge made for a covered service in the geographic area by those of similar professional standing.

Voluntary eligibility—All individuals in a defined class, such as "all students," will have the option to enroll in the institution-sponsored insurance plan. The covered class may be specifically defined to meet the needs of the institution or benefit plan. Enrollment is handled on an individual basis, with each member directly submitting an application and appropriate premium to the insurance carrier or plan administrator.

REFERENCES

1. Caulfield SC. "Emerging Trends in Managed Care," Journal of the American Society of CLU & ChFC. Sept. 1997, 46–54.

2. Mercer/Foster Higgins. *National Survey of Employer-Sponsored Health Plans*, February 2000.

3. Reschovsky JD et al. Do HMOs Make a Difference?" Issue Brief, Health System Change, Number 28. March 2000.

4. *National Institute for Health Care Management*, "Factors Affecting the Growth of Prescription Drug Expenditures," July 9, 1999.

5. Anderson GF and Poullier J, "Health Spending, Access and Outcomes: Trends in Industrialized Countries," Health Affairs, 18:3:178, May–June 1998.

6. Pear R. "Still Uninsured, and Still a Campaign Issue," New York Times, June 25, 2000.

7. Satcher D. "The Surgeon General's Prescription for a Healthy Nation," Keynote address, ACHA 2000 annual meeting, Toronto, Ontario, May 31, 2000.

8. Caper P. Testimony Before the Year 2000 Blue Ribbon Commission on Health Care, State of Maine. March 7, 2000.

9. Waid WC. "Third Party Payment to Fund Student Health Services," presented at the Leadership Meeting of Student Health Services at Academic Medical Centers, San Francisco. January 30, 1999.

10. Caper, op. cit.

11. ACHA Standards for Student Health Insurance, 1999.

12. Revised ACHA Guidelines for Student Health Insurance, adopted at the ACHA Annual Meeting 2000, Toronto, Ontario, May 31, 2000.

13. Ibid.

14. Pear, op. cit.

15. Boehm S, Selves EJ, Raleigh, E, et al. "College Students' Perception of Vulnerability/Susceptibility and Desire for Health Information," Patient Education Counseling. 1993; 21:77–87.

16. Kronick R, Gilmer T. "Explaining the Decline in Health Insurance Coverage, 1979–1995," Health Affairs, March/April 1999; 18:2:30–47.

17. Ibid.

18. Corson-Rikert J, Lyon V, Molnar J. "A Report on an Audit of the Hard Waiver Program at Cornell," Hot Topics Session, ACHA annual meeting 2000, Toronto, Ontario, June 1, 2000.

19. Silva PV. "QSHIP in Review," Student Health Spectrum, Spring 1999; Vol. 2, Number 1.

20. Corson-Rikert, Lyon, Molnar, op. cit.

21. University of California, UC Newswire, "UC Meeting Student Health Needs through Mandatory Health Insurance," Sept. 14, 2000.

22. Personal Communication between S. Caulfield and Linda J. Rice, Risk Manager, Clemson University, April 2000.

23. Harker C. *Self-Funding of Health Care Benefits,* International Foundation of Employee Benefit Plans, 4th Edition, USA, 1998, pg 1.

24. Pierog MB. "Graduate Student Health Insurance: Why Graduate Students Are Different from Undergraduates," Student Health Spectrum. Spring 2000; Vol. 4, Number 1.

25. Davies J, McRae B, et al. "Identifying Male College Students' Perceived Health Needs, Barriers to Seeking Help, and Recommendations to Help Men Adopt Healthier Lifestyles," Journal of the American College Health Association. 48:6:259–267; May 2000.

26. Egdahl RH, Walsh DC, eds. *Containing Health Benefit Costs: The Self-Insurance Option,* Springer-Verlag, New York; 1979. See particularly Chapter 3: "Shaving Percentage Points off Administrative Costs."

27. Ibid., p. 20.

28. Ibid., p. 29.

29. Harker, op. cit., p. 29.

30. Ibid., p. 27.

31. Caper, op. cit.

32. Gillespie G. "Transactions Role to State HIPAA Ball Rolling," *Health Data Management,* Volume 8, Number 7, July 2000, pp. 12–18.

33. Mercer/Foster Higgins, op. cit.

34. Pierog, op. cit.

CHAPTER 18

IMMUNIZATIONS AND TUBERCULIN TESTING

Mark R. Gardner, MD, and H. Spencer Turner, MD, MS, FACPM

INTRODUCTION

Among the most important public health accomplishments during the 20th century were the steps made toward the control of infectious diseases.[1] From a level in 1900 of about 800 deaths per 100,000 population per year caused by infectious disease, a rather precipitous decline began in this death rate,[*] which, even with the introduction of penicillin in about 1940, and the Salk polio vaccine in the early 1950s, continued at the same rate until a leveling-off point about 1960. This decline reflected a sharp drop in infant/child mortality and resulted in nearly a 30-year increase in life expectancy. In 1900, 30% of all deaths occurred among children younger than five; by 1997, that percentage was only 1.4%. In 1900, the three leading causes of death in the United States were pneumonia, tuberculosis, and enteritis—causing one-third of all deaths. By 1997, only 4.5% were attributable to infectious diseases, notably, pneumonia, influenza, and HIV infection.

Without question this decline in death from infectious disease was related to the control of these diseases, which became possible following the 19th century discovery of microorganisms as their cause. With the application of this knowledge, subsequent disease control resulted from improvements in sanitation and hygiene, the development of vaccines during the 20th century, the discovery of antibiotics (to some extent) and, importantly for this discussion, the implementation of universal childhood vaccination programs.

Fortunately, timing could not have been better, with the population shift during the 19th century resulting from increased industrialization and immigration beginning to

---

[*]With the single exception of the influenza pandemic of 1918 which killed 20 million people worldwide and one half a million in one year in the United States—more than died in a similar period of time during any war or epidemic in recorded history.

occur from the country to the city. Both of these led to crowding in housing and inadequate or nonexistent public water supplies and waste disposal systems, with repeated outbreaks of cholera, TB, typhoid, influenza, measles, varicella, and other childhood diseases. Thus, improvements in public health activities related to sanitation and hygiene by local, state, and federal programs enforced the concept of a collective "public health," one result of which was the provision of clean drinking water, which by extension also led to more effective sewage disposal. Also, there is evidence that the beginning of modern college health programs as we know them today (which had begun in a nominal way associated with physical education programs, about 1860) actually occurred as the result of outbreaks of certain infectious diseases, causing university administrators to realize that campuses, where large numbers of people studied, ate, slept, and lived together, needed some sort of medical support.

By 1900, 40 of the 45 states had established health departments; county health departments followed shortly thereafter; and from then to the mid part of the 20th century, state and local health departments made major steps in disease prevention activities, particularly related to sewage disposal, water treatment, chlorination of drinking-water supplies and, not to be neglected, public education as to hygienic practices, particularly food-handling and hand-washing.

Further, the incidence of tuberculosis declined as improvement in housing reduced crowding, and TB control programs were initiated. Whereas 194 of every 100,000 U.S. residents died from tuberculosis in 1900 (most inhabitants of urban areas), by 1940—and before the introduction of antibiotic therapy—although TB remained the leading cause of death in the United States, the crude annual death rate had decreased by 75% to 46 per 100,000.

Also important—and of major continuing importance—was the introduction during the 20th century of vaccination campaigns in the United States, which have virtually eliminated previously common diseases, including diphtheria, tetanus, polio, smallpox (considered to be eliminated worldwide), measles, mumps, rubella, and haemophilus influenzae meningitis. In the mid-1940s, state and local health departments, which had been formed initially to deal with issues related to sewage and waste (as previously mentioned), instituted vaccination programs aimed primarily at poor children. In the mid-1950s, the introduction of the Salk vaccine for polio made a major impact on the public health, and by the mid-1960s, a federally coordinated vaccination program was established through the passage of the Vaccination Act, which became truly landmark legislation. While many individual state public health departments had developed immunization requirements for children entering schools prior to that act, the act provided a major impetus not only to encourage childhood immunizations but to encourage the passage of laws requiring a certain series of immunizations for school children before entering public education. By extension, many individual states also began to establish prematriculation immunization requirements (PIRs) for postsecondary schools (colleges and universities). Because of the success of immunization programs even where there are no state requirements, many institutions have now established their own PIRs.

Immunization requirements and tuberculin testing which are required for matriculation (whether by the state or by the institution) can provide a solid foundation for disease prevention on college and university campuses, even in those without an organized student health service. The rationale behind establishing PIRs is that many entering college students, domestic and foreign, have not completed the currently recommended schedule for childhood immunizations. Moreover, tuberculosis remains a serious potential health problem globally on college campuses, because of the large number of students coming from countries where tuberculosis is common. Institutional PIRs serve as a public health "checkpoint" to help minimize future interruptions in students' academic pursuits, while at the same time, decreasing healthcare and administrative costs and the resultant disruption to normal campus life associated with outbreaks of preventable infectious diseases.

TUBERCULIN TESTING

Mycobacterium tuberculosis, the causative agent of TB, is spread primarily via tiny airborne particles ejected during coughing by a person with active disease. If another person inhales these droplets (for example, under crowded conditions in classrooms or residence halls), infection may occur. Two to ten weeks are required for a newly infected person to develop a positive tuberculin skin test, and, further, within the same two-to-ten-week period the immune system is usually able to halt multiplication of the tubercle bacillus and, therefore, prevent further spread throughout the body. Such persons who are TB-infected, but without symptoms and not contagious, are considered to have latent tuberculosis. However, left untreated, approximately 10% of individuals with latent tuberculosis will at some time during their lifetime develop active TB disease.[2] The risk for developing active TB disease is greatly increased for persons who are immunosuppressed. Those with HIV infection appear to be most at risk and have up to a hundredfold increase in the likelihood of developing active TB.[2]

The purpose of a TB screening requirement for college and university students is to identify individuals with either active or latent TB infection in order to reduce the transmission of the disease on campus. Optimally, only persons who are at high risk for having TB infection should be tested to maximize the cost-benefit ratio of the requirement.[2] Persons not at increased risk for TB infection are statistically less likely to be infected and are therefore less cost-effective to test. Dixon and Collins, in pointing out the concern on college campuses regarding active tuberculosis, recommend that in order to maximize the benefit of a testing program, health services should administer tuberculin skin tests to high-risk students *only*.[3] In addition, they point out the importance of appreciation of the criteria which identify students as being high-risk, especially those born outside the United States, noting that by understanding these criteria and employing a consistent approach, college health professionals can make correct screening decisions and thereby reduce risk to their campus communities.

This cost-benefit approach of screening only high-risk students has also been confirmed in a study by Hennessey et al.[4] This study examined the tuberculin skin-test screening practices and the results of the screenings in colleges and universities throughout the United States, using a self-administered mail and telephone questionnaire. Seven hundred ninety-six schools were surveyed, with 624 (78%) responding. Three hundred seventy-eight schools (61%) required some sort of tuberculin screening. It was required for all new students (U.S. citizens and international students) at 161 (26%) of the total schools, of only new international students in 53 (8%), and only in students in specific academic programs in 294 (47%). Of the 378 schools with screening requirements, unfortunately, 25% accepted a tine (multiple-puncture) test. "Of the 168 (27%) of 624 schools accepting only Mantoux skin tests and reporting results for school years 1992–1993 through 1995–1996, 3.1% of the 348,368 students screened had positive skin test results ... while international students had a significantly higher case rate for active tuberculosis [than] their U.S. residents (35.2 versus 1.1 per 100,000 students screened)."[4,p.1]

Nonetheless, the specifics of a program for TB testing should also address the unique administrative needs of each institution implementing the requirement. For some colleges and universities, TB screening of either all students or all international students may be less onerous and require less time and human resources than trying to carefully identify and test only verified "high-risk" individuals before or after their arrival on campus.

Whatever the decision about whom to test, TB testing of the target population should be done within 3 months but no more than 12 months prior to first day of classes and include (at the least) all of individuals who fit the "high-risk" profile by being either at higher risk for TB exposure or at higher risk for TB disease once infected (Table 1).

All screening for TB should begin with an evaluation for the symptoms and signs of active disease. In addition to skin testing, persons suspected of having active TB disease should undergo chest radiography and sputum evaluation, as some may skin-test falsely negative due to immunosuppression. The Mantoux test remains the preferred tuberculin skin test and is performed by intradermal injection, into the volar surface of the forearm, of 0.1 cc of purified protein derivative (PPD) tuberculin containing 5 tuberculin units (TU) of PPD. If annual testing is to be performed (e.g., for health science students), the same manufacturer's preparation of testing material should be used, as different preparations may vary in the degree of induration produced. Prior immunization with BCG does not obviate TB skin testing. A reaction of 10 mm induration to PPD in a past BCG recipient is nearly always due to active or latent TB infection and not to a prior remote immunization with BCG.[2]

Interpretation of the tuberculin skin test is based on both the millimeters of skin induration—the palpable raised hardened area—and the individual's risk for TB infection (Table 2); erythema (redness) is not measured. The diameter of the indurated area should be measured across the forearm, perpendicular to the long axis of the arm, at 48 to 72 hours after injection. Patients who miss their appointment for reading and return later than 72 hours with no reaction must be retested. Those who return later than 72 hours with positive reactions (induration) may be measured up to 7 days after placement. TB skin test results should be recorded in millimeters of induration. If no induration is found, "0 mm" should be recorded as the result.

Infection with nontuberculous mycobacteria can cause false-positive reactions. Anergy, an absence of a delayed hypersensitivity reaction, is the most common reason for false-negative reactions. False negative tests are most commonly associated with HIV infection, overwhelming TB disease, severe febrile illness, viral infections, recent live-

Table 1. Persons and Groups That Should Be Tested for TB

Persons at higher risk for either TB exposure or infection . . .
- Presence of symptoms or signs suggestive of active TB
- Chest radiograph suggestive of current or prior TB
- Household or close contacts of persons with known or suspected active TB disease
- Foreign-born persons, including children, from areas with a high TB prevalence or incidence (e.g., Asia, Africa, Latin America, Eastern Europe, Russia)
- Residents or employees of high-risk, group-living establishments, such as nursing homes, correctional institutions, mental institutions, other long-term residential facilities, and homeless shelters
- Healthcare workers who work with high-risk clients
- Certain medically underserved, low-income populations who are locally defined to be at high risk
- High-risk racial or ethnic minority populations, locally defined as having an increased prevalence of TB (e.g., homeless persons, migrant farm workers, Asians and Pacific Islanders, Hispanics, Native Americans, African Americans)
- Substance abuse, particularly use of either injectable drugs or crack cocaine
- Infants, children, and adolescents exposed to adults belonging to one or more high-risk categories

Persons at higher risk for active TB disease once infected . . .
- Confirmed or suspected HIV infection
- Persons who have become infected with TB within the last two years, particularly infants and very young children
- Individuals with certain medical conditions such as the following: diabetes mellitus, low body weight (90% of ideal), end-stage renal disease, silicosis, prolonged corticosteroid therapy, other immunosuppressive therapy, head and neck cancer, hematologic and reticuloendothelial diseases (e.g., Hodgkin's disease, leukemia), gastrectomy or intestinal bypass, chronic malabsorption syndromes
- Substance abuse, particularly use of either injectable drugs or crack cocaine
- Persons with a history of inadequately treated active TB

Adapted from the Centers for Disease Control, Core Curriculum on Tuberculosis: What the Clinician Should Know, Fourth Edition, 2000.[2]

virus immunizations, or immunosuppressive therapy. In the college setting, TB skin testing should be done before or no later than the same day as measles or other live-virus vaccinations, otherwise the testing will need to be delayed for 4–6 weeks after immunization.

Entering students with a past history of either TB disease or a positive TB skin test *should not be retested,* due to the risk of an adversely large reaction with potential skin compromise. Careful history should be obtained concerning the exact circumstances of

Table 2. Reading the Mantoux Tuberculin Skin Test

Induration of 0–4 mm is generally considered negative.

Induration of 5–9 mm is considered positive in . . .
* household or close contacts of a person with active TB
* persons with known or suspected HIV infection
* persons with a chest radiograph suggestive of TB
* persons who inject drugs (if HIV status unknown)

Induration of 10–14 mm is considered positive in . . .
* persons with certain clinical conditions, excluding HIV infection, that make them high-risk for TB (see Table 1)
* persons who inject drugs (if HIV-negative)
* foreign-born persons or travelers who have recently arrived (<5 years) from high-prevalence countries
* medically underserved, low-income populations, including high-risk racial and ethnic groups
* residents of long-term care facilities
* locally identified high-prevalence groups (e.g., homeless persons or migrant farm workers)

Induration of 15 mm or greater is considered positive in . . .
* all persons with no known risk factors for TB

Adapted from the Centers for Disease Control, Core Curriculum on Tuberculosis: What the Clinician Should Know, Fourth Edition, 2000.[2]

prior disease, testing, current health, and receipt of adequate treatment or prophylaxis. A recent chest radiograph should be reviewed or, if unavailable, a new study ordered. Ultimately, drug therapy may be needed for those patients with prior inadequate treatment of active disease or incomplete prophylaxis.

If an exposure to TB occurs, the individual should be given a tuberculin test if there is no history of prior positivity. If the test is positive (in absence of a prior known positive), this person should be considered to have become infected with tuberculosis and be referred for appropriate clinical follow-up, including, to the extent necessary, X-rays, sputum culturing, and treatment. If the initial test is negative, the person should be rechecked three months from the first tuberculin test. If that test is positive, the individual should be handled as just described; if negative, the individual may be released from regular follow-up unless required by his or her school curriculum, e.g., health professions students.

IMMUNIZATIONS

"The ultimate goal of immunization is eradication of disease; the immediate goal is prevention of disease in individuals or groups. To accomplish these goals, physicians must maintain timely immunization, including both active and passive immuno-prophylaxis, as a high priority in the care of infants, children, adolescents, and adults. The global eradication of smallpox in 1977 and elimination of poliomyelitis from the Americas in 1991, serve as models for control of disease through immunization. Both of these accomplishments were achieved by combining an effective immunization program with intensive surveillance and effective public health control measures."[5,p.1]

Further, the use of routine immunizations, particularly in childhood, has significantly reduced the prevalence of many vaccine-preventable diseases worldwide. This current decade fosters the possibility of the worldwide elimination of polio, measles, rubella, and other previously common infectious diseases. Many of the currently licensed vaccines available for use in the United States are important for all college students or to specific subsets of college students based on the subsets' individual risks (Table 3). Other, less common vaccines may be important but most relevant only to individual students based on their individual risks (Table 4).

The American College Health Association has established recommendations for institutional prematriculation immunizations[6] through its Vaccine-Preventable Diseases Task Force. The Task Force notes that ". . . recommendations are provided to colleges and universities to facilitate the implementation of a comprehensive institutional prematriculation immunization policy. . . . The Task Force recognizes that many colleges and universities are mandated by state law to require certain vaccinations for matriculating students. States and educational institutions may require fewer or more vaccines, while some may only recommend certain vaccinations."[6,p.1]

The development of PIRs for vaccine preventable diseases at a specific institution of higher education requires careful consideration of many variables. These include:

- Applicable state immunization laws and public health regulations for students attending postsecondary schools
- Requirements established by the board of regents for state (public) institutions
- Recommendations and guidelines from recognized groups in the healthcare community, including the Advisory Committee on Immunization Practices (ACIP) from the CDC, the American College Health Association (see above), the American Academy of Pediatrics (*The Red Book*) and others
- The risk demographics of enrolled students
- Types of academic and research programs on and off campus
- Prevalence data for preventable diseases on campus

While certain immunizations are important for an individual (tetanus toxoid being a good example), more specifically important for a college or university are those immunizations for infectious diseases which pose a public health menace. Important among this latter group are measles, mumps, rubella (MMR), diphtheria, pertussis, and tetanus (DPTs—discussed together because of the inclusion of diphtheria and pertussis), polio, varicella, hepatitis B, and a recent recommendation (which remains somewhat controversial), meningococcal quadrivalent polysaccharide vaccine.

Because of the importance of these particular diseases on the college campus, issues related to immunization for these diseases are discussed individually.

Measles, Mumps, Rubella vaccine

The ACIP and ACHA currently recommend two doses of measles, mumps, and rubella (MMR) vaccine for all college students born after 1956.[6] This recommendation is based on the established need for at least two doses of measles vaccine to produce acceptable disease prevention. Although a safe and effective live-virus measles vaccine has been available since the late 1960s, outbreaks occurred at college and university campuses in the late 1980s and early 1990s. Adoption of a two-dose measles immunization requirement by many states and institutions has been successful at effectively eliminating this problem. At present, 32 states require at least one dose and 27 require two doses of either measles or combined MMR vaccines. Measles transmission in the U.S. is now primarily related to cases imported from countries where immunization levels are sub-optimal.

Tetanus, Diphtheria and Pertussis

Ordinarily, the DPT immunization series has been completed in childhood, with a booster at age 11 or 12. Subsequently, an adult tetanus-diphtheria booster (Td) should be given every 10 years.

Because tetanus does not typically rate a public health concern as regards person-to-person spread, and with the rarity of diphtheria on college campuses at this time, the important public health component of the DPT vaccine is related to pertussis. The *Red Book* reports that in 1997 adolescents and adults accounted for as much as 46% of reported cases of pertussis.[5] With effective vaccination programs, significant decline has occurred in pertussis outbreaks during the past half century. However, during the decade of the 1980s, an average of 2800 cases were reported annually in the United States, while this number increased during the early part of the 1990s to an average of 4500 cases annually. Pertussis seen in recent years in the United States in adolescents and young adults has varied from an atypical respiratory illness to full-blown disease.[7] Many of these cases have occurred in previously immunized persons, suggesting a waning immunity.[6] The relative rarity of the disease in college students may frequently allow pertussis to go unrecognized. However, because of its highly communicable nature, particularly in the early stages, early recognition and treatment with erythromycin is important. While erythromycin does shorten the period of communicability, it does not reduce symptoms except when given during the incubation period or very early in the course of the disease. Of particular importance, however, is that *pertussis vaccine should **not** be given beyond age seven.*

Polio Vaccine

Routine vaccination of adults who are citizens of the United States is not considered necessary, since most adults are already immune because of the widespread immunization programs carried out beginning with the first use of the polio vaccine in the early 1950s. Further, because of the relative absence of unimmunized adults in the United States, there is very little risk of exposure to naturally occurring polio virus.

Unvaccinated adults can receive polio vaccine, preferably using inactivated poliovi-rus vaccine (IPV), because the risk of vaccine-associated paralysis following oral polio vaccine (OPV) is higher in adults than in children. Even though vaccination is not rou-tinely recommended, if it has not already been accomplished, it should be remembered in the setting of a college or university that certain adults may be at increased risk of infection with poliovirus. It is particularly important to include those who may be work-ing with poliovirus in the laboratory or travelers to areas of the world where poliomyeli-tis is endemic or epidemic. If a student has not received poliovirus vaccine, the schedule for unvaccinated adults using IPV should be followed. If the student has received a pri-mary course of OPV, another dose of OPV may be given, since these students are not at increased risk for vaccine acquired poliomyelitis. Students who have not previously re-ceived a full primary course of polio vaccine, but who by virtue of traveling may be at increased risk, should be given the remaining doses regardless of the interval since the last dose was given.[8]

Varicella

While the majority of cases of varicella (85%) occur among children younger than 15, adults 20 years of age or older account for 7% of the cases.[9] About 10,000 persons with varicella require hospitalization each year, with the higher hospitalization rate occurring among young adults (8/100,000 cases). Death occurs in 1 per 60,000 cases.[9] Complica-tions are much higher in persons over 15 years of age with a fatality rate of 2.7 per 100,000 cases among persons 15–19. A history of varicella is accepted as documentation of having had the disease. Most authorities estimate that 90% of people questioned about a history of varicella will answer affirmatively. With the remaining 10%, approximately 90% will be found to have a positive antibody titer. The remaining 1% should be consid-ered for immunization with varicella vaccine. The vaccine is particularly recommended for health science students or healthcare workers.[9]

Hepatitis B Vaccine

While hepatitis has been a reportable disease in the United States for many years, hepa-titis B became reportable as a specific diagnosis during the 1970s, after its differentia-tion from other types of hepatitis. Reports of hepatitis B reached a high point in the mid-1980s, with about 26,000 cases reported annually. Reported cases have fallen since that time and were below 10,000 in 1996; in 1998, this number fell below 9000. This decline is believed to be primarily due to the reduction in transmission among homo-sexual men and drug users associated with the HIV outbreak.[9]

However, reported cases of hepatitis B probably represent only a small portion of those that actually occur. Better data derived from areas of clinical and serologic surveil-lance for hepatitis suggests that 100,000–150,000 persons in the United States become infected with hepatitis B each year. Further, it is estimated that between 1 million and 1.25 million persons are chronically infected with hepatitis B and that an additional 10,000–15,000 persons become chronically infected each year.[9]

The most common risk factor for hepatitis B infection in the United States is sexual contact (heterosexual–41%, homosexual–14%), while injected drug use is responsible for 12%, household contact with a chronic carrier, 4%; and healthcare workers, 2% of cases.[9] Since the most important mechanism of transmission in the United States is by sexual contact, particularly in situations where there is exposure to multiple sexual partners, this vaccine is important for individuals of college age.

Properly administered, hepatitis B vaccine has an excellent immunogenicity after three doses. Over 90% of adults develop protective antibody responses. Further, the vaccine appears to be 80–100% effective in preventing infection with clinical hepatitis in those who have received a complete course of the vaccine.[9] The high immunogenicity and the high efficacy of the vaccine are important for the college-age population, since at this time it appears the vaccine gives long-term (perhaps lifelong) immunity. It also fulfills another requirement of a good vaccine in that it creates "herd immunity," i.e., decreases the number of susceptibles and thereby decreases the risk of spread of the disease throughout the population.

For all these reasons, the American College Health Association's Vaccine-Preventable Disease Task Force has included hepatitis B as a PIR. Further, for the same reasons, many institutions who do not have PIRs have held annual hepatitis B vaccination weeks, which have been, in most cases, highly successful.[10]

Meningococcal Quadrivalent Polysaccharide Vaccine

Perhaps few issues in college health have caused as much controversy as the discussions and recommendations from the ACHA Vaccine-Preventable Disease Task Force on the issue of meningococcal vaccine. In September of 1997, the Task Force issued the following press release: "For the first time, the American College Health Association (ACHA) is recommending that college students consider vaccination against potentially fatal meningococcal disease. This represents a departure from ACHA's previous policy to recommend the vaccination of students only after a college outbreak has been discovered."[11] Specifically, the recommendations made were that:

- College health services take a more proactive role in alerting students and their parents about the dangers of meningococcal disease
- College students consider vaccination against potentially fatal meningococcal disease
- Colleges and universities insure all students have access to a vaccination program for those who want to be vaccinated

In 1998, ACHA and CDC collaborated on a study of risk factors for meningococcal disease in college students. The study indicated that the incidence of meningococcal disease among undergraduate college students was 0.7 per 100,000 (lower than the rate for the general population of 18–23-year-old non-students of 1.5 per 100,000). However, it was documented that rates were higher among freshmen and among students living in residence halls—specifically, an incidence of 4.6 pr 100,000. Thus, the CDC, through its

Advisory Committee on Immunization Practices, published the following recommendations for college students in *MMWR* in June 2000:

1. Medical practitioners who provide medical care to freshmen, particularly those who live
    in or plan to live in dormitories or residence halls, should discuss the meningococcal
    disease and the benefits of vaccination with those students and their parents and make
    immunization readily available to those freshmen who wish to reduce their disease risk.
2. Colleges should provide information about meningococcal disease and the availability
    of a safe and effective vaccine to freshmen, particularly those who plan to live in dormi-
    tories.
3. Public health agencies should serve as a technical resource regarding meningococcal
    disease and vaccine for colleges and providers, including serving as a resource of infor-
    mation regarding how to obtain vaccine.
4. College students who are at higher risk for meningococcal disease due to underlying
    immune deficiencies, travel or occupational exposure should also be considered for vac-
    cination.[12]

These recommendations notwithstanding, several concerns have been expressed by
many college health professionals regarding the recommendation for the use of meningococcal vaccine on a widespread basis. These concerns have taken several forms. First,
there are currently about five known different serotypes of meningococcus: A, B, C, Y,
and W-135. The currently available vaccine in the U.S. is effective against A, C, Y, and
W-135, and has an immunogenicity of 80–90%; in the ACHA/CDC study just cited,
approximately 70% of the cases were considered to be potentially vaccine-preventable.
The efficacy of the vaccine appears to fall off fairly rapidly and may be under 70% by the
end of the third year; thus, there is concern that the duration of protection for a college
student immunized as a freshman will perhaps not cover even his or her entire college
career. Also important is the fact that the vaccine does not appear to provide "herd immunity," since it does not decrease the carrier rate, estimated in many different studies at
about 10% of the general population. Further, at this time, the vaccine is quite expensive,
at least $60–$70 per dose.

In the CDC/ACHA study just discussed, 90 cases of meningococcal disease were
identified in college students during a one-year period from September 1998 through August 1999. And, as in previous studies, the incidence was calculated to be less than half that
among the general population of 18–23-year-olds throughout the United States. Thus, college health professionals are faced with a dilemma for the use of meningitis vaccine:

*   an expensive vaccine for a relatively rare disease, rarer among college students than
    among the general population of the same age
*   a vaccine which may have a fairly short efficacy
*   a vaccine which is effective against only about two-thirds of the various strains of men-
    ingitis that would cause infection
*   a vaccine which does not appear to affect the carrier state

Various college health officials have calculated and reported through personal communications to one of the chapter authors (HST), as well as to the Student Health Service electronic mailing list (see Chapter 2) that calculations indicate that if meningitis vaccination were required of all freshmen living in residence halls, between one and two deaths would be prevented annually, at a cost of up to $30,000,000 per death (personal calculations of HST).

Further, at this time, many other national and professional organizations, including the American Academy of Family Practice, do not endorse the ACHA or the ACIP recommendation from CDC, noting, as have many college health professionals, that there are a large number of public health issues which are of considerably greater importance for the college-age population (i.e., young adults), such as use and abuse of alcohol and other drugs, including tobacco, accident prevention, and the prevention of sexually transmitted disease.[5]

Unfortunately, not only does controversy continue, but confusion concerning ACHA's actual recommendation continues as well. For example, even the classic *Red Book* indicates in the discussion of immunization under special clinical circumstances that "immunization of college students is recommended by the ACHA."[5,p.74] That, of course, as just discussed, is not, and has never been, ACHA's recommendation. Rather, based on more recent studies mentioned earlier, ACHA continues to recommend that college students receive information about the availability of meningococcal vaccine for reducing the risk of meningococcal disease, with the effort aimed primarily at freshmen living in residence halls. Nonetheless, it is probably fair to say at this point in time that although required mass vaccination of all college students or college freshmen is clearly not cost effective, individual students and parents should be given the information necessary for making an informed decision about whether or not to receive meningococcal vaccine and where to obtain it, if desired.

Influenza

Although influenza is not recommended as a PIR by the American College Health Association (for obvious reasons), it is worth discussion in this text. Influenza is a highly infectious viral disease with two important subtypes which cause disease in humans: influenza A and influenza B. Influenza vaccine is composed of viruses closely related antigenically to the "current" circulating strains of influenza A and B. In the past several years, the vaccine has contained three inactivated viruses—two type A and one type B. The efficacy of the vaccine varies by how closely the vaccine strain matches the circulating strain, and the age and health status of the recipient. With young, healthy adults, vaccines appear to be up to 90% effective in preventing illness when the vaccine strain is similar to the circulating strain.[9] Protection following the vaccination cannot be considered to be effective beyond one year, in part because of the changing antigenic nature of the circulating influenza viruses.

CDC recommends consideration of influenza vaccination for "students or others in institutional settings"[9] to "minimize disruption of routine activities during outbreaks."[9,p.257] For this reason, many colleges and universities institute each fall an influenza vaccine campaign to reach as many students as possible. Not only do these students have an excellent chance of prevention, if the vaccine strain matches the circulating strain of influenza, but, further, because the vaccine is so efficacious, a "barrier of immunes" is created to further help prevent the spread of the disease.

Caveats

There is an innate risk in including in any textbook a discussion of tuberculin testing and immunization. Because of changes in technology, the epidemiology of disease, mutations in disease-causing organisms themselves, and changes in the regulatory environment, any discussion of immunizations must include a caveat with such a dynamic state.

Thus, while the discussions above are current and valid at the time they are written, they may with little warning no longer represent "best practice" or at the worst, may become obsolete, with changes in any of the conditions mentioned above. Therefore, it behooves the reader to be aware of the necessity to stay abreast of specifics of any immunization program and to be aware of resources for this information. Thus, attention is directed to the list of suggested resources at the end of this chapter which the authors believe to be useful for college health practitioners. Even this list, however, deserves a caveat. With the explosion of information sources through the Internet, new software appears regularly with specific information related to immunization recommendations. Therefore, the reader is advised to keep abreast of not only standard reference sources but also those new sites of information which may become available.

RESOURCES

As stated in the text of this chapter, it is imperative that any college health professional who administers a tuberculin testing program, administers either single doses of vaccines or mass immunization programs, or particularly one who runs a travel clinic, be aware of changes and recommendations for immunizations which may occur on a regular basis.

The following list of resources may be helpful in this regard, with at least two important provisos. First, names of texts are given, but dates and editions are not. As a general rule, most of the texts cited below have a long history and will likely be available in some form for many years to come. Therefore, the reader is advised to always consult the most recent edition of the text.

In addition, a list of websites which may be useful is given. However, again, the reader is advised that given the relatively recent history of the web as a source of information and communication, it would not be surprising if website addresses changed.

Finally, though not listed here, many excellent commercial software products are available for immunization recommendations. Some of these provide the user with regular updates and therefore remain quite current.

Websites

Morbidity and Mortality Weekly Report (MMWR). http://www.cdc.gov/mmwr/
Advisory Committee on Immunization Practices. http://www.acip.org/new/
National Immunization Program. http://www.cdc.gov/nip/

Texts

Red Book: Report of the Committee on Infectious Diseases. American Academy of Pediatrics, 141 North West Point Blvd., Elk Grove Village, IL 60009.

Morbidity and Mortality Weekly Report (MMWR). Advisory Committee on Immunization Practices (ACIP). Statements (ACIP statements are published in MMWR).

Epidemiology and Prevention of Vaccine Preventable Diseases (The Pink Book). Centers for Disease Control and Prevention, National Immunization Program.

Control of Communicable Diseases Manual, 17th edition, 2000. Washington, D.C.: American Public Health Association.

Health Information for International Travel (The Yellow Book). Centers for Disease Control and Prevention.

Finally, resources that are often very helpful are the state and local health departments. Most have immunization program managers, who nearly always have current information on vaccines and immunization programs.

Table 3. Summary of Imunizations Commonly Recommended for College Students

AGENT	INDICATIONS	PRIMARY SCHEDULE	CONTRAINDICATIONS
Measles, Mumps, Rubella Vaccine (MMR)	All entering college students born after 1956 without either written documentation of vaccination or positive serology (In some states, physician documentation of date of conclusive diagnosis of disease is acceptable as proof of immunity for either measles or mumps, but not for rubella.)	2 doses of live vaccine: Dose 1, on or after 1st birthday Dose 2, 30 days or more after 1st dose	Avoid if a) pregnant (and avoid pregnancy for 3 months after each dose); b) history of anaphylactic or anaphylactoid reaction to a prior dose, gelatin, or neomycin (egg allergy is no longer a contraindication since 1997, per ACIP); c) moderate or severe acute febrile illness; d) active untreated TB; e) on immunosuppressive therapy; f) blood dyscrasia or malignancy affecting the bone marrow or lymphatic system; g) acquired or congenital immunodeficiency or severe immunosuppression (appropriate for HIV-infected persons without marked immunosuppression); h) family history of first-degree relative with congenital immunodeficiency, unless immune competence of the intended vaccine recipient has been verified; i) recipient of blood or blood product in preceding 3–11 months.
Tetanus & Diphtheria Toxoids combined for adult use (Td)	All college students should have previously received primary series of at least 3 doses of vaccine(s) containing tetanus and diphtheria toxoids, with last dose within <10 years.	For unvaccinated persons give 3 doses of Td vaccine: Dose 1 now Dose 2, 4–8 weeks after 1st Dose 3, 6–12 months after 2nd For persons who previously completed a primary series: Booster dose every 10 years (Booster dose in 5 years if a tetanus-prone wound occurs or if in an occupation with regular and frequent tetanus-prone wounds)	Avoid if a) either neurological or severe hypersensitivity reaction to the previous dose; b) moderate or severe acute febrile illness.

(continued)

Table 3. Summary of Imunizations Commonly Recommended for College Students *(cont)*

AGENT	INDICATIONS	PRIMARY SCHEDULE	CONTRAINDICATIONS
Hepatitis B Vaccine	All college students not previously vaccinated	3 doses of vaccine: Dose 1 nowDose 2, 1 month after 1stDose 3, 4–6 months after 2nd	Avoid if a) anaphylactic allergy to yeast or the previous dose; b) moderate or severe acute febrile illness.
Varicella Vaccine	All entering college students without either a) history of the disease, b) evidence of appropriate immunization, or c) positive serology	For persons <13 years: One dose on or after 1st birthday; For persons ≥13 years: Dose 1, on or after 1st birthday Dose 2, 4–8 weeks after 1st	Avoid if a) pregnant and avoid pregnancy for 1 month after each dose; b) history of anaphylactic or anaphylactoid reaction to prior dose, gelatin, or neomycin; c) moderate or severe acute febrile illness; d) active untreated TB; e) on immunosuppressive therapy; f) blood dyscrasia or malignancy affecting the bone marrow or lymphatic system; g) acquired or congenital immunodeficiency or HIV infection; h) family history of first-degree relative with congenital immunodeficiency, unless immune competence of the intended vaccine recipient has been verified; i) recipient of blood or blood product in preceding 5 months.
Meningococc-al Quadrivalent Polysaccharide Vaccine	Certain high-risk groups, including persons with terminal complement deficiencies, functional or anatomic asplenia, risk of occupational exposure in research or laboratory settings, foreign travel to certain destinations, military recruits risk of being affected during an outbreak of certain types of the disease.	One dose every 3–5 years as long as the indication persists	Avoid if a) moderate or severe acute febrile illness or b) severe hypersensitivity reaction to either previous dose or thimerosal.

(continued)

Table 3. Summary of Imunizations Commonly Recommended for College Students *(cont)*

AGENT	INDICATIONS	PRIMARY SCHEDULE	CONTRAINDICATIONS

ACIP recommendations for information and access to vaccine:
1. Providers of medical care to incoming or current college freshmen, particularly those who plan to or already live in dormitories and residence halls, should, during routine medical care, inform these students and their parents about meningococcal disease and the benefits of vaccination. ACIP does not recommend that the level of increased risk among freshmen warrants any specific changes in living situations for freshmen.
2. College freshmen who want to reduce their risk for meningococcal disease should either be administered vaccine (by a doctor's office or student health service) or directed to a site where vaccine is available.
3. The risk for meningococcal disease among non-freshmen college students is similar to that for the general population. However, the vaccine is safe and efficacious and therefore can be provided to non-freshmen undergraduates who want to reduce their risk for meningococcal disease. Colleges and universities should inform incoming and/or current freshmen, particularly those who plan to live or already live in dormitories or residence halls, about the availability of a safe and effective vaccine.
4. Public health agencies should provide colleges and health-care providers with information about meningococcal disease and the vaccine as well as information regarding how to obtain vaccine. (Excerpt from Centers for Disease Control, Prevention and Control of Meningococcal Disease and Meningococcal Disease and College Students, MMWR, Vol. 29 No. RR-7, June 30, 2000.)

AGENT	INDICATIONS	PRIMARY SCHEDULE	CONTRAINDICATIONS
Poliovirus Vaccine: IPV —Inactivated OPV—Oral (Live)	Routine vaccination of college students ≥18 years of age. Residing in the U.S. is not necessary. Vaccination is recommended for students who are a) traveling to certain international destinations where risk of poliovirus exists, b) working in the laboratory with live poliovirus, or c) working in a healthcare setting and are exposed to a patient who is currently contagious with wild poliovirus infection.	For previously unvaccinated students with current risk: IPV is the preferred vaccine; OPV is not recommended for use in the U.S. because of the risk for vaccine-associated paralytic polio. Give 3 doses of IPV vaccine. Dose 1 now. Dose 2, 4–8 weeks after 1st. Dose 3, 6–12 months after 2nd. For persons who were previously vaccinated with a complete series (3 doses) of either IPV or OPV and are at current risk: one adult booster dose with IPV is indicated.	Avoid OPV if a) anaphylactic reaction to prior dose; b) immunocompromised, pregnant, or HIV-infected; c) moderate or severe acute febrile illness. Avoid IPV a) if anaphylactic reaction to prior dose or to streptomycin, polymyxin B, or neomycin; b) moderate or severe acute febrile illness.

(continued)

Table 3. Summary of Imunizations Commonly Recommended for College Students *(cont)*

AGENT	INDICATIONS	PRIMARY SCHEDULE	CONTRAINDICATIONS
Pneumococcal Polysaccharide Vaccine (PPV)	Certain high-risk groups, including persons with diabetes, sickle cell disease, functional or anatomic asplenia, age 65 or older, heart disease, lung disease, alcoholism, cirrhosis, cerebrospinal fluid leaks, renal failure, nephrotic syndrome, organ transplant, hematologic or other malignancies, immuno-suppression from any cause.	One dose for most persons. Second dose 5 years after 1st for certain persons at high risk. Routine booster dose is indicated at age 65 for persons vaccinated 5 or more years prior.	Avoid if a) neurological or hypersensitivity reaction to a prior dose; b) history of hypersensitivity reaction to thimerosal (Pnu-Imune 23) or phenol (Pneumovax 23); c) moderate or severe acute febrile illness.
Hepatitis A Vaccine (HAV)	Certain high-risk groups, including men who have sex with men, locally defined high-risk communities in the U.S., persons traveling to most foreign destinations, individuals with chronic liver disease, persons who use illicit drugs, individuals who receive clotting factor concentrates.	Two doses of vaccine: Dose 1 now Dose 2, 6 months after 1st	Avoid if a) history of hypersensitivity to a prior dose, alum, or the preservative 2-phenoxyethanol; b) moderate or severe acute febrile illness.

(continued)

Table 3. Summary of Imunizations Commonly Recommended for College Students *(cont)*

AGENT	INDICATIONS	PRIMARY SCHEDULE	CONTRAINDICATIONS
Influenza Vaccine	All persons/ groups at high risk for developing severe complications from influenza, including the following: age 50 or older, respiratory or cardiac diseases (e.g., asthma, CHF, COPD, cystic fibrosis, etc.), age ≤18 on long-term aspirin therapy and at risk for Reye's syndrome, diabetes or other chronic metabolic diseases, sickle-cell anemia or other hemoglobi-nopathy, immuno- suppression from any cause, pregnant women who have other medical conditions that increase their risks for complications from influenza after consultation with their obstetrician. Other valid reasons for vaccination include:attend or live with high-risk persons, provide essential community services, wish to reduce the chance of acquiring the influenza infection, students and other persons in schools and colleges if outbreaks would cause major disruptions of school activities, traveling to the tropics any month or to either hemisphere during their respective influenza transmission seasons.	One dose annually, either in mid-fall or 4 weeks prior to international travel.	Avoid if hypersensitivity reaction to a prior dose, anaphylactic allergy to eggs** or thimerosal, moderate or severe acute febrile illness, or history of Guillain-Barré Syndrome. Persons with a history of other neurologic diseases, such as amyotrophic lateral sclerosis (ALS) or multiple sclerosis (MS), should consult with their neurologist before receiving this vaccine.

*Adapted from the recommendations of the U.S. Centers for Disease Control and Prevention and the Advisory Committee on Immunization Practices (ACIP), and guidelines from the American College Health Association (ACHA).

Table 4. Summary of Imunizations Recommended for Specific Individuals at Risk

AGENT	INDICATIONS
Anthrax Vaccine	Individuals age 18 to 65 years of age potentially exposed to large amounts of B. anthracis on the job, such as laboratory workers or military personnel.
BCG Vaccine	Individuals with regular ongoing occupational exposure to patients with active multidrug-resistant TB (resistant to isoniazid and rifampin at a minimum).
Cholera Vaccine	Individuals with travel to certain foreign destinations who are either living or working in less sanitary conditions where medical care is unavailable. The current heat-inactivated vaccine is considered to be only about 50% effective and is presently being discontinued. Currently, there are no countries requiring this vaccine for entry. However, a minimum of one dose may be needed for foreign travel to certain destinations to circumvent administrative encumbrances with local authorities during border crossings in remote areas. Recommendations will likely be updated once the more efficacious vaccines in development are approved for general use in the U.S.
Haemophilus Influenza Type B Vaccine (Hib)	Some individuals with special health concerns, including sickle cell disease, HIV/AIDS, splenectomy, bone marrow transplant, or cancer chemotherapy.
Japanese B Encephalitis Vaccine	Individuals traveling to certain foreign destinations with moderate or high risk during peak disease transmission season.
Lyme Vaccine	Individuals with frequent or prolonged exposure to tick-infested habitat or animals in areas of high or moderate risk during Lyme disease transmission season.
Plague Vaccine*	Individuals regularly working with Y. pestis in a laboratory setting or those with prolonged direct contact with animals in geographic areas of high risk for disease transmission.
Rabies Vaccine	Preexposure: veterinary medical and other students regularly working with either rabies virus in a laboratory setting or animals capable of transmitting rabies virus. Postexposure: persons with significant exposure to infected animals or to animals capable of disease transmission but not available for examination to exclude rabies infection.
Smallpox Vaccine*	Persons directly working in laboratory settings with vaccinia, closely related orthopox viruses, or research animals infected with these viruses.
Typhoid Vaccine	Individuals either working regularly with S. typhi in a laboratory setting or traveling to certain foreign destinations where infection with typhoid is a serious risk.
Yellow Fever Vaccine	Individuals traveling to certain foreign destinations that present risk of disease transmission.

Adapted from the recommendations of the U.S. Centers for Disease Control and Prevention.
* Vaccine must be ordered directly through the U.S. Centers for Disease Control and Prevention.

REFERENCES

1. Centers for Disease Control and Prevention. Ten Great Public Health Achievements—United States, 1900–1999. MMWR. April 2, 1999;48(12).

2. Centers for Disease Control and Prevention. Core Curriculum on Tuberculosis: What the Clinician Should Know, Fourth Edition, 2000.

3. Dixon WC, Collins M. Screening and Chemoprophylaxis for Tuberculosis Infection in College Populations. J Am Coll Health. January 1998;46:171–175.

4. Hennessey, KA, Schulte JM, Cooke L, Collins M, Onorato IM, Valway SE. Tuberculin Skin Test Screening Practices among U.S. Colleges and Universities. JAMA. December 16, 1998; 280(23):2008–2012.

5. American Academy of Pediatrics. Pickering LK, Editor. Active and Passive Immunization. Red Book, 25th edition. Elk Grove Village, IL, American Academy of Pediatrics, 2000.

6. American College Health Association. Recommendations for Institutional Prematriculation Immunizations, Vaccine-Preventable Diseases Task Force, January 2000.

7. Centers for Disease Control and Prevention, Health Information for International Travel, 1999–2000.

8. Chin J, Editor. Control of Communicable Diseases Manual, 17th Edition, Washington, D.C., American Public Health Association., 2000.

9. Atkinson W, Humiston S, Wolfe C, Nelson R, Editors. Epidemiology and Prevention of Vaccine-Preventable Disease, N.p., 1999. Fifth Edition. Atlanta: Centers for Disease Control and Prevention.

10. Hurley JL, Turner HS, Butler KM. Planning and Execution of a Successful Hepatitis B Immunization Program. J Am Coll Health. 2001; 49:109–191.

11. American College Health Association. American College Health Association now recommends that college students consider pre-exposure vaccination against meningococcal meningitis. Press Release, September 30, 1997.

12. Centers for Disease Control and Prevention. Prevention and Control of Meningococcal Disease and Meningococcal Disease; in College Students. MMWR 49, RR-7, June 2000.

CHAPTER 19

INTEGRATING PUBLIC HEALTH AND CLINICAL PREVENTIVE MEDICINE INTO COLLEGE HEALTH

Ted W. Grace, MD, MPH

INTRODUCTION

The origins of college health are traceable to movements in the early 1800s that incorporated physical education and hygiene into the college curriculum, but it was an emphasis on the control of communicable diseases in the 1900s that first brought public health issues onto college campuses.[1] An increasing interest in intercollegiate athletics further strengthened the emphasis on physical activity, and athletic medicine began to gradually separate from student health services at many universities. The onset of World War I led to increased attention to the health status of the youth of the United States and to the creation of another traditional role for college health—the diagnosis and treatment of venereal diseases. While health education was gradually incorporated into the mission of college health, it was the geometric expansion of medical science and technology in the latter half of the twentieth century that solidified the medical model approach to disease that persists at most student health centers to this day.

There has been intense pressure from parents and the surrounding community in recent years for higher education to address the newly developing health issues associated with the profound changes occurring in our society. Alcohol and drug abuse, sexuality issues, campus violence, and other such disturbing problems have not been as readily embraced as have traditional intervention programs focusing on physical fitness and nutrition. Federal mandates have attempted to redirect the emphasis of campus programs towards HIV and alcohol-related problems, but the results have been discouraging. As new developments in modifying unhealthy risk behaviors occur, it will become progressively more difficult to justify spending the majority of health care resources on treating the sick. More global health-enhancing programs that include environmental approaches to health promotion are already being integrated into and aligned with many student health centers' programs.

PUBLIC HEALTH

Public health applies community-based strategies of health promotion and disease prevention to defined groups of individuals. Accordingly, the fundamental unit of public health on a college campus is the *population* as defined by age, sex, race, social characteristics, living places, location, susceptibility, and exposures to specific agents over time. As the basic science and foundation for the practice of public health and preventive medicine, *epidemiology* studies the distribution and determinants of health and disease in a population, and uses this information to resolve any health problems.[2] Such information has important applications to the college health field in directing epidemiological investigation and control of communicable diseases, program operation, policy development, and the creation of a campus environment in which faculty, staff, students, and visitors can remain healthy.

Since many campus-based health centers originated in the first half of the twentieth century to specifically address the problems associated with communicable diseases, it is not surprising that student health service directors or designated providers are often assigned public health officer duties on campus, either directly or by default. Working in close collaboration with local health department agencies, they might investigate foodborne-illness outbreaks in residence halls, conduct screening and contact tracing for serious communicable diseases (e.g., tuberculosis, meningococcal meningitis, and measles), and provide immunizations and/or treatment when indicated. Such efforts have led to many new partnerships over the years between campus-based health centers, academic medical centers, and local public health organizations and agencies.

Some student health centers provide occupational and environmental health care services, although with increasing state and federal regulations, these responsibilities are often shifted to other campus departments. Many student health centers continue to provide outpatient medical care for university employees, including pre-employment assessment, work-site monitoring, injury care, and rehabilitation.

COMPREHENSIVE SCHOOL HEALTH PROGRAMS

The effectiveness of preventive health services in school settings has been disappointing because of its limited impact on health outcomes such as morbidity and mortality. Substance abuse and sexually transmitted diseases are increasing, injuries from automobile accidents and violence are highest in the secondary school age group, and the 15- to 24-year age group was the only age group in the United States to experience an increased death rate in recent decades. Health care services and school health education services were not able to solve these problems alone, but partnering these groups with community social and environmental efforts has been shown to have a measurable impact on knowledge, attitudes, and skills that impact students' health behaviors.[3]

The Comprehensive School Health Program model also more closely addresses the primary function of schools—the academic success of their students. By combining educational objectives, school and community health services, and environmental interventions, the emphasis is being shifted toward health as a means to academic success. This model has already demonstrated the link between educational performance and such short-term behavioral factors as sleep, exercise, diet, and stress, but it will be much more difficult to show an association between lifestyle behaviors and long-term health outcomes.[4]

CAMPUS-ORIENTED HEALTH CARE

Many public health authorities believe that societal or community-level interventions offer the only effective solution to a lasting change in health-related behaviors. Community-oriented primary care (COPC) uses a team of health professionals working in collaboration with community members to systematically identify and address the health problems of a defined population.[5] Combining principles of primary care, epidemiology, and public health, COPC focuses on population-based risk as a whole rather than on the care of individual patients.

The original operational model for COPC, published by the Institute of Medicine, included four steps: 1) define and characterize the community; 2) identify the community's health problems; 3) develop an intervention; and 4) monitor the impact of the intervention.[6] While traditional epidemiological studies can take years to complete, COPC offers immediate feedback through repeated population-based measurement. This allows the health care team to modify the intervention within months if beneficial change has not occurred. Later authors have emphasized the importance of community involvement by adding "involve the community" as a fifth step to the model. This group health concept has gradually been incorporated into college health through comprehensive health promotion and campus wellness programs.

Some would suggest that college health has always been a community-based, community-responsive network practice. Campus wellness programs often work together in a team effort with leaders from academic planning, residence life, student life, student health, health education, physical education, recreational sports, disability services, food services, counseling, student affairs, campus security, etc., to address such issues as alcohol and drug abuse, sexuality issues, and campus violence. In reality, such behavior patterns are so interrelated that addressing them must involve a much more comprehensive approach. Using community-based interventions, these programs reach out to students who may not present to the student health center, guiding whole populations of students toward healthier lifestyles.

One group of leaders from higher education clearly recognized the importance of treating communities when they wrote: "The health of the campus and the health of the community become ever more interdependent. In various ways institutions of higher education create a health environment for their students. That environment affects students' educational outcomes, as well as the quality of life of everyone on campus and the health of the surrounding community."[7]

APPLYING EPIDEMIOLOGY TO COLLEGE HEALTH

Epidemiological Information Cycle

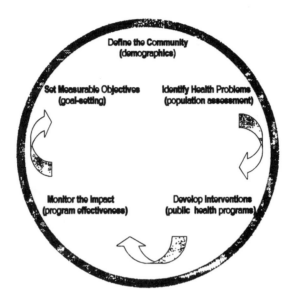

Campus Demographics

Understanding the dramatic shift in age, health status, core values, and distinctive characteristics of the college student population over the past several decades is necessary for interventionists to be able to reach them with effective health promotion programs. Born during a surge in birth rate that demographers locate between 1979 and 1994, the current generation of college students has been called Generation Y, Echo Boomers, or the Millennium Generation. At 60 million strong, they are the second-largest birth cohort in American history—after the 72 million baby boomers. This generation is much more racially diverse, with one in three not being Caucasian. One in four lives in a single-parent household, and three in four have working mothers. Today's traditional-age college student grew up in a time when the nation's worsening economy was coupled with a technological revolution. In short, they came of age when everything around them was changing. Just as importantly, they lived in this environment of economic, political, social, and psychological upheaval without much of the support that had been afforded to students in prior generations by family, church, schools, and youth groups.

On college campuses, the nontraditional students of past decades became the traditional students of today. This more heterogeneous student body challenges college health professionals to find new ways to serve a larger number of students who are older, financially independent, and more likely to be uninsured or underinsured. The average college student is now 26 years of age, and female students are in the majority. Minority students, international students, and students with spouses and/or families represent an increasing proportion of the college population, and the commuter campus has become the norm at a number of colleges and universities. Many students live at home longer and/or find part-time or full-time jobs to help finance their college fees. Balancing school, family, and job responsibilities, today's students spend relatively less time on campus outside of the classroom. Since access to health care is often limited for these students, they continue to challenge college health professionals to find better methods to meet their unique health care needs.

Population Assessment

Public health and prevention efforts are traditionally based on scientific studies of morbidity and mortality factors, but it has been the definition and measurement of indices of risk status that has had the greatest influence on the practice of college health. As the foundation of epidemiological practice, *surveillance* is "the ongoing systematic collection, analysis, and interpretation of health data essential to the planning, implementation, and evaluation of public health practice."[8] Health surveys provide one type of data that is especially valuable to health professionals. The Centers for Disease Control and Prevention's National Center for Health Statistics (NCHS) has conducted nationwide household interview surveys since 1957. They have subsequently initiated a number of other surveys, such as the National Health and Nutrition Examination Survey (NHANES), the National Ambulatory Medical Care Survey (NAMCS), and the National Health Interview Survey (NHIS). Unfortunately, the epidemiology of health risk behaviors in the college-age population was not being captured by these data.

When the epidemic of high-risk health behaviors in adolescents became apparent to public health officials, the Centers for Disease Control and Prevention (CDC) developed a Youth Risk Behavior Surveillance System (YRBS) to collect data on 9th- through 12th-

Figure 2. Health-risk Behaviors of College Students Monitored by the National College Health Risk Behavior Survey (NCHRBS)

1. Safety-Belt Use	19. Other Illegal-Drug Use
2. Motorcycle-Helmet Use	20. Combined Illegal Drug and Alcohol Use
3. Bicycle-Helmet Use	21. Sexual Intercourse
4. Riding with a Driver Who has Been Drinking	22. Contraceptive Use
5. Driving After Drinking Alcohol	23. Condom Use
6. Drinking Alcohol When Boating or Swimming	24. Alcohol and Drug Use at Last Sexual Intercourse
7. Carrying a Weapon	25. Pregnancy
8. Forced Sexual Intercourse	26. Consumption of Fruits and Vegetables
9. Engaging in a Physical Fight	27. Consumption of Foods Typically High in Fat Content
10. Suicide Ideation and Attempts	28. Overweight
11. Cigarette Use	29. Attempted Weight Loss
12. Smokeless-Tobacco Use	30. Vigorous and Moderate Physical Activity
13. Alcohol Use	31. Stretching Exercises
14. Marijuana Use	32. Strengthening Exercises
15. Cocaine Use	33. Participation in Physical Education Class
16. Inhalant Use	34. Participation on Sports Teams
17. Steroid Use	
18. Injecting-Drug Use	

grade students, followed later by an additional component that monitored all 12- to 21-year-old youth regardless of school status. More significantly for college health, the Youth Risk Behavior Surveillance System: National College Health Risk Behavior Survey (NCHRBS) became the first national college-based surveillance system to monitor priority health-risk behaviors among representative samples of undergraduate college students. (Figure 2)

Public Health Programs

After the health risk behaviors were identified, a number of national programs were initiated to specifically address behavioral risk factors in the college-age population. One of the first initiatives to address a preventable health problem in a college-age population was by the Division of Adolescent and School Health of the U.S. Public Health Service, implementing a major nationwide initiative focused on HIV-related risk factor surveillance and health promotion activities. The Fund for the Improvement of Postsecondary Education (FIPSE) of the U.S. Department of Education has also financed many innovative programs on college campuses to combat alcohol and drug abuse, and the American Medical Association developed a comprehensive set of Guidelines for Adolescent Preventive Services (GAPS).[9]

Program Effectiveness

The recent emphasis on practice guidelines has shifted the public health field toward outcome measures as indicators of community health. One of the earliest reviews was performed by the Canadian Task Force on the Periodic Health Examination, followed closely by the 1989 release of the U.S. Preventive Services Task Force.[10,11] This report established the first set of national guidelines for prevention based on a rigorous review of the scientific evidence of the effectiveness of 169 clinical preventive services. The American College of Physicians also evaluated available preventive services in adults over the age of 18.[12]

Goal-Setting

In the past decade, there have been considerable efforts made to establish goals for communities to use in measuring improvements in health status. While much of this work has been done at the national level, many campus communities are setting local goals based on differing priorities, needs, and perceptions, and in so doing, are redirecting the use of their limited health care resources.

The most important development in the promotion of public health and prevention interventions over the past two decades has been the release of the landmark *Healthy People* goals and objectives for the nation that not only documented the current health status of the U.S. population, but also established population-based goals for the nation to attain by the year 2000. In *Healthy People 2000: National Health Promotion and Disease Prevention Objectives for the Year 2000,* young people were recognized as a special population that experienced higher rates of morbidity, disability, and mortality than did the general population from certain health risk behaviors.[13] The American Medical Association excerpted the *Healthy Youth 2000* objectives for adolescents from this work.[14] While student health professionals were involved in the initial development of these goals, they were subsequently adapted more specifically to college health in the *Healthy Campus 2000* document.[15] *Healthy People 2010* and *Healthy Campus 2010* objectives are being developed at the time of this writing.

HEALTH PROMOTION AND DISEASE PREVENTION

As college health professionals become more adept at behavioral change skills, they have an increasing opportunity to favorably alter risk factors for many causes of premature morbidity and mortality. The goal of many student health centers is to integrate these behavior change processes into an ambulatory care arena, and ultimately into community-based health promotion programs.

Depending on how broadly it is defined, most patient contacts in clinical medicine involve some form of prevention activity. Prevention efforts are often classified by the stage of disease toward which they are directed. Traditional private medical practices focus primarily on *tertiary prevention,* or those clinical activities that minimize the progression and/or reduce the complications after a disease has become symptomatic.[16] As the prevalence of chronic disease continues to rise in an aging population, this form of prevention directed toward the disease stage will continue to consume a disproportionate amount of human and fiscal resources. Since most of the recipients of this high-technology-based or curative medicine are the very sick and/or the very old, the average student health center spends proportionally many fewer resources on tertiary prevention.

SECONDARY PREVENTION

Secondary prevention is directed toward the asymptomatic or subclinical stage of disease in an attempt to reduce its expression or severity through specific preventive interventions or definitive treatment.[16]

Screening

As a major tool for the early detection of disease, *screening* is one of the cornerstones of secondary prevention. An effective medical screening program identifies individuals with unrecognized disease by applying rapid and cost-effective tests or examinations to differentiate asymptomatic persons who may have a disease from those who do not.[17] The best screening programs are those involving relatively common conditions for which there are acceptable, available, and affordable tests and treatments.

Student health centers have traditionally used screening programs to prevent the spread of communicable diseases on campus, but a number of college health centers are now screening for chronic diseases and/or their risk factors. Campus screening programs can include patients presenting to college health providers for other problems, or mass screening tests applied to larger segments of the population.

Tuberculosis

The intermittent resurgence of tuberculosis (TB) cases in the U.S. college-age population has been attributed to a number of factors, including the transmission of *Mycobacterium tuberculosis* in the close social structure of college settings and the increased prevalence of TB in immigrants and foreign-born students. The rate of positive skin test results among foreign-born or international students has been reported by various colleges over the past two decades to range from 23 to 50 percent.[18, 19, 20, 21] Six percent of all tuberculosis cases reported in the United States from 1993 to 1997 were among persons aged 18 through 24 years, and 62% of these individuals were foreign-born.[18]

Some two-thirds of U.S. colleges currently screen for tuberculosis, as a traditional public health function at academic institutions. Tuberculosis screening using the Mantoux method for groups at high risk of infection as defined by the Centers for Disease Control and Prevention reduces both the expenses and the medical risks associated with such skin-testing programs.[22]

Patients with positive tuberculin skin tests need to be further evaluated to identify those with active disease who will require multiple-drug therapy. Those individuals with inactive or latent infection should generally receive prophylaxis using monotherapy. One of the major challenges to college health practitioners is convincing international students that a positive TB skin test is not solely attributable to having been innoculated previously with bacille Calmette-Guerin (BCG).

Sexually Transmitted Diseases

Early detection of sexually transmitted diseases (STDs) through screening is a principal component of most prevention strategies. Screening affects primary prevention by decreasing the period of infectiousness, and secondary prevention by resulting in treatment before complications can occur. While screening has a central role in the control of gonorrhea, syphilis, human immunodeficiency virus (HIV) infections, and chlamydial infections, its value in controlling herpes simplex virus (HSV) infections, human papillomavirus (HPV) infections, and other STDs remains to be determined. Screening is especially important for students at risk for sexually transmitted diseases who may lack clinical evidence of infection. One study of college women found that 79 percent of those who tested positive for chlamydia had no symptoms of disease.[23]

While universal screening for STDs is impractical in most settings, screening for *C. trachomatis* in female college students was previously found to be cost-effective when the prevalence rate in the population exceeded 7 percent.[24] The prevalence rate of genital infections with *C. trachomatis* in female adolescents has been reported to exceed 20 percent in some high-risk populations.[25] Since *C. trachomatis* infections are responsible for at least half of all infection-related tubal infertility and have a long period of potential transmission, routine annual screening is currently recommended for all sexually active adolescent females younger than 20 years, as well as for older women at risk.[26] In other settings where the prevalence of chlamydial infection is higher, raising the routine screening age to 25 or 30 is necessary to increase the yield of screening and decrease the occurrence of infections.[27]

The American College of Obstetricians and Gynecologists (ACOG) also recommends routine gonorrhea screening for all sexually active adolescents and other asymptomatic women at high risk for sexually transmitted infections.

Data to guide STD screening and treatment programs in adolescent males are more limited, but the CDC recommends routinely screening young, sexually active men for chlamydial and gonococcal infections.[28]

The enhanced sensitivity of newer diagnostic tests using first-voided urine samples from men and women, as well as vaginal swabs collected by female patients, is making community-based screening a more popular alternative to conventional screening programs that use cervical or urethral swabs to collect specimens.

Cancer

An annual pelvic examination and Pap smear for women who are sexually active or over the age of 18 are the key to early detection of cervical neoplasia. Epidemiologic studies convincingly demonstrate that the major risk factor for development of pre-invasive or invasive carcinoma of the cervix is HPV infection. The patient with an abnormal cervical cytology of a high-risk type should be thoroughly evaluated with colposcopy and biopsy. Patients with low-risk cytology or cytology of unclear abnormality, such as atypical squamous cells of undetermined significance (ASCUS), using the Bethesda System, may or may not have pre-invasive or micro-invasive cancer. While studies are ongoing to determine how HPV typing can be used to help stratify these women into follow-up and treatment groups, at least one study has suggested HPV DNA typing may aid in differentiating which patients to evaluate intensively and which to follow more conservatively.[29]

Breast cancer mortality is decreasing for the first time in the six decades for which statistics are available, this at least partially attributable to the growing acceptance by the U.S. public of mammography screening.[30] The lower prevalence of breast cancer in younger women and the decreased sensitivity of mammography in younger women with denser breast tissue lead many authorities not to recommend routine screening mammography below the age of 50. Others recommend mammography screening be offered to women who have substantial risk factors at age 40 years, particularly a family history, and to those with no risk factors between the ages of 45 and 50 years.[30]

Testicular cancer accounts for only 1% of all cancers in men, but is most common in college-age males. In white men, it is the most common cancer between 20 and 34 years of age, the second most common from 35 to 39 years of age, and the third most common from 15 to 19 years of age. Most testicular cancers are discovered by the patient, either unintentionally or by self-examination, although some are discovered on routine physical examination. However, no studies to date have been able to document a decrease in mortality associated with screening programs, probably because testicular cancer is curable at advanced stages and there are relatively few cases.

Cardiovascular Disease

Hypercholesterolemia and hypertension are largely asymptomatic risk factors for coronary heart disease that are modifiable in adolescents and young adults through lifestyle interventions when identified early by screening programs. Current guidelines from the

National Cholesterol Education Program (NCEP) of the National Heart, Lung, and Blood Institute recommend universal total blood cholesterol and HDL-cholesterol screening of adults aged 20 and above at least once every five years.[31] The American College of Physicians later proposed guidelines using only a total cholesterol level, and excluding men younger than age 35, women younger than age 45, and many persons 65 years and older;[32] however, some experts feel these recommendations are flawed.[33,34] Data indicating that effective therapy of hypercholesterolemia can limit the progression of atherosclerosis, the primary and secondary prevention trials, and evidence that cholesterol levels in young adults can predict midlife coronary heart disease all suggest the importance of early detection and therapy in a college-age population.

Recommendations regarding hypertension screening are not as controversial, as most major authorities recommend measuring blood pressure in people of all ages in order to reduce cardiovascular-related morbidity and mortality.[35,36,37] The recommended frequency of blood pressure screening varies from every "clinical visit" or "every one to two years," to guidelines as vague as "periodically" and "the optimal interval is left to clinical discretion."

Primary Prevention

Directed toward the susceptibility stage of disease, *primary prevention* reduces the severity, or even the likelihood, of a disease or injury.[16] Unlike screening programs aimed at the early detection of disease for secondary prevention, primary prevention programs often target high-risk health behaviors or lifestyle factors. Caring for a relatively young and healthy population, college health practitioners devote a substantially greater proportion of their efforts toward these primary preventive activities.

Vaccine-preventable Diseases

Despite current recommendations for effective prevention programs, vaccine-preventable diseases continue to have an adverse health and economic impact on college campuses today.[38] The American College Health Association's (ACHA) Vaccine-Preventable Diseases Task Force currently recommends that all college and university students receive the following immunizations prior to matriculation: measles, mumps, rubella (MMR), two doses at least one month apart for students born after 1956; diphtheria, pertussis, tetanus (DPT), primary series in childhood, followed by Td booster at age 11–12 years, then every 10 years; polio, primary series in childhood, with booster only if needed for travel after age 18 years, with inactivated form (IPV); varicella, two doses one month apart if over age 13 years for students with no history of disease or with a negative antibody titer; and hepatitis B, in a series of three doses given at 0, 1–2 months, and 6–12 months.[39] The task force also encourages all college students, particularly high-risk individuals or those living in dormitories, to receive influenza vaccine annually during autumn; and the Centers for Disease Control and Prevention's Advisory Committee on Immunization Practices recommends that freshmen, particularly those living in dormitories, be informed about meningococcal disease and the benefits of vaccination. Institutions that train health care professionals may impose additional immunization requirements, such as rabies vaccine for veterinary students or varicella vaccine. Hepatitis A vaccine may be indicated in selected geographic areas.

Health Risk Behaviors

Promising developments in the field of medical behavioral psychology have convinced many health authorities that it is more cost-effective to reduce the modifiable risk factors for chronic disease than to treat the disease once it occurs. Those interventions designed to reinforce individual and collective behaviors are thought to be much more effective during the critical late-adolescent period, before the unhealthy lifestyles have had an opportunity to become more fully developed and extend into adulthood.

Alcohol and Other Drugs

Alcohol abuse continues to be identified as the number one health-risk factor on college campuses today. In the report from the 1999 Harvard School of Public Health College Alcohol Study, Henry Wechsler and colleagues found that heavy episodic or binge drinking rates in college students continue to exceed 40 percent, in spite of the increased attention given to this problem since their first survey in 1993.[40] This report is particularly alarming because the students most likely to experience alcohol-related problems—the frequent binge drinkers—increased by nearly 5 percent in the six years since the Harvard Study began. The misuse of alcohol and other drugs also affects the peers of heavy drinkers, who encounter the secondhand effects of the problem. Heavy drinking is associated with increased campus violence, physical injuries, emotional difficulties, poor academic performance, unplanned and unsafe sexual activity, and motor vehicle fatalities.[41–46]

In their prior study, the Harvard researchers postulated that the overall decline in drinking in U.S. society was not being reflected on college campuses, suggesting that colleges and universities were inadvertently perpetuating their own drinking cultures through selection, tradition, ambivalence in establishing and enforcing campus alcohol policies, and other strategies that reinforce the wrong types of behavior.[47] While most residential colleges and universities today have a campus alcohol program, educator, and/or treatment specialist, the recent data raise serious concern that the interventions undertaken so far may not be adequate. Some colleges and universities are responding to alcohol-related incidents with reflexive reactions intended to punish rather than help, such as zero tolerance policies that remove the problem students from the campus and surrounding community, where the resources these students need for help are most likely to exist. Such policies run counter to the models of student development and community-based interventions that are used to address other serious behavioral problems on campus. It is still too early to tell if the fact that binge drinking is decreasing among students living on campus is because our newer prevention methods are working, or because we are removing students with alcohol problems from the campus environment.

After alcohol and tobacco, marijuana remains the most frequently used drug of abuse among college students. In 1996, the New York State Office of Alcoholism and Substance Abuse Services (OASAS) conducted a major survey of alcohol and other drug use among undergraduate students in the state of New York.[48] This study, consistent with data from other areas of the country, found that about one in five college students is a current marijuana user, and that 14 percent of the students use marijuana at least weekly. Cocaine, hallucinogens, and amphetamines were reportedly used by smaller percentages of students, with sedatives, opiates, inhalants, designer drugs, and steroids being the least-used drugs.[49]

Smoking

The negative health consequences of tobacco consumption are well known, and cigarette smoking is the single most preventable cause of premature death in the United States. Smoking usually starts during adolescence and young adulthood; cigarette use increased by 32 percent in high school students between 1991 and 1997.[50] This undoubtedly translates into increasing smoking rates among college students. The monthly prevalence rate of cigarette use in college students reached 28 percent in a 1997 study.[51] Another group of researchers reported that among undergraduates in the Florida State University system, white students were more likely than minority students to try cigarettes, women more likely than men to smoke regularly, and married students the most likely to smoke regularly and less likely to have tried to quit.[52] While alcohol and other drug use usually decreases with age, smoking does not, and this rise in youth smoking will almost certainly be reflected in rising smoking rates among future generations of adults.

Sexual Behavior

One of the primary national health objectives for the college-age population is a reduction in unintended pregnancy and transmission of sexually transmitted diseases and HIV infection. Despite successful efforts to educate college and university students about risky sexual activities, there is widespread evidence that this knowledge does not necessarily result in preventive behavior changes. Numerous studies provide insight on the extent that high-risk sexual behaviors exist on college campuses today. A survey at one large midwestern university found that 80 percent of males and 73 percent of females reported being sexually active, with eight and six lifetime partners, respectively.[53] Another major study of female college students examined trends in sexual behavior during 1975, 1986, and 1989.[54] While the percentage of sexually active women who reported condom use increased from 12 percent to 41 percent, there were no other significant changes in other high-risk sexual practices, such as number of partners.

A survey of university students in Hawaii found that 21 percent of women and 16 percent of men reported a past history of a sexually transmitted disease.[55] In other studies, one found that nearly half of female college students tested had evidence of genital human papillomavirus (HPV) infection,[56] while another reported that the cumulative 36-month incidence of HPV infection in study participants was 43 percent.[57] The prevalence of herpes simplex virus (HSV) type 2 has increased by 30 percent since the late 1970s, and now is detectable in about one in five persons nationwide who are 12 years of age or older.[58] The prevalence rate of chlamydia infection exceeds 20 percent in some high-risk adolescent populations,[25] while a recent study in female military recruits 25 years of age or less reported an overall prevalence rate of 9.2 percent.[59] Although the overall prevalence of human immunodeficiency virus infection (HIV) is low in college students,[60] the occurrence of behaviors that facilitate sexual transmission of HIV is obviously increasing. Studies have indicated at least a twofold to fivefold increased risk for HIV infection among persons who have other STDs, including genital ulcer diseases and non-ulcerative, inflammatory STDs.[61] Consequently, the Advisory Committee for HIV and STD Prevention (ACHSP) is advising early detection and treatment of other STDs as an effective strategy for preventing sexually transmitted HIV infection.

Eighteen- to twenty-four-year-old women also account for more than one-third of reported pregnancy terminations,[62] and past studies suggest a significant proportion of sexually active college students use contraceptives inconsistently. One study reported that during an initial interview nearly one in five female college students reported using an unreliable contraceptive method, and that 60 percent of the women used unreliable contraception over the next six months.[63] This suggests that interventions to improve contraceptive and barrier method use must emphasize the consistency of use.

Injuries and Violence

The three leading causes of death among school-age youth and young adults are motor vehicle crashes and other unintentional injuries, homicide, and suicide.[64] This is unique in comparison to adults age 25 or older, where the leading causes of mortality and morbidity are heart disease, cancer, and stroke. Injury may be the most under-recognized major public health problem in the nation today, since the burden of injury falls disproportionately on the young.[65] Unintentional injuries remain the leading cause of years of potential life lost, surpassing the rates for both cancer and cardiovascular disease.[66]

Concern grew about violence at the nation's postsecondary institutions in the 1980s, following several high-profile incidents of campus violence. Such concerns led Congress to pass legislation regarding campus security and crime reporting, including the Student Right to Know and Campus Security Act of 1990, which required universities to publish statistics about criminal victimization on campus.[67] In 1992, the Buckley Amendment ruled that records kept by campus police and security for law enforcement purposes were not confidential "education" records under federal law. The Foley Amendment in 1998 determined that the final results of school disciplinary cases involving a crime of violence or non-forcible sex offense are not protected from disclosure under federal student privacy laws.

Such laws destroyed the past perceptions of colleges and universities as "safe havens" and led to surveys that provided the first national estimates on campus crime statistics. One such survey in 1996, conducted on a diverse sample of postsecondary institutions, reported a total of about 10,000 violent crimes and almost 40,000 property crimes during the preceding three years. For 1994 alone, the crime composition was about 20 murders, 1,300 forcible sex offenses, 3,100 individual robberies, 5,100 cases of aggravated assault, 28,800 burglaries, and 9,000 motor vehicle thefts.[68] This converts to an overall violent crime rate on college campuses of 0.65 per 1,000 students, but these ratios are decreased by the large number of schools in the survey that are "for-profit, less-than-two-year" institutions, without campus housing, and having less than 10,000 students. In other surveys of college-age students, 53.7 percent of college women indicated they had experienced some form of sexual victimization since the age of 14, including 15.4 percent rape and 12.1 percent attempted rape.[69] A random sample of undergraduate students from 130 four-year colleges found that approximately 3.5 percent of students reported they had a working firearm at college.[70] As with injuries and suicide, the incidence of sexual assault and other violent crimes is increased by alcohol and other drug use.

Suicide involves violence directed against self. In the past four decades, suicide rates among younger age groups have increased dramatically.[71] In particular, the suicide rate has more than tripled in the 15-to-24-year-old age group. The suicide rate for this group was 4.5 per 100,000 in 1950, but had increased to nearly 14 percent by 1994.[72] The National College Health Risk Behavior Survey found that one in ten U.S. college students seriously considered suicide in the preceding 12 months.[73] Respondents reported to be more likely to have considered suicide tended to be under 25 years old, freshmen or sophomores, and non-white. Roughly twice as many people with suicidal ideations drank alcohol, used illegal drugs, and/or smoked cigarettes.

Nutrition and Physical Activity

Students gain total independence in many areas of their lives for the first time when they go away to college, and making healthy food choices may be the responsibility for which they are least prepared. While the college years present a distinct set of nutritional priorities, it is not uncommon for poor eating habits to develop that will last a lifetime. A recent study reported that the dietary patterns of college students are well short of the recommended number of servings for all four food categories, but that students perceive themselves as being healthy eaters.[74] This incongruity between perceptions and reality can be a significant barrier to future dietary improvements.

The incidence of eating disorders is estimated to have increased two to five times in the past 30 years, making it the third most common chronic illness in teenagers today.[75] Most typical in adolescent girls and young women, an estimated 3 percent of this population have an eating disorder, and at least twice that number may have clinically important variants.[76] Some 5 to 15 percent of these cases occur in boys and men.[76] The mortality rate associated with anorexia nervosa alone is more than 12 times as high as the mortality rate among young women in the general population.[76] Body image disorders can also manifest themselves through other risky behaviors such as obsessive exercise and/or weight training, steroid use, cosmetic surgery, and others.

Increased concern about problems of inadequate calories among college women has probably resulted in too little attention being paid to the other end of the spectrum of eating disorders—the overeaters. The National Health and Nutrition Examination Survey (NHANES III) reported that one-third of Americans are now overweight.[77] Such changes will undoubtedly have marked adverse effects on future health care expenditures, since obesity is strongly associated with cardiovascular disease, hypercholesterolemia, diabetes, and other chronic diseases.[78]

Adding to the problem, studies suggest that a substantial proportion of young adults on a college campus today are adopting sedentary lifestyles.[79] Surveys suggest that the fitness levels of young Americans may be declining, and that the most rapid reduction in physical activity levels is occurring between the ages of 18 and 24.[80] This is particularly concerning given the strong epidemiological evidence supporting a positive relationship between physical activity, physical health, and psychological health.[81-88]

Recreational programs focusing on behavioral maintenance strategies for physically active students should not overlook the different set of intervention strategies that is necessary to motivate more sedentary groups to begin exercising. While late adolescents and young adults often perceive themselves to be physically fit, high levels of muscle strength associated with an emphasis on weight-training activities to improve appearance may actually be accompanied by low levels of both muscle endurance and cardio-respiratory fitness.

Behavioral Change

Considering the epidemic of unhealthy lifestyles in college students today, it is no wonder the majority of the Healthy People Objectives addressed individual behaviors. Modifiable health-related behaviors contribute significantly to many chronic diseases, and individual decision-making determines which behaviors will be adopted. Consequently, many researchers in college health are beginning to focus on models of health behavior intervention.

A number of such models have been developed to explain health-related behavior from an individualistic perspective. The Health Belief Model, Theory of Reasoned Action, Social Learning Theory, Social Norms Theory, Transtheoretical or Stages of Change Model, Relapse Prevention Model, and Decision-Making Theory all offer unique approaches to changing health behaviors.[89, 90] The decision of which model to apply in a given intervention depends largely on the nature of the problem, the focus of the intervention, and the attributes of the population.

Social Norms Theory

The *Social Norms Theory* describes situations in which individuals incorrectly perceive the attitudes and/or behaviors of peers and other community members to be different from their own; these misperceptions about peer attitudes or lifestyles may inappropriately guide their behaviors in the wrong, less healthful direction.[90] While this pattern has been demonstrated to influence eating, sexual health, and sexual assault behaviors, most social norms research has targeted high-risk drinking.[91, 92, 93] The Social Norms Model can also be applied to an individual's peers in an effort to change the "bystander attitudes" that promote tolerance for unhealthy behaviors.

Interventions that are successful in promoting one type of health outcome may not be effective in addressing other types, and interventions that succeed on one campus may not work on another. Each campus has unique cultural and historical issues that affect the campus social norms, and these must be taken into consideration during the early research analysis and planning stages. In addition, a social norms campaign is not always adequate by itself to address certain complex problem behaviors, and may require other skill-building steps or interventions as part of the campaign.

Social Marketing

Social marketing holds considerable promise in college health for addressing a variety of public health issues. This approach to behavior change involves the application of basic marketing principles to the design and implementation of programs and information campaigns that reinforce selective behaviors in a target population. While it often involves an advertising campaign to advance a social cause or a change in the social environment, it is the consumer-oriented component that defines it. The success of mass-media prevention campaigns is again dependent on conducting extensive preliminary research on the problem behavior of concern and the target audience.

Stages of Change Model

The *Stages of Change Model* has been used extensively in health behavior research because it offers a unique approach to behavior change that is not static. In smoking cessation, for example, this model identifies a pre-contemplation stage, a contemplation stage, a preparation stage, an action stage, and a maintenance stage. Individuals move from one stage to another based on their assessment of the pros and cons of a particular action, termed "decision balance."[89] The relative strengths of these pros and cons differ for various behaviors and at different stages.

Putting Prevention into Practice at College Health Centers

It is widely assumed that college health providers, compared to community providers caring for older populations, spend less time on illness-related complaints and more time on clinical prevention. Even if there were data available to support this assumption (which there are not), it does not justify the lower productivity rates by providers at many student health centers. Community providers can spend considerable time providing secondary and tertiary prevention during a routine office visit. Some would argue that college health providers even have more time available to address prevention, because they are dealing with relatively minor problems in a healthy college-age population.

The difference is that most private medical resources emphasize the physical components of health and the treatment of existing symptomatic disease, with less emphasis on primary preventive approaches such as screening and counseling for high-risk behaviors. (Figure 3) This is not surprising, since the time providers spend addressing these behavior-related issues is usually not covered by third party payers under the current health care financing system and, therefore, is not reimbursable.

The comprehensive college health model in which basic primary medical services and community-based health promotion are linked and funded through a prepaid, universal health fee provides an ideal opportunity to successfully intervene in the natural history of many chronic and disabling diseases. However, college health providers must adapt to this era of rapidly rising medical costs and decreases in public funding by using the limited time available during routine office visits to efficiently and systematically provide preventive services. Hopefully, more health center administrators will review their time-honored practices and begin shifting their limited resources toward evidence-based interventions that have measurable outcomes.

Periodic Physical Examinations

Prematriculation health histories, physical examinations, and even laboratory studies are

Figure 3

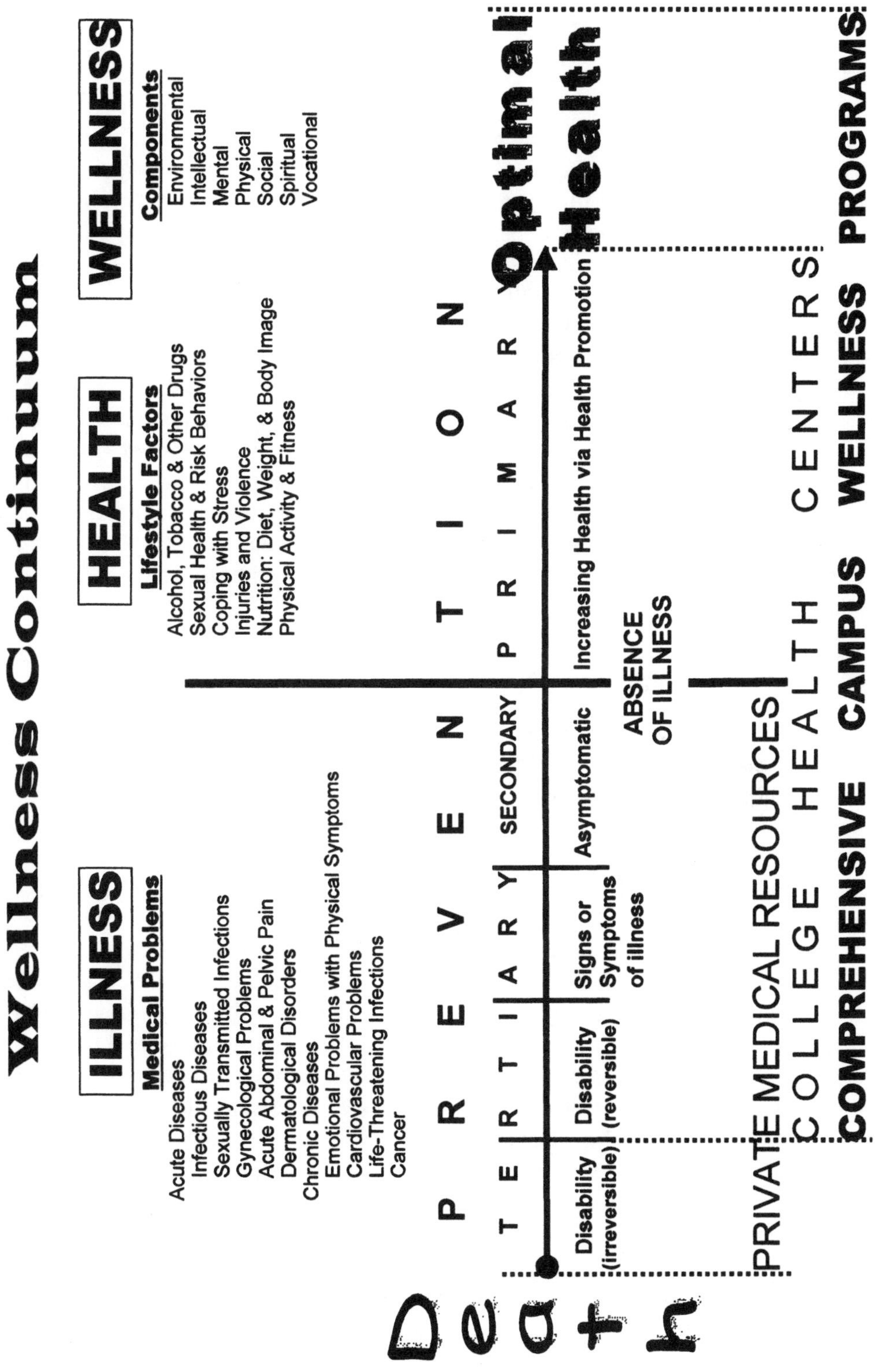

Wellness Continuum

ILLNESS

Medical Problems

Acute Diseases
Infectious Diseases
Sexually Transmitted Infections
Gynecological Problems
Acute Abdominal & Pelvic Pain
Dermatological Disorders
Chronic Diseases
Emotional Problems with Physical Symptoms
Cardiovascular Problems
Life-Threatening Infections
Cancer

HEALTH

Lifestyle Factors

Alcohol, Tobacco & Other Drugs
Sexual Health & Risk Behaviors
Coping with Stress
Injuries and Violence
Nutrition: Diet, Weight, & Body Image
Physical Activity & Fitness

WELLNESS

Components

Environmental
Intellectual
Mental
Physical
Social
Spiritual
Vocational

P R E V E N T I O N

TERTIARY | SECONDARY | PRIMARY

Disability (irreversible) | Disability (reversible) | Signs or Symptoms of illness | Asymptomatic | Increasing Health via Health Promotion

ABSENCE OF ILLNESS

Optimal Health

Death

PRIVATE MEDICAL RESOURCES
COLLEGE HEALTH CENTERS
COMPREHENSIVE CAMPUS WELLNESS PROGRAMS

still required by many universities. Except for pre-participation examinations for inter-collegiate athletes required by the National Collegiate Athletic Association (NCAA), other colleges and universities are eliminating these health requirements for a number of reasons. The costs of complete physical examinations and other prematriculation health requirements, either to the student or to the university through support of student health centers, adds another layer of expense for college students. In addition, prematriculation requirements involve costs to the university, such as administrative overhead expenses associated with placing and removing registration holds to enforce compliance. These records also represent potential risk-management problems for campus health authorities.

A number of other college health centers are starting to limit or restrict comprehensive physical examinations. Based on age and health risk, periodic physicals have not been found to be effective in a non-pregnant, college-age population by a number of expert panels, including the Canadian Task Force on Periodic Health Examination, the U.S. Preventive Services Task Force, and the American College of Physicians. The American Academy of Pediatrics and the American Medical Association (AMA) Guidelines for Adolescent Preventive Services (GAPS) both suggest annual preventive visits for adolescents, and the latter recommends a comprehensive physical examination be completed during visits in the early, middle, and late adolescent periods. No groups have found routine physicals to be a cost-effective method of disease prevention in young adults.

Brief Office Interventions

While college health providers have always found it a challenge to persuade students to have periodic health examinations or preventive visits, there are recommendations by the various panels for preventive services that have been found to be effective in decreasing morbidity or mortality in a college-age population. Many college health professionals find these recommendations to be woefully incomplete, but they do represent a starting point for the provision of preventive services for college students during a routine office visit.

Several national groups have addressed the effectiveness of counseling for behavior change in primary care, including The U.S. Preventive Services Task Force.[94] Primary care providers actually have a unique opportunity that other health professionals do not to screen for risky lifestyle behaviors during visits for minor illnesses. It is important to stress the brevity of the intervention, since detailed discussions of diets, smoking cessation, safer sex, etc., can more cost-effectively be referred to nutritionists, health educators, counselors, and other interventionists. In order to close the loop between interventions and assessment, however, providers need to be sure to document their preventive care efforts in the medical record.

There is evidence from a number of studies that visit-planning tools and teamwork improve the rate of behavior-change counseling by primary care providers.[95] A preventive care profile is one such tool that consolidates the patient's preventive care history and makes it easier to determine when tests or counseling are needed. (Figure 4) With standing orders, support staff can initiate many routine screenings and immunizations without having to consult a medical provider. The average student visits the student health center between two to three times per year, so there should be ample opportunity through coordinated efforts to address many high-risk behaviors.

One major drawback in combining preventive care services into an office visit for acute medical problems is that it reaches only students utilizing the health center. On the average campus, this varies somewhere between 50 and 80 percent of students per year. The other students could be reminded via telephone calls, mailings, or e-mail messages to come in for preventive care, reached through outreach events, such as health risk appraisal tools administered at health fairs or other group interventions, or to obtain the services from their private community providers.

The real controversy exists around deciding what components to include in a health-screening visit for college students. National authorities vary widely on their recommended frequency and appropriateness of various screening techniques based on scientific proof of effectiveness. The challenge often comes from university professionals who are narrowly focused on a particular discipline or risk factor, or from campus health policies that have been institutionalized over decades with scant attention to assessing outcomes.

The U.S. Preventive Services Task Force recommendations are not a complete list of all preventive services that should be offered during a periodic office visit, but rather an evidence-based approach to identifying those services that have been demonstrated to be effective. Many of the activities that college health professionals take for granted, such as counseling on nutrition and physical activity, have not been demonstrated to be effective. This is not to say they are not effective, but only that research has not yet proven them to be. The empirical evidence supporting the causal link between some health behaviors and outcomes has been tenuous because it is not experimental and nearly impossible to establish. With these caveats in mind, college health providers must make individual decisions based on their own campus risk assessments and values.

SUMMARY

With one exception, the 22 areas covered by the Healthy People 2000 objectives all include components pertaining to individual behavior.[13] Many college health care delivery systems have taken the lead in addressing these modifiable health-related behaviors, but are running short on resources. At the beginning of a new millennium, it is appropriate to reassess our priorities and to scrutinize the effectiveness of traditional campus prevention activities and their relationship to improving health outcomes. When many states mandate various immunizations throughout the K–12 school years, does it continue to be cost-effective in domestic students to track them into their college years? Even if tuberculosis screening requirements are restricted to international students from selected high-risk areas of the world, how much disease is prevented if a high proportion of the students with positive tests refuse chemoprophylaxis? Are mandatory health history forms and physical examinations the most effective method of detecting asymptomatic disease in a college-age group? Perhaps some of these resources should be redirected toward community-based behavioral change models and the creation of healthier campus environments.

Figure 4

College Health Preventive Care Profile

(Review at each visit and document preventive care given)

NAME: _____   SSN: _____

BIRTHDATE: _____   E-MAIL: _____

SCREENING	RECOMMENDATIONS	DATES OF PREVENTIVE CARE					
Blood Pressure	yearly						
Height/Weight	every 1-2 years (or BMI)						
Pap test	yearly in females						
Chlamydia screen	yearly in sexually active females						
Rubella serology/vaccination hx.	females >12 years						
PPD Skin Test	pos. exposure, from endemic area, or immunocompromised						
Breast Examination	females yearly > age 40						
Mammography, Baseline	females age 40						
Mammography Screening	females every 1-2 years ages 40-49; yearly ages 50-60						
Total Cholesterol	every 5 years > age 20						
Gonorrhea Screen (females)	high-risk sex/another STD						
HIV Screen	high-risk sex or IV drugs						
RPR/VDRL	high-risk sex or IV drugs						

IMMUNIZATIONS

Tetanus Diphtheria (Td)	age 11-16, then every 10 years						
Hepatitis A	at risk*						
Hepatitis B (titer in 1-2 mos.)	<age 25 or medical professions						
Hepatitis C	IV drugs						
Influenza	yearly, especially if at risk						
MMR	2 doses at least 1 mo. apart						
Varicella	susceptible persons >13 yrs**						

COUNSELING

Meningococcal Vaccine	freshmen in residence halls						
Problem Drinking	Attempt to address						
Illicit Drug Use	3-4 behavioral factors						
Alcohol/Drug Use & Driving	at each visit, and record						
Tobacco Use	the date discussed.						
Sexual Behavior	High-risk behaviors						
Abstinence/# partners	should be recorded						
Use of condoms	in the problem list						
Effective contraception	so they can be						
Limit Intake of Dietary Fat	followed up at future						
Calcium Intake (females)	office visits.						
Regular Physical Activity							
Lap and Shoulder Belts	Screening tools are						
Use of Helmets	available for alcohol						
Affective Disorders/Suicide	abuse, depression/						
Eating Disorders	suicide, and eating						
Sunscreens/Avoid Sun & UV	disorders.						

*at risk = men who have sex with men, travel to endemic countries, lab workers, etc.

**susceptible = negative history or titer

Cigarette smoking has been identified as the most significant cause of preventable morbidity and premature death,[96] but alcohol abuse is reported by college presidents to be the number one problem on college campuses today. This apparent incongruity occurs because the adverse health effects from tobacco may take years to occur, and are not associated with the disruptive behavior and adverse publicity that accompanies alcohol abuse on campus. By concentrating only on health outcomes that enhance retention and graduation, institutions of higher education are missing a golden opportunity to practice what they teach, to protect the state's investment in education, and to benefit the health of future generations. As new research continues to identify the increasing complexity and interactions of behavioral factors responsible for chronic disease, who better to develop effective intervention models than centers of higher education? Society continues to challenge our institutional leaders to become more involved in improving the health of our youth by assuring that programs exist on campus to keep students healthy at all levels—both during their academic years and beyond.

REFERENCES

1. Patrick K: The History and Current Status of College Health. In *Principles and Practices of Student Health,* Oakland, CA: Third Party Publishing Company, 1992.

2. Tyler CW, Last, JM: Epidemiology. In *Public Health & Preventive Medicine.* Stamford, CT: Appleton & Lange, 1998.

3. Green, LW: Prevention and Health Education in Clinical, School, and Community Settings. In *Public Health & Preventive Medicine.* Stamford, CT: Appleton & Lange, 1998.

4. Kolbe LJ, Green LW, Foreyt J, et al.: Appropriate Functions of Health Education in Schools. In *Child Health Behavior.* New York: John Wiley & Sons, 1985.

5. Rhyne R, Bogue R, Kukulka G, et al.: *Community-Oriented Primary Care: Health Care for the 21st Century.* Washington, DC: American Public Health Association, 1998.

6. Nutting PA, Connor EM: Institute of Medicine. *Community-Oriented Primary Care: A Practical Assessment.* Washington, DC: National Academy Press, 1984.

7. Harvard University and The Centers for Disease Control and Prevention: Higher Education and the Health of Youth: Charting a National Course in a Changing Environment. Harvard Project on Schooling and Children, Cambridge, MA, 1995.

8. Centers for Disease Control: Comprehensive Plan for Epidemiologic Surveillance. Atlanta Centers for Disease Control, 1986.

9. American Medical Association: *AMA Guidelines for Adolescent Preventive Services (GAPS): Recommendations and Rationale.* Chicago, IL: American Medical Association, 1994.

10. Canadian Task Force on the Periodic Health Examination: The Periodic Health Examination. *Can Med Assoc J,* 121:1194–1254, 1979.

11. U.S. Preventive Services Task Force: *Guide to Clinical Preventive Services: An Assessment of the Effectiveness of 169 Interventions.* Baltimore: Williams & Wilkins, 1989.

12. American College of Physicians. Guidelines. In Eddy DM, ed. *Common Screening Tests.* Philadelphia, PA: American College of Physicians, 1991.

13. U.S. Department of Health and Human Services, Public Health Service. *Healthy People 2000: National Health Promotion and Disease Prevention Objectives.* Washington, DC: PHS 91–50213, 1991.

14. American Medical Association, Department of Adolescent Health: *Healthy Youth 2000, National Health Promotion, Disease Prevention Objectives for Adolescents (10–24 years).* Chicago, IL: American Medical Association, 1990.

15. American College Health Association, Task Force on National Health Objectives in Higher Education. *Healthy Campus 2000: Making It Happen.* Baltimore, MD: American College Health Association, 1992.

16. Gerstman BB: *Epidemiology Kept Simple: An Introduction to Classic and Modern Epidemiology.* New York: John Wiley & Sons, 1998.

17. Wallace RB: Screening for Early and Asymptomatic Conditions. In *Public Health & Preventive Medicine.* Stamford, CT: Appleton & Lange, 1998.

18. Hennessey KA, Schulte JM, Cook L, et al.: Tuberculin Skin Test Screening Practices Among US Colleges and Universities. *JAMA* 280:2008–2012, 1998.

19. Nelson ME, Fingar AR. Tuberculosis Screening and Prevention for Foreign-born Students: Eight Years Experience at Ohio University. *Am J Prev Med* 11:48–54, 1995.

20. Susmano S: Testing International Students for Tuberculosis. *J Am Coll Health* 39:287–290, 1990.

21. Quillan S, Malotte K, Shlian D: Evaluation of a Tuberculosis Screening and Prophylaxis Program for International Students. *J Am Coll Health* 38:165–170, 1990.

22. Dixon, WC, Collins M: Screening and Chemoprophylaxis for Tuberculosis Infection in College Populations. *J Am Coll Health* 46:171–175, 1998.

23. Keim J, Woodard MP, Anderson MK: Screening for *Chlamydia trachomatis* in College Women on Routine Gynecological Exams. *J Am Coll Health* 41:17–23, 1992.

24. Phillips RS, Aronson MD, Taylor WC, et al.: Should Tests for *Chlamydia trachomatis* Cervical Infection Be Done During Routine Gynecologic Visits? An Analysis of the Costs of Alternative Strategies. *Ann Intern Med* 107:188–194, 1987.

25. Burstein GR, Gaydos CA, Diener-West M, et al.: Incident *Chlamydia trachomatis* Infections Among Inner-city Adolescent Females. *JAMA* 280:521–526, 1998.

26. Centers for Disease Control. 1998 Guidelines for Treatment of Sexually Transmitted Diseases. *MMWR* 47:1–116, 1998.

27. Howell MR, Quinn TC, Gaydos CA: Screening for *Chlamydia trachomatis* in Asymptomatic Women Attending Family Planning Clinics: A Cost-Effectiveness Analysis of Three Strategies. *Ann Intern Med.* 128:277–284, 1998.

28. Centers for Disease Control. HIV Prevention Through Early Detection and Treatment of Other Sexually Transmitted Diseases—United States. *MMWR.* 47/No.RR-12, July 31, 1998.

29. Manos MM, Kinney WK, Hurley LB, et al.: Identifying Women with Cervical Neoplasia. *JAMA,* 281:1605–1610, 1999.

30. Antman K, Shea S: Screening Mammography Under Age 50. *JAMA,* 281:1470–1472, 1999.

31. National Cholesterol Education Program: Second Report of the National Cholesterol Education Program Expert Panel on Detection, Evaluation, and Treatment of High Blood Cholesterol in Adults (Adult Treatment Panel II). *Circulation* 89:1329–1445, 1994.

32. American College of Physicians: Guidelines for Using Serum Cholesterol, High-Density Lipoprotein Cholesterol, and Triglyceride Levels as Screening Tests for Preventing Coronary Heart Disease in Adults. *Ann Intern Med* 124:515–517, 1996.

33. Cleeman JI, and Grundy SM: National Cholesterol Education Program Recommendations for Cholesterol Testing in Young Adults. *Circulation* 95:1646–1650, 1997.

34. Task Force on Risk Reduction, American Heart Association: Cholesterol Screening in Asymptomatic Adults: No Cause to Change. *Circulation* 93:1067–1068, 1996.

35. American Medical Association: Rationale and Recommendation: Hypertension. In *AMA Guidelines for Adolescent Preventive Services (GAPS): Recommendations and Rationale.* Chicago, IL: American Medical Association; 1994: chap 8.

36. Joint National Committee on Prevention, Detection, Evaluation, and Treatment of High Blood Pressure: The Sixth Report of the Joint National Committee on Prevention, Detection, Evaluation, and Treatment of High Blood Pressure. *Arch Intern Med* 157:2413–2446, 1997.

37. U.S. Preventive Services Task Force: Screening for hypertension. In *Guide to Clinical Preventive Services.* 2nd ed. Washington, DC: US Department of Health and Human Services; 1996; chap 3.

38. Cook LG, Collins M, Williams WW, et al.: Prematriculation Immunization Requirements of American Colleges and Universities. *J Am Coll Health* 42:91–98, 1993.

39. American College Health Association. Vaccine-Preventable Diseases Task Force: Recommendations for Institutional Prematriculation Immunizations. Baltimore, MD: American College Health Association; January 2000.

40. Wechsler H, Lee JE, Kuo M, et al.: College Binge Drinking in the 1990s: A Continuing Problem. *J Am Coll Health* 48:199–210, 2000.

41. Hanson DJ, Engs RC: College Students' Drinking Problems: A National Study, 1982–1991. *Psychol Rep* 71:39–42, 1992.

42. Johnston LD, O'Malley PM, Bachman JG: *National Survey Results on Drug Use from the Monitoring the Future Study, 1975–1992. Vol. II: College Students and Young Adults,* Rockville, MD: National Institute on Drug Abuse, NIH Pub. No. 93–3598, 1993.

43. Prendergast ML: Substance Use and Abuse Among College Students: A Review of Recent Literature. *J Am Coll Health* 43:99–111, 1994.

44. The Higher Education Center for Alcohol and Other Drug Prevention. College Academic Performance and Alcohol and Other Drug Use. Newton, MA: Infofacts Resources, 1997.

45. The Higher Education Center for Alcohol and Other Drug Prevention: Sexual Assault and Alcohol and Other Drug Use. Newton, MA: Infofacts Resources, 1997.

46. Wechsler H, Isaac N: "Binge" Drinkers at Massachusetts Colleges: Prevalence, Drinking Styles, Time Trends, and Associated Problems. *JAMA* 267:2929–2931, 1992.

47. Wechsler H, Davenport A, Dowdall G, et al.: Health and Behavioral Consequences of Binge Drinking in College: A National Survey of Students at 140 Campuses. *JAMA* 272:1672–1677, 1994.

48. New York State Office of Alcoholism and Substance Abuse Services (OASAS): Alcohol and Other Drug Use Among College Students in New York State: Findings from a Statewide College Survey, 1996. www.oasas.state.ny.us/pio/col-exec.htm

49. Presley CA, et al.: *Alcohol and Drugs on American College Campuses: Use, Consequences, and Perceptions of the Campus Environment. Volume IV: 1992–94,* Carbondale: The Core Institute, Southern Illinois University-Carbondale, 1996.

50. Centers for Disease Control. Tobacco Use among High School students—United States, 1997. *MMWR* 47:229–233, 1998.

51. Wechsler H, Rigotti NA, Gledhill-Hoyt J, et al.: Increased Levels of Cigarette Use Among College Students: A Cause for National Concern. *JAMA* 280:1673–1678, 1998.

52. Moskal PD, Dziuban CD, West GB: Examining the Use of Tobacco on College Campuses. *J Am Coll Health* 47:260–265, 1999.

53. Reinisch JM, Hill CA, Sanders S, et al.: High-Risk Sexual Behavior at a Midwestern University: A Confirmatory Study. *Fam Plann Perspect* 27:79–82, 1995.

54. DeBuono BA, Zinner SH, Daamen M, et al.: Sexual Behavior of College Women in 1975, 1986, and 1989. *N Engl J Med,* 322:821–825, 1990.

55. Hale RW, Char DF, Nagy K, et al.: Seventeen-Year Review of Sexual and Contraceptive Behavior on a College Campus. *Am J Obstet Gynecol* 168:1833–1837, 1993.

56. Bauer HM, Ting Y, Greer CE, et al.: Genital Human Papillomavirus Infection in Female University Students as Determined by a PCR-based Method. *JAMA* 265:472–477, 1991.

57. Ho GYF, Bierman R, Beardsley L, et al.: Natural History of Cervicovaginal Papillomavirus Infection in Young Women. *N Eng J Med* 338:423–428, 1998.

58. Fleming DT, McQuillan GM, Johnson RE, et al.: Herpes Simplex Virus Type 2 in the United States, 1976–1994. *N Eng J Med* 337:1105–1111, 1997.

59. Gaydos CA, Howell MR, Pare, B, et al.: *Chlamydia Trachomatis* Infections in Female Military Recruits. *N Eng J Med,* 339:739–744, 1998.

60. Gayle HD, Keeling RP, Garcia-Tunon M, et al.: Prevalence of the Human Immunodeficiency Virus among University Students. *N Eng J Med* 323:1538–1541, 1990.

61. Centers for Disease Control. HIV Prevention through Early Detection and Treatment of Other Sexually Transmitted Diseases—United States. *MMWR, Recommendations and Reports,* 47/No.RR-12:1–24, 1998.

62. Koonin LM, Smith JC, Ramick M, et al.: Abortion Surveillance—United States, 1989. *MMWR CDC Surveill Summ* 41:1–33, 1992.

63. Kusseling FS, Wenger NS, Shapiro MF: Inconsistent Contraceptive Use Among Female College Students: Implications for Intervention. *J Am Coll Health* 43:191–195, 1995.

64. Centers for Disease Control. Update: Youth Risk Behavior Surveillance—United States, 1993. *MMWR,* 44:1–58, 1995.

65. The National Committee for Injury Prevention and Control: Injury Prevention: Meeting the Challenge, *Am J of Prev Med* 5(3) suppl, 1989.

66. Centers for Disease Control. Years of Potential Life Lost before Age 65—United States, 1990 and 1991. *MMWR,* 42:251–253, 1993.

67. Hoffmann, AM, Schuh, JH, Fenske, RH: *Violence on Campus: Defining the Problems, Strategies for Action.* Gaithersburg, MD: Aspen, 1998.

68. United States Department of Education, National Center for Education Statistics. Statistical Analysis Report: Campus Crime and Security at Postsecondary Education Institutions, January 1997.

69. Koss P, Gidycz A, Wisniewski N: The Scope of Rape: Incidence and Prevalence of Sexual Aggression and Victimization in a National Sample of Higher Education Students. *J Consult Clin Psychol* 55:162–170, 1987.

70. Miller M, Hemenway D, Wechsler H: Guns at College. *J Am Coll Health* 48:7–12, 1999.

71. Rosenberg ML, Smith JC, Davidson LE, et. al.: The Emergence of Youth Suicide: An Epidemiologic Analysis and Public Health Perspective. *Ann Rev Public Health* 8:417–440, 1987.

72. Singh GK, Kochanek KD, MacDorman MF: Advance Report of Final Mortality Statistics, 1994. *Mon Vital Stat Rep* 45(3), 1996.

73. Centers for Disease Control. Youth Risk Behavior Surveillance: National College Health Risk Behavior Survey—United States, 1995. *MMWR* 46(SS-6):1–54, 1997.

74. Stonecipher L, et al.: Students Think They Eat Well, but They Don't. *J of Am Coll of Nutri 1999.*

75. Levine RL: Eating Disorders in Adolescents: A Comprehensive Update. *Int Pediatr.* 10(4):327–335, 1995.

76. Becker AE, Grinspoon SK, Klibanski A, et al.: Eating Disorders. *N Eng J Med* 340:1092–1098, 1999.

77. Andersen RE, Wadden TA, Bartlett SJ, et al.: Effects of Lifestyle Activity vs. Structured Aerobic Exercise in Obese Women. *JAMA* 281:335–340, 1999.

78. Mokdad AH, Serdula MK, Dietz WH, et al.: The Spread of the Obesity Epidemic in the United States, 1991–1998. *JAMA* 282:1519–1522, 1999.

79. Pinto BM, Marcus BH: A Stages of Change Approach to Understanding College Students' Physical Activity. *J Am Coll Health* 44:27–31, 1995.

80. Stephens T, Jacobs DR, White CC: A Descriptive Epidemiology of Leisure-time Physical Activity. *Public Health Rep* 100:147–158, 1985.

81. Smith JK, Dykes R, Douglas JE, et al.: Long-Term Exercise and Atherogenic Activity of Blood Mononuclear Cells in Persons at Risk of Developing Ischemic Heart Disease. *JAMA* 281:1722–1727, 1999.

82. Wei M, Kampert JB, Barlow CE, et al.: Relationship between Low Cardiorespiratory Fitness and Mortality in Normal-Weight, Overweight, and Obese Men. *JAMA* 282:1547–1553, 1999.

83. Kujala UM, Kaprio J, Sarna S, et al.: Relationship of Leisure-Time Physical Activity and Mortality. *JAMA* 279:440–444, 1998.

84. U.S. Department of Health and Human Resources. Physical Activity and Health: A Report of the Surgeon General. *MMWR* 45:591–592, 1996.

85. Pinto BM, Marcus BH: Physical Activity, Exercise, and Cancer in Women. *Med Exerc Nutr Health* 3:102–111, 1994.

86. LaFontaine TP, DiLorenzo TM, Frensch PA, et al: Aerobic Exercise andMood: A Brief Review. *Sports Med* 13:160–170, 1992.

87. Plante TG, Rodin J: Physical Fitness and Enhanced Psychological Health. *Curr Psychol: Res Rev* 9:3–24, 1990.

88. Raglin JS: Exercise and Mental Health: Beneficial and Detrimental Effects. *Sports Med* 9:323–329, 1990.

89. Ferguson KJ: Health Behavior. In *Public Health & Preventive Medicine.* Stamford, CT: Appleton & Lange, 1998.

90. Berkowitz AD: Applications of Social Norms Theory to Other Health and Social Justice Issues. In *The Social Norms Approach to Prevention,* H. Wesley Perkins, ed. In publication. Available from the author at alan@fltg.net.

91. Perkins HW, Meilman PW, Leichliter JS, et al.: Misperceptions of the Norms for the Frequency of Alcohol and Other Drug Use on College Campuses. *J Am Coll Health* 47:253–258, 1999.

92. Haines M, Spear SF: Changing the Perception of the Norm: A Strategy to Decrease Binge Drinking Among College Students. *J Am Coll Health* 45:134–140, 1996

93. Perkins HW, Berkowitz AD: Perceiving the Community Norms of Alcohol Use among Students:

Some Research Implications for Campus Alcohol Education Programming. *Int J Addictions* 21:961<n>976, 1986.

94. U.S. Preventive Services Task Force. *Guide to Clinical Preventive Services,* 2nd ed. Washington D.C.: U.S. Department of Health Human Services, 1996.

95. Dickey LL, Gemson DH, Carney P: Office System Interventions Supporting Primary Care-Based Health Behavior Change Counseling. *Am J Prev Med* 17:299<n>308, 1999.

96. McGinnis JM, Foege WH: Actual Causes of Death in the United States. *JAMA* 270:2207<n>2212, 1993.

CHAPTER 20

NON-STUDENT MEDICAL PROGRAMS IN STUDENT HEALTH SERVICES

H. Spencer Turner, MD, MS, FACPM, and Janet L. Hurley, PhD

From their beginnings, student health services directly or indirectly offered services for faculty and staff, thereby extending their parameters beyond student care. This extension was usually related to public health activities, which were often the impetus for the development of college health services in the first place. Obviously, when an epidemic required treatment and isolation of students, the effects of this treatment and isolation extended beyond the student body, and, in fact, helped protect faculty and staff. While this institutional public health role for student health services was traditionally unrecognized (or at least not acknowledged) by institutions of higher education, it definitely impacted all who attended or worked at the institution. There are numerous examples of such early programs; notable are typhoid outbreaks at Cornell University in 1903 and the University of Wisconsin in 1907.[1] In addition, the extensive tuberculosis control programs carried out by college health services to protect students, offered (and continue to offer) protection for faculty and staff as well.

It is also clear through anecdotal evidence that many of the health promotion programs sponsored by college health services in the early part of the century were utilized by faculty and staff, including screening programs for hypertension, diabetes, and others. Also, it is known that student health services professionals were (and are) frequently asked to provide emergency care. Nonetheless, despite considerable activity during the last half of the 19th century and the early part of the 20th century, there was little formal documentation or acknowledgment of the inclusion of faculty, staff, or students' families into medical care programs by student health services.

One of the pioneers in college health who first formally extended care to faculty and staff was Dr. Dana L. Farnsworth, director at Harvard from 1954 until 1971. Farnsworth was an early advocate of the importance of college health services and believed one of the goals of a program was to provide care at the highest possible professional level. To encourage this goal, while at the Massachusetts Institute of Technology, shortly after

World War II, he developed a program that integrated student health care with services provided to faculty and employees.[2] By developing such a program, Farnsworth was able to attract physicians who might wish a broader range of patients, and, by developing a larger patient base, make feasible a wider range of specialty services. In 1954, on the assumption of the directorship at Harvard, Farnsworth further advanced these ideas by expanding services to faculty, employee, and retirees, and "integrating the program with a specially designed indemnity insurance plan that covered services not provided on site."[3]

Later in the century, in 1975, Dr. Warren Wacker, also of Harvard, went one step further by establishing a health maintenance organization that provided care for dependents of faculty, retirees, and their dependents. Wacker observed that it is "somewhat surprising to me that the idea of broadening the population base of college and university health services has not been more extensive. At present, only MIT, Yale and the University of Massachusetts at Amherst have similar programs."[3*]

Despite the public health activities of the early part of the century, and the documentation of excellent clinical programs in two or three health services in the 1970s, there were few programs which, in any formal, recognized way, performed employee health services in the traditional sense. Thus, in 1981, Turner could still observe that "our survival during the next two decades will reflect how well we have responded to the challenge of . . . environmental health and safety on our respective campuses, [and it will be necessary to make] clear to our administration that these activities affect the entire campus—student, staff and visitors . . ."[4]

Fortunately, by the mid-eighties, there had been some progress to a more formal involvement of college health services with their respective campuses, particularly in the area of occupational and environmental health care services. Patrick reported that " . . . the one with the greatest continued overlap . . . is that of outpatient medical care for university employees. Services here may range from the immediate care of individuals injured on the job to full scale occupational health units dealing with pre-employment worker assessment, work site monitoring, injury care, and rehabilitation."[5]

Even more recently, since the advent in the 1990s of the Occupational Safety and Health Administration's bloodborne pathogen legislation, many college health services, particularly those at academic medical centers, have assumed responsibilities in bloodborne pathogen control programs for the entire campus. A good example of this activity is the program at the University of Kentucky Chandler Medical Center.[6]

CURRENT STATUS

With the variable nature, size, and assigned responsibilities of college health services, it is exceedingly difficult to document with any precision those activities currently performed by health services which extend beyond student care. Such services include "in-

---

* For those who are interested in further discussion of certain aspects of the early development of the inclusion of employees for regular medical care in the college health service, the reader is directed to College Health Administration, D. L. Farnsworth, Editor, New York, Appleton-Century-Crofts, 1964.

direct" programs in areas of public health, such as mentioned previously, or direct medical care programs, including routine clinical care or occupational health. The complex nature of college health services today allows for marked variability in programs offered for employees, students' spouses, or, for that matter, students' or employees' families.

It would probably take an approach similar to the historic Moore-Summerskill Report (previously mentioned, in the first chapter of this text) to ascertain the level of these "non-student" activities with certainty. Nonetheless, it is clear from anecdotal information that, indeed, college health services are often assigned, or assume, responsibilities well beyond those directly related to student care. In fact, the "Guidelines for a College Health Program" published by the American College Health Association, includes a specific section covering issues related to environmental health and safety and to occupational health services.[7]

Because of the scarcity of information in the literature on activities of student health services that offer medical care to other than students, the decision was made by the authors of this chapter to gather data which have not previously been available. In the fall of 1999, a general question was distributed via the Student Health Services electronic mailing list that reaches college health professionals in over 500 institutions to determine the extent to which medical programs were offered in college and university health services to populations other than students. Although a large number of responses were received, the responses were so varied that it was difficult to glean any details about the type and extent of the programs. Thus, the decision was made to develop a survey questionnaire and post the survey via the Student Health Services list in April 2000 (Figure 1).

This survey was sent to list subscribers three separate times over a period of approximately seven to ten days. At the time of the second and third requests, an appeal was made specifically for institutions that did *not* perform non-student care in their health services to understand that it was also appropriate and important for them to respond to the survey.

At the time the survey was conducted, there were approximately 530 different colleges and universities participating in the Student Health Service list. Responses were received from 194 institutions, representing a 36.6% response rate. As a further reference point, the American College Health Association reports approximately 950 institutional members. Approximately 1,500 health services exist in four-year institutions.

The responses to the survey were divided into seven categories based on FTE enrollment size: institutions with student populations of 2,000 or less; 2,001–5,000; 5,001–10,000; 10,001–20,000; 20,001–30,000; and over 30,000. In addition, cumulative data for all respondents were calculated. The data for the overall view of activities are presented in Table 1. (Percentage of total respondents by institution size is indicated on Table 1, as well as in subsequent tables.)*

---

* An attempt was made to compare the percentages of respondents with the percentages overall of similar sized institutions throughout the United States. However, data available from the American Council of Education, as well as data on the institutions known to have college health services, were not available to make this comparison

Figure 1

1. What is the approximate full-time enrollment of your institution? _____

2. Does your health service provide clinical care of any type for non-students? (faculty, staff, or others)
Yes ____ Please continue questionnaire.
No ____ (No need to continue questionnaire. Thanks for your help.)

3. What type of clinical care do you provide? **Check all that apply. In the blank following the type of care, list what type of people qualify for this care (i.e., employees, dependents).**

	Student	Students' Spouses	Students' Children	Employees	Employee Dependents
a.___ Complete ambulatory medical care	___	___	___	___	
b.___ Acute care only	___	___	___	___	
c.___ Workers' Compensation	___	___	___	___	
d.___ Allergy shots	___	___	___	___	
e.___ Immunizations	___	___	___	___	
f. ___ TB screening	___	___	___	___	
g.___ Travel Clinic	___	___	___	___	
h.___ Mental Health counseling	___	___	___	___	
i. ___ Drug and alcohol counseling	___	___	___	___	
j. ___ Physical examinations	___	___	___	___	
k.___ Employee health. (If yes, be sure and answer questions in # 5 below.)					

4. Does your clinic treat patients not affiliated with the university?
____ Yes   ____ No

5. Does your clinic have contracts to provide medical care for groups of individuals who are not part of the university?
____ Yes   ____ No
If yes: ___ clinical care
        ___ occupational health only

6. Do you perform Employee Health functions of any sort?
____ Yes   ____ No
If yes: ___ pre-employment/pre-placement physical exams
       ___ evaluation of acute illness/injury
       ___ fit for duty/return to work evaluations
       ___ bloodborne pathogen exposure control programs
       ___ respirator fitting
Other specific clinical programs related to general campus immunization programs, health fairs, and such activities.
____ Yes   ____ No
If yes, please explain: _____
_____
_____

Table 1 — Overview							
Enrollment	2000 or less	2001- 5000	5001- 10,000	10,001- 20,000	20,001- 30,000	>30,000	All Respondents
Number in category % of all respondents	N=46 23/7%	N=30 15.5%	N=33 17.0%	N=51 26.3%	N=22 11.3%	N=12 6.2%	N=194 100%
SHS provides:							
clinical care for non-students	78.3%	80.0%	75.8%	78.4%	100.0%	83.3%	80.9%
clinical care for patients not affliated with the university	19.6%	13.3%	15.2%	43.1%	54.5%	33.3%	28.9%
contacts for groups	8.7%	3.3%	3.0%	17.6%	27.3%	33.3%	12.9%
employee health functions	63.0%	60.0%	54.5%	64.7%	72.7%	75.0%	63.4%
campus-wide programs	58.7%	63.3%	51.5%	60.8%	68.2%	58.3%	59.8%

To the question "Does your student health service provide clinical care for non-students," over 80% of all respondents answered affirmatively. That percentage was remarkably constant regardless of the size of the institution. Further, over one-fourth of the institutions provided patient care for individuals not affiliated with their college or university, and over 10% indicated contracts for medical care with groups outside their institution. And, of major significance, nearly two-thirds indicated that they performed employee health functions.

In addition, 60% indicated they conducted campus wide activities which can be categorized as health promotion and public health programs for faculty and staff. The list of these activities was remarkably consistent and recurring, regardless of the size of the institution. They included such programs as influenza immunization; screening for many diseases, including hypertension, diabetes, hypercholesterolemia, hyperlipidemia; health fairs of all varieties; weight screening and weight management programs; evaluation for modified work assignments; ergonomic assessments; mammography screening programs; CPR training; blood pressure clinics; alcohol and depression screening; "smoke-out days"; exercise program evaluations and body composition measurements; nutrition and eating disorder screening and classes; and many others. In short, it is clear that public health programs and health screening activities performed by college and university health services were truly limited only by the imagination of the health care providers and the specific needs of the university communities.

Of particular interest is the observation that the smallest institutions (< 2000), which might be presumed to have small health services and, therefore, small clinical staffs, still indicated program activities for non-student care on a level as extensive as in larger institutions, in nearly all areas about which inquiries were made.

Table 2 reflects responses to questions regarding "complete ambulatory care for non-students." Over one-fifth of respondents indicated they furnished such care; in the larger institutions (above 10,000) one-third offered this care for students' spouses. Overall, nearly 9% of all colleges and universities offered "complete ambulatory care" for students' children, while over 12% offered such care for employees and 4% for employees' children.

Table 2 — Complete Ambulatory Care							
Enrollment	2000 or less	2001-5000	5001-10,000	10,001-20,000	20,001-30,000	>30,000	All Respondents
Number in category % of all respondents	N=46 23.7%	N=30 15.5%	N=33 17.0%	N=51 26.3%	N=22 11.3%	N=12 6.2%	N=194 100%
Students' spouses	10.9%	3.3%	21.2%	31.4%	45.5%	33.3%	22.2%
Students' children	6.5%	3.3%	9.1%	9.8%	18.2%	8.3%	8.8%
Employees	15.2%	6.7%	18.2%	9.8%	9.1%	16.7%	12.4%
Employees' dependents	4.3%	3.3%	3.0%	2.0%	4.5%	16.7%	4.1%

Table 3 includes programs regarding the provision of acute care only. Approximately 9% of the institutions (but one-fourth of institutions over 20,000) offered this service to students' spouses and slightly over 6% offered the service to students' children. Approximately 35% offered acute care services to employees and nearly 5% offered the service to employees' children.

Table 3 — Acute Care Only							
Enrollment	2000 or less	2001-5000	5001-10,000	10,001-20,000	20,001-30,000	>30,000	All Respondents
Number in category % of all respondents	N=46 23.7%	N=30 15.5%	N=33 17.0%	N=51 26.3%	N=22 11.3%	N=12 6.2%	N=194 100%
Students' spouses	4.3%	3.3%	3.0%	9.8%	27.3%	25.0%	9.3%
Students' children	6.5%	3.3%	0%	9.8%	9.1%	8.3%	6.2%
Employees	15.2%	40.0%	24.2%	25.5%	36.4%	25.0%	35.6%
Employees' children	4.3%	6.7%	0%	3.9%	0%	16.7%	4.6%

One particularly interesting concern addressed was the delivery of workers' compensation care for campuses by student health services (Table 4). Such care was often provided; with 30% of the health services indicating they had a responsibility for workers' compensation clinical activities. Not surprisingly, very few (1 to 3 percent) indicated they perform such care for students' spouses, children, or employees' children.

Table 4 — Workers' Compensation							
Enrollment	2000 or less	2001-5000	5001-10,000	10,001-20,000	20,001-30,000	>30,000	All Respondents
Number in category % of all respondents	N=46 23.7%	N=30 15.5%	N=33 17.0%	N=51 26.3%	N=22 11.3%	N=12 6.2%	N=194 100%
Students' spouses	0%	0%	0%	5.9%	9.1%	8.3%	3.1%
Students' children	0%	0%	0%	2.0%	4.5%	8.3%	1.5%
Employees	23.9%	20.0%	27.3%	41.2%	18.2%	58.3%	29.2%
Employees' children	0%	3.3%	0%	2.0%	0%	8.3%	1.5%

Inquiries were made as to whether allergy shots, immunizations and tuberculin testing were available to non-students. Allergy shots were provided for family members by a small percentage of institutions, but one-third provided this service for employees (Table 5). Somewhat higher numbers were noted for the performance of immunizations (Table 6); one of ten for students' children or approximately one of four employees' children, but well over half for employees. The availability of tuberculin testing (Table 7) was similar to the availability of immunizations.

Table 5 — Allergy Shots							
Enrollment	2000 or less	2001-5000	5001-10,000	10,001-20,000	20,001-30,000	>30,000	All Respondents
Number in category % of all respondents	N=46 23.7%	N=30 15.5%	N=33 17.0%	N=51 26.3%	N=22 11.3%	N=12 6.2%	N=194 100%
Students' spouses	8.7%	6.7%	12.1%	2.0%	45.5%	25.0%	12.4%
Students' children	2.2%	0%	9.1%	9.8%	13.6%	0%	6.2%
Employees	28.3%	36.7%	18.2%	43.1%	31.8%	16.7%	31.4%
Employees' children	2.2%	10.0%	3.0%	3.9%	4.5%	8.3%	4.6%

Table 6 — Immunizations							
Enrollment	2000 or less	2001-5000	5001-10,000	10,001-20,000	20,001-30,000	>30,000	All Respondents
Number in category % of all respondents	N=46 23.7%	N=30 15.5%	N=33 17.0%	N=51 26.3%	N=22 11.3%	N=12 6.2%	N=194 100%
Students' spouses	17.4%	10.0%	18.2%	35.3%	50.0%	33.3%	25.8%
Students' children	13.0%	0%	9.1%	13.7%	22.7%	8.3%	11.3%
Employees	56.5%	60.0%	51.5%	64.7%	54.5%	41.7%	57.2%
Employees' children	10.9%	13.3%	6.1%	11.8%	9.1%	25.0%	11.3%

Table 7 — TB Screening							
Enrollment	**2000 or less**	**2001- 5000**	**5001- 10,000**	**10,001- 20,000**	**20,001- 30,000**	**>30,000**	**All Respondents**
Number in category % of all respondents	N=46 23.7%	N=30 15.5%	N=33 17.0%	N=51 26.3%	N=22 11.3%	N=12 6.2%	N=194 100%
Students' spouses	13.0%	10.0%	24.2%	33.3%	40.9%	25.0%	23.7%
Students' children	6.5%	0%	6.1%	11.8%	13.6%	8.3%	7.7%
Employees	50.0%	53.3%	36.4%	58.8%	31.8%	50.0%	48.5%
Employees' children	6.5%	13.3%	3.0%	3.9%	4.5%	8.3%	6.2%

Table 8 reports the availability of travel clinics for non-students. Nearly one in five offered this service for student spouses; about one in ten for students' and employees' children; and over one-third for employees. Of note was a general trend for the larger institutions to be more likely to offer travel clinics than the smaller institutions.

Table 8 — Travel Clinics							
Enrollment	**2000 or less**	**2001- 5000**	**5001- 10,000**	**10,001- 20,000**	**20,001- 30,000**	**>30,000**	**All Respondents**
Number in category % of all respondents	N=46 23.7%	N=30 15.5%	N=33 17.0%	N=51 26.3%	N=22 11.3%	N=12 6.2%	N=194 100%
Students' spouses	6.5%	6.7%	9.1%	29.4%	54.5%	25.0%	19.6%
Students' children	2.2%	3.3%	6.1%	7.8%	22.7%	16.7%	7.7%
Employees	23.9%	30.0%	18.2%	45.1%	63.6%	66.7%	36.6%
Employees' children	2.2%	13.3%	6.0%	13.7%	18.2%	25.0%	10.8%

Queries were also made as to whether or not mental health counseling was offered for non-students (Table 9). Overall, 11% of student spouses were afforded such care. Very few institutions offered this care for students' or employees' children. Employees, on the other hand, received such care in 12% of the cases. The smaller institutions seemed to offer this service as commonly as larger institutions.

Table 9 — Mental Health Counseling							
Enrollment	**2000 or less**	**2001- 5000**	**5001- 10,000**	**10,001- 20,000**	**20,001- 30,000**	**>30,000**	**All Respondents**
Number in category % of all respondents	N=46 23.7%	N=30 15.5%	N=33 17.0%	N=51 26.3%	N=22 11.3%	N=12 6.2%	N=194 100%
Students' spouses	6.5%	6.7%	12.1%	9.8%	31.8%	8.3%	11.3%
Students' children	0%	3.3%	9.1%	2.0%	4.5%	8.3%	3.6%
Employees	13.0%	16.7%	15.2%	7.8%	4.5%	16.7%	11.6%
Employees' children	2.2%	10.0%	3.0%	0%	0%	8.3%	3.1%

A similar question was asked about drug and alcohol counseling (Table 10), and the results were nearly identical to those for mental health counseling in terms of overall percentages, but the tendency of smaller institutions was to have this service less available than general mental health counseling.

Table 10 — Drug and Alcohol Counseling						
Enrollment	2000 or less	2001-5000	5001-10,000	10,001-20,000	20,001-30,000	>30,000	All Respondents
Number in category % of all respondents	N=46 23.7%	N=30 15.5%	N=33 17.0%	N=51 26.3%	N=22 11.3%	N=12 6.2%	N=194 100%
Students' spouses	4.3%	3.3%	9.1%	15.7%	31.8%	8.3%	11.3%
Students' children	0%	3.3%	6.1%	2.0%	4.5%	0%	2.6%
Employees	8.7%	10.0%	18.2%	7.8%	9.1%	16.7%	10.8%
Employees' children	0%	6.7%	3.0%	0%	0%	0%	1.5%

Provision of physical examination services is reported in Table 11. Physicals were available overall to 19% of spouses; 6% of students' children; 5% of employees' children; and 16% of employees.

Table 11 — Physical Examination						
Enrollment	2000 or less	2001-5000	5001-10,000	10,001-20,000	20,001-30,000	>30,000	All Respondents
Number in category % of all respondents	N=46 23.7%	N=30 15.5%	N=33 17.0%	N=51 26.3%	N=22 11.3%	N=12 6.2%	N=194 100%
Students' spouses	8.7%	6.7%	15.2%	25.5%	45.5%	25.0%	19.1%
Students' children	4.3%	6.7%	3.0%	3.9%	18.2%	8.3%	6.2%
Employees	13.0%	16.7%	3.0%	21.6%	27.3%	25.0%	16.5%
Employees' children	6.5%	6.7%	3.0%	2.0%	4.5%	16.7%	5.2%

It was believed important in this brief survey to determine specifically what type of employee health functions were performed by student health services. Sixteen and a half percent provided pre-employment and pre-placement exams. There was a clear progression of the frequency of this activity from smaller to larger institutions, with nearly half of the latter commonly involved with this service. A different pattern was seen, however, on the responsibility for evaluation of acute illness and injury. Nearly 46% of all respondents reported acute care as a responsibility, and the frequency across institutions, regardless of size, was generally similar. Nearly 28% of institutions indicated they were assigned the responsibility of "fitness for duty" and "return to work" evaluations, but, as indicated in Table 12, there was no clear pattern based on institutional size. Bloodborne pathogen control programs were the responsibility of nearly 40% of the institutions, with, again, variability in the frequency across institutional size, as well as a slight tendency towards this responsibility being more common, the larger the institution. Finally, in the employee health category, a question was posed regarding responsibility for respirator fitting. About one of ten of the institutions had this responsibility; the general trend was for this activity to be more common in larger rather than smaller institutions.

Table 12 — Employee Health Functions Performed							
Enrollment	2000 or less	2001- 5000	5001- 10,000	10,001- 20,000	20,001- 30,000	>30,000	All Respondents
Number in category % of all respondents	N=46 23.7%	N=30 15.5%	N=33 17.0%	N=51 26.3%	N=22 11.3%	N=12 6.2%	N=194 100%
Pre-employment / pre-placement exam	2.2%	10.0%	12.1%	21.6%	36.4%	41.7%	16.5%
Evaluation of acute illness/ injury	47.8%	53.3%	45.5%	37.3%	45.5%	58.3%	45.9%
Fit for duty/return to work evaluation	30.4%	13.3%	18.2%	29.4%	36.4%	58.3%	27.8%
Blood-borne pathogen exposure control program	30.4%	43.3%	30.3%	43.1%	50.0%	58.3%	39.7%
Respirator fittings	6.5%	3.3%	12.1%	18.7%	22.7%	25.0%	12.4%

COMMENTS

This survey represents, as nearly as the authors are able to ascertain, the first documentation of the extent to which non-student health activities are performed in so-called student health services. It is apparent that such activities are not only common, but that they are much more common than previously realized and that they are exceedingly common without regard to the size of the institution.

Subsequent to the survey, at the June 2000 meeting of the American College Health Association, the committee on Benchmarking, DataShare I reported the results of its first benchmarking survey. At least two of the benchmarks dealt with the issue of non-student patient visits to student health services. The first was "the number of non-student patient visits as a percentage of total patient visits," defining "the extent to which non-students utilize the services of the college health center." One hundred eighty-two institutions responded to this particular question, indicating a mean of 6.8% (range 0–60%) of their visits were non-student visits. The second relevant benchmark was the number of non-student patient visits for a full-time equivalent provider during a year's period of time. The range was 0–5,996 patients annually, with a mean number of visits of 187 and a median of 62.[8] While these data represent a first attempt to develop a series of specific relevant benchmarks for college health, they are somewhat complicated by reporting difficulties, according to personal conversations with the authors of the study. Nonetheless, the data offer additional confirmation of the activity of college health services which extends beyond student care.

In many respects, these data raise more questions than they supply answers. No inquiries were made as regards funding of these activities, space allocated for non-student activities, or whether or not these activities add to the overall budget of the student health service. Perhaps the most obvious, but important, question to be asked is "why?" Why have student health services expanded beyond medical care for students? Part of that question was answered at the outset of this chapter and relates to the very existence of health services for students on college campuses. However, the authors believe that there are more critical, timely issues involved, as well. These relate to better integration of the "student" health service into the university community. The recognition that college health services are frequently more efficient in terms of timeliness of health care delivery and are frequently less costly than outside sources (e.g., care of workers' compensation injuries—seeing individuals promptly, returning them to work, and doing so at modest costs—offers an excellent example). Important, too, is the recognition by many college health professionals that limiting their programs to clearly defined boundaries of "only student" care is risky in terms of program survival and, in fact, opens the door for student health care being delivered by others than the campus health service. Clearly, this whole issue needs further study (particularly with a large sample). Hopefully, the inclusion of the information in this text not heretofore available will generate interest in others pursuing this topic.

REFERENCES

1. Boynton RE. Historical Development of College Health Services, Student Medicine 1962; 10(3):294–305.

2. Wacker WEC. College Health: A Harvard Experience. J Am Coll Health 1995;43(6):289.

3. Ibid.

4. Turner HS, New Realities: The Challenge to Change. J Am Coll Health 1981;30(6):7

5. Patrick K. Student Health Medical Care within Institutions of Higher Education. J Am Med Assoc. 1988;260(22):3302.

6. Turner HS, Hurley JL, Butler KM, Hill J. Accidental Exposures to Blood and Other Bodily Fluids in a Large Academic Medical Center. J Am Coll Health 1999;47(2):199–206.

7. Standards Revision Work Group, Guidelines for a College Health Program, Sixth Edition. J Am Coll Health, 1999.

8. Fredericksen G, Wiener E. 1998–99, Data Share I, American College Health Association, May 31, 2000.

CHAPTER 21

PHYSICAL PLANT: CONSTRUCTION, MAINTENANCE, AND SAFETY

J. Robert Wirag, HSD, and
Robert Watson, EdD, FACHE, Col. USA (Ret.)

CONSTRUCTION

The purpose of this chapter is to orient the reader to the process involved in new construction or major renovation of a campus health care facility and to highlight the various aspects of building maintenance. Given the heterogeneity of college campuses, it will be necessary for the reader to "tailor to fit" the information contained in this chapter according to "at-home" realities.

The first part of the chapter posits a new paradigm . . . call it the NASH facility (for New Age Student Health). As a new framework for thinking about the kind of facility one envisions working in and in which students receive care, consider the NASH facility as the foundation for a student health service for the future. For some, it may mean a major renovation of, or a major addition to, an existing facility. For others, it may mean new construction. The chapter is completed with practical considerations about maintaining a medical facility to assure an environment for care which promotes safety, infection control, and provider and consumer satisfaction alike.

New Age Student Health (NASH)

Many health service facilities on today's college campuses were built 30–40 years ago and no longer meet provider and patient needs. Some are functionally obsolete. Of great

The authors express thanks to the Architecture and Engineering Department, Physical Plant Division, University of Florida, for the use of the Project Manual in writing parts of this chapter.

concern is the impression the facility makes and how the facility affects one's perception of quality. Students complain about how bad a building looks and, as a result, may relate what they see to their perception of quality—if it doesn't look like quality care is provided, students become convinced it isn't.

Fortunately, a new era of renovation and replacement of college health physical facilities seems to have begun. In the early-to-mid-'90s the college health community began to see a changing face of health service facilities on many college campuses. Substantial additions to existing buildings were at various stages of construction. Major renovation projects were undertaken. And on other campuses, planning was underway to replace the old with the new. The "look" of student health facilities was beginning to resemble the "look" of community-based health care facilities to which our students have become accustomed. Many of the new facilities resulted from a combination of a vision for change and a willingness to "make it happen," a trend that continues to gather momentum.

Key features included in a NASH facility are: a patient-centered design; a technology-enriched environment; a cost-effective and easy-to-maintain facility; an environmentally safe and attractive physical plant; and programs which are outcomes-oriented in terms of both clinical care promotion and patient satisfaction. Patient flow will be designed more for the convenience of patients than for staff. "Point of service" will be emphasized, so patients are not hassled with unnecessary movement from one part of the facility to another. The "outside will be brought in" to move from a traditional institutional look to visually appealing and comfortable surroundings. Real-time data entry will be done electronically. Delayed entry of progress notes will be more the exception than the rule. And paper will be virtually eliminated. Work station sites, nursing stations, exam rooms, and more must reflect these changes.

Consider, as well, how much more complex our patients are. They are more knowledgeable, have higher expectations, are more diverse than ever, and present more challenging medical complaints than students of 30 or 40 years ago. Student health facilities of the future must enable a health center to house a program of services reflecting consumers' needs and expectations.

Since no two campuses are alike, no facility or program will be a carbon copy of another. Each will have its own uniqueness and pace of change. Each facility will make a statement about what it's like to work there and about what it's like to receive care there. While the design must be patient-focused, caregivers and other health care workers must also be afforded consideration, from recruitment to training to retention. Therefore, during the planning stage, thought must be given as to how the facility can be designed to be part of the strategy to become the employer of choice in the local market area, as our student health facilities must be attractive to those who provide the services, in order to stay competitive with the health care marketplace. Finally, student health service facilities must resemble the state-of-the-art facilities to which students will have access following graduation. In short, the building must look good, feel good, and be relatively hassle-free in terms of access and service.

Determining the Need and the Viability

If the need for a new student health facility is clear, it should be relatively easy to document and articulate. Such documentation and justification might include: the location is poor; confidentiality is compromised because of cramped quarters and paper-thin walls; patient flow is confusing; the cost of upgrading the HVAC is prohibitive; no space is available to house newly hired staff to meet increasing patient demand; the current wiring can't meet demands of new technology; too few exam rooms per provider compromise efficiency and productivity; architectural barriers prohibit renovation to increase the number of exam rooms; or standards leading to accreditation cannot be met in the current facility. Collectively, these needs constitute the basis of the "case" for a suitable remedy, which may be a major renovation project, an addition to the current facility, or the construction of a new facility tailored to fit the health needs of students and others eligible for services. The need(s) drive the change. Any change expresses itself in ways determined by the viability of the proposed need(s).

Considerations outside the health service also impact the viability of the idea. How involved and supportive are students, particularly student leaders? How supportive are higher administration officials? What are the funding options, and how likely is it the project can be funded? Will the current "footprint" allow expansion or replacement of the current facility? Can a large enough "footprint" be found elsewhere on campus to build the new health center? If so, how accessible and convenient will it be for students?

Planning the Plan

Showcasing the Vision

Sharing the vision with others to elicit feedback helps refine the concept and stimulates a wider base of support. Curbstone conversations, discussions at staff meetings, idea-sharing during division meetings with other director-level colleagues, and an agenda item at a student health advisory board meeting are a few of the ways to begin to showcase the idea. Student leaders or advisory board members may choose to feature the idea with a story in the campus newspaper. Using such a medium with campus-wide visibility may serve to interest a wider group of faculty, staff and students. The risk, of course, is to elicit a negative reaction from those who may be opposed to the idea, think it is premature in its development, or simply feel blind-sided if they were not preconditioned to consider the possibility of a capital investment to build a new student health service facility. At some point, however, finding the right means to showcase the idea serves to condition the community to the possibility and, hopefully, begin to generate support.

Assessing the Political Climate

Ideas remain "just ideas" until there is a fertile environment to allow them to become reality. Knowing who has the decision-making authority and identifying individuals from whom one may anticipate resistance (and why) are elements of the political process that impact transforming an idea into something tangible. Garnering the support of one's associates, discussing the idea with immediate superiors, enlisting the interest and support of key students (student advisory board members or student government leaders) are essential steps, and, ultimately, support must be obtained from senior administration, specifically those who have final decision-making authority. Getting the "pulse" of these groups of individuals is an essential first step in moving the idea forward. However, if the idea has merit, the needs are legitimate, and attention is paid to timing, the process will move forward.

Considering the Alternatives

Even with documented need and excellent support, at times the idea of a new facility will be rejected by higher authorities within the institution. This is the time to consider other alternatives and to communicate them to those in authority. These might include a major renovation or even a recommendation to close the existing facility and have students fend for themselves as a better alternative than continuing to provide services in a sub-optimal facility that does not meet accreditation standards. Outsourcing may be another option. What makes sense?; what is feasible?; what is affordable?; what is in students' best interests?

Concept Design

Once a general sense of support is clear, then the idea can begin to be transformed into reality—to be put on paper. This first stage of this process is the most creative, but the vision must be rooted in reality. Early in the process it is more important to focus on program elements than to be overly concerned about space requirements; this stage provides the opportunity for the health service staff to convey the features any new construction or renovation should include. It is during this first phase of the planning project that the architect spends considerable time determining the requirements of the project and preparing schematic studies, consisting of drawings and other documents illustrating the scale and relationships of the project components. However, concept designs should be driven by the current and projected needs:

- Are the demographics of students changing on your campus?
- What are the ratios of females to males; graduate students to undergraduate students; students in on-campus housing to students living off-campus; traditional age to nontraditional/older students?
- What are the enrollment projections for the next 5, 10, 15, and 20 years?
- What programs do you offer?
- What new programs should you offer?

If capital investments are to be taken seriously, they require good data from past and current programs and vision to reflect a longer-term view to justify the expenditure. To neglect the prognostications for future change is akin to planning with blinders. Further, concept design requires identifying the pieces that will be put together—where contiguous relationships of the program elements are discussed and agreed upon. It is at this stage that space requirements begin to take shape and a cost projection for the project can be derived.

Design Development

During design development, plans become more concrete. The architect prepares more detailed drawings and finalizes the design plan, showing correct sizes and shapes for rooms. Also included is an outline of the construction specifications, listing the major materials to be used. All health service staff can and should have a role in design development. This is the time to determine what fills the workspace occupied by staff. Furnishings (moveable or permanent), floor coverings, cabinetry, storage, lighting, special HVAC requirements, plumbing, and electrical are among the many details which must be addressed.

Depending on the size and scope of the project and the campus resources (professional staff) available, both concept design and design development may be done in-house (internally, using campus resources) before an architect is selected.

Committing to Proceed

Delegation of Project Management

The size of a project for either a renovation or a new construction project determines *who* manages the project and *how* it is managed. Large campuses usually have an office of facilities planning and construction or a campus facilities planning agency. This office provides the oversight for a major project involving new construction, with the campus physical plant officials delegated the responsibility for more hands-on involvement with the project. University officials should work closely with health service personnel to secure an appropriate architect. Smaller projects may be managed by campus physical plant architects and engineers, with limited or no involvement by other offices.

Early on, it is important that a health service contact person be designated; i.e., someone who is responsible for decision making as it relates to the overall renovation/ construction project. This person serves as the coordinator for all activities focusing on the project. Appointed committees within the student health service working on renovation and construction activities should funnel their concerns and actions through this coordinator. The project manager should be the official health service spokesperson when addressing activities, agencies, or organizations that are external to the student health service. If a new building is to include other tenants because it is a multi-use facility, the project manager should coordinate the planning with the various tenants.

Choosing the Architect for Construction

The size, cost, and complexity of the renovation or new construction project determine whether in-house architectural expertise is adequate and appropriate or if an external architecture firm should be utilized. (For this discussion it is assumed that the scope of the project requires the services of an outside architectural firm.) Although campus or system policies and procedures typically govern the process of selecting an architect, the health service director must have some understanding of the process at the beginning of a successful architect-client relationship, since the architect, the health service director, and health service staff spend considerable time discussing various aspects of the project. An excellent resource available through the American Institute of Architects is "You and Your Architect."[1] The document features helpful tips on getting started, selecting an architect, identifying the services you need, and negotiating the formal agreement between owner and architect.

While the size and scope of the proposed project may extend beyond campus resources in terms of staff, expertise, and the time required to manage the project, some combination of architectural services by individuals on and off campus may be advisable and, at times, required by your institution. The basic expectations of the architect include preliminary designs (usually called concept or schematic designs); design development (more detailed drawings, showing correct sizes and shapes for rooms); preparation of construction documents (drawings and specifications); assistance in the bidding or negotiation process; and facilitating interaction between the university and the builder or contractor.[1] Thus, it is important that what needs to be provided by an outside architect and what can be provided by campus staff be clarified and agreed upon at the outset. Some campuses have considerable project planning, design, and construction expertise and may be able to manage many of the project tasks themselves. Therefore, it is essential that the campus facility's planning agency be involved in architect selection to insure adherence to all campus policies related to design and construction.

There may be a requirement for a bid or request for proposal for architectural service. The appropriate campus agency—facilities planning or purchasing—usually takes the lead in calling for bids from various architectural firms for the renovation or new construction project. In selecting the architect, it is important to underscore accepting bids from those specializing in medical facilities.

Interviewing and Selection Consideration

Officials from an appropriate office at the campus or system level may be responsible for identifying architects or architectural firms as eligible candidates for the project, and will schedule interviews. However, the health service director may request an architect recognized for work with health care facilities and recommend the architect be considered as a candidate. It is ideal if the health service director, or representative, participates in the interviewing/selection process of the architect.

Questions need to be asked to elicit information about the kind of relationship or partnership that will lead to a successful outcome. The following considerations are important:[1]

- How will the team the architect has assembled approach your project?
- How will the architect gather information, establish priorities, and make decisions?
- What does the architect see as important issues or considerations in the project?
- What does the architect expect from the project?
- How does the architect set priorities and make decisions?
- Who in the firm will work directly with you, the client?
- How will the engineering or other design services be provided?
- How will the firm provide quality control during design?

- What is the firm's construction-cost experience?
- Are the architect's style, personality, and approach compatible with the health service director/staff?

Additionally, the interview should be a two-way process; the architect should be inquisitive as well. A thoughtful architect must be as careful in selecting a client as the client is in selecting the architect. The architect also has a vested interest in the success of the project. If the architect and the client are compatible, the prospects for a successful outcome are enhanced.

Agreement between Institution and Architect

Negotiating the final agreement between the institution's representative(s) and the representative(s) of the architectural firm is an opportunity to assure that both agree and are clear on the project before them and that both agree on requirements and expectations. Before finalizing the agreement, the following four steps should be addressed to a level of mutual satisfaction and understanding:

- Establish specific project requirements—project scope; project site; levels of design quality; target completion date; budget estimate and sources of financing; and codes, regulations, and required design reviews.
- Describe project tasks and assign responsibility for each.
- Develop a preliminary schedule with timelines for the various tasks and responsibilities, and determine whether or not the schedule is reasonable, given the project's requirements and budget.
- Use the planning work as a basis for establishing the architect's compensation; ask the architect to provide a compensation proposal.[2]

Partnering with the Architect

Creating a Project Team

A project team consists of any or all of the following: the university's designated representative(s), individuals or entities required to review the architect's submittals, the university's other consultants and contractors, the architect's designated representative(s), and the consultants retained by the architect for engineering and other specialty services.

Refining the Project's Scope

At some point a "wish list" must be grounded in a realistic and tangible plan. What may have begun as an individual interest may grow to include the interests of many others. For example, the notion of a freestanding student health center may evolve into a multipurpose facility to serve several campus needs. (Examples include the facilities of the University of Texas at Austin, Illinois State University, and the University of Arizona.) Separately, various service units on campus may be experiencing similar concerns to that of the health service (an antiquated building, an undesirable location, and excessive maintenance costs). Economies of scale that can be achieved by combining the interests of several programs may make a new facility affordable.

Defining the Responsibilities of the Parties

The size and scope of the building project determine how many people will represent the university. If it is a stand-alone health service project, the number will be fewer than if the health service is part of a multiservice facility. The more entities to be included, the more challenging it is to determine the placement of services and the contiguous relationship of services, either on the same floor or on different floors. One can expect team members to vie for position to secure the most suitable space to facilitate students' access to their service(s). The health service representative will be no exception, arguing for high visibility and appropriate positioning to allow easy access to essential services.

The chair of the project team plays a critical role in setting the ground rules for clarifying the roles and responsibilities of various team members. The most important and time-consuming part of the entire process is during the concept design and design development phases of the project, when the tenants are most intimately involved with the architect and other members of the planning team. While it is the chair who typically manages the discussion, it is usually the campus or system representative for facilities, planning, and construction who keeps the discussion within boundaries dictated by budget, footprint, codes, regulatory requirements, and campus-wide policies and procedures governing such activity. Among the items to be considered and "assigned" to the various members of the project team are:

- Analysis of remodeling/renovation vs. new construction
- Economic feasibility studies
- Regulatory approvals
- Site analysis and selection
- Project and financing
- Architecture and engineering
- Estimating costs
- Interior design
- Construction

Other points of discussion may include:

- Structural configuration: what it should look like
- Space usage: dedicated space for what purpose(s); relationship of one space to another; types of activities/functions/individuals to be assigned
- Patient and staff traffic patterns: for whose convenience . . . patients' or staff's
- Essential equipment: what and where; special reinforcements (weight-bearing)
- Signage: way-finding
- Technology: hard wire, wireless; locations/placements; flexibility for future applications

Maintaining a Professional Relationship

Participating in the planning of a building project is serious business. The quality of the outcome is directly related to the quality of the interpersonal relationships among the principals on the project team. An atmosphere that is respectful of different viewpoints and various disciplines represented on the project team is critical to success. The chair sets the standard and serves as the model for the behavior of others.

Coordination

The usual custom is for the architect, the campus planning office official, and the project manager and/or student health service representative to meet periodically to review the details during the design development stage of the project. Included in this review should be the architect's study and review of factors such as patient flow, ancillary medical equipment, practice habits, patient statistics, fiscal operation, services provided, scope of practice/service, projected future patient population, and future medical and business technology trends.

The final stage of architectural planning focuses on coordinating the schematic design and the design development phases of the project with the budget allocation for the project. If the projected costs exceed the allocation of funds for the project, alternatives need to be discussed to either trim back the scope of the project or find additional funds to support the project as designed. When design features and financial issues are resolved to the satisfaction of the respective parties, working drawings can be completed, specifications can be described and finalized, and the complete packet known as the "contract document" can be produced. The contractor's price is based on this document and is part of the contract which the university signs with the builder.[3]

Call for Bids from Contractors

The invitation for contractors to bid on the project is normally orchestrated by the campus facilities planning office or the purchasing office, as the responsible agent for the university/college. A call for bids usually states the qualifications for bidders, the date, times, and place where the sealed bids are to be received, the name of the architectural firm, any pre-solicitation/pre-bid meetings, deposit needed for each set of drawings and project manual, and bid opening date.

Coordination with Campus Facilities Planning Office

The campus facilities planning office or the campus physical plant division is the university/college agency responsible for coordinating all issues focusing on new construction and major renovation. It is this campus office which coordinates the meetings between the health service project manager, architect, contractor, subcontractors, other involved campus organizations, and utility representatives. It is usually the responsibility of the campus faculties planning office to assemble the data and publish the project manual and to negotiate the contract papers. The university legal counsel should review the contract papers and documents.

Review Bids and Select Contractor

Bids which have been received in good order and prior to the designated time must be considered and acted upon in accordance with the university's own internal requirements and/or state regulations. Bids received after the designated time should not be accepted. Bids should be opened publicly and read aloud at the time and location stated in the "Call for Bids" invitation. On the day of the opening and reading of bids, a tabulation of the bids should be done and posted at the site where the bids were opened. More then one bid from a firm should not be allowed, and the university/college should reserve the right to reject a bid if there appears to be falsification, collusion, or any other irregularity.

In awarding the contract, again, subject to state statutes and/or university regulations, the low aggregate bidder is the winner. It is important to specify to the contract winner that work shall commence on a certain date and be completed within a certain number of calendar days. There should be a provision for liquidated damages if the specified work is not completed by a stated time. The official document that becomes the work contract is called the "Proposal Form." The form will usually be negotiated by the university/college general counsel or the campus facilities planning office.

Identify Subcontractors

Subcontractors should be listed on a separate form prepared by the winning bidder. This listing of subcontractors and alternates normally accompanies the proposal form, which is presented to the university/college. A subcontractor is an individual who has a direct contract with the contractor to perform a portion of the work at the job site.

Change Orders

During renovation/construction the architect visits the job site at agreed-upon times. Frequently, the architectural firm will appoint an on-site architect to be available on a daily basis for consultation and to ascertain if the contractor is fulfilling his contractual obligations in a proper manner. This individual discusses project changes which involve changes in cost. The architect will formally draw up these changes and present the recommendation to the contractor, the health service, or the campus facilities planning office. Changes which involve costs are called "change orders." Change orders, when approved by the appropriate campus authority, are returned immediately to the architect, so that the contractor can be informed. Change orders are costly and should be kept to a minimum. Careful pre-construction planning helps reduce the total number of change orders.

Project Manual

The backbone of the renovation/construction project is the project manual. It is the guide which contains the architect's instructions for building. In short, it is the "cookbook" for the project. The project manual should have several important sections, including:

- General provisions of the contract
- Administration of the contract

- Work order changes
- Time for completion of work plans
- Payments, completion, inspection, and warranty agreement
- Protection of persons and property
- Insurance and bonds
- Correcting work requirements
- Miscellaneous provisions
- Termination of contract conditions

Pre-Construction Conference

A pre-construction conference is essential before any construction project begins. Arrangements should be assured for the contractor to have a field office to include telephone service, electricity, and electronic equipment normally expected in today's business, portable toilets, a storage area for equipment, supplies and vehicles, and fencing material to enclose the area to insure public safety as well as safety of the construction equipment and materials.

It may be useful, as well, to have more working knowledge of basic architectural terms. A good source of information for this terminology is that furnished by the American Institute of Architecture.[4]

MAINTENANCE

Introduction

The care and maintenance of a health service's physical plant and related services are paramount to the provision of quality medical care. While it is important that directors and administrators be familiar with the operation of physical plant activities, in most large student health services the housekeeping supervisor or equivalent is responsible for actual physical plant operations and functions. As such, this individual should be accorded a status parallel to other department supervisors. The department supervisor should have experience and skills in mechanical systems, be able to read a blueprint, and be proficient in housekeeping responsibilities, as well as providing leadership.

Building Structure

The National Fire Protection Association (NFPA) 101 Life Safety Code Manual classifies health services according to inpatient or outpatient capability.[5*] The purpose of the Life Safety Code is to provide minimum requirements for the design, operation, and maintenance of buildings and structures for safety to life from fire and similar emergen-

---

* For those health services facilities that offer in-patient services to four or more occupants, Chapter 12 and Chapter 13 of the manual are applicable. For those ambulatory outpatient student health services, Chapter 26 and Chapter 27 apply. Facilities with inpatients are identified as health care occupancies while those offering ambulatory outpatient services are identified under the business classification.

cies.[6] Directors, administrators, and housekeeping supervisors should be familiar with the NFPA manual, as it describes the safety measures needed to meet accreditation standards of the Joint Commission on Accreditation of Healthcare Organizations (JCAHO) and the Accreditation Association for Ambulatory Health Care, Inc. (AAAHC).

Student health administrators should have points of contact in the campus physical plant division and the campus facilities planning office, so that repairs, scheduled maintenance, equipment calibration, remodeling, renovation, and emergency mechanical services can be obtained in a timely manner. The health service should schedule a qualified representative from the campus physical plant division to provide a detailed "walkthrough" inspection of the health service facility, pointing out the operation of all mechanical equipment, steam and hot-water lines, chilled-water lines, plumbing and wastewater lines, the electrical system (including emergency lighting and the emergency generator), elevator operation, fire alarms and emergency water sprinkler systems, and telephone and other intercom or communication systems. It is important to know how to turn off the building water supply and to shut off electrical power. Further, it is wise to have a complete set of blueprints available. These drawings should include, by floor, heating, ventilation and air conditioning systems, plumbing and sewer lines, electrical and communication lines, construction drawings, sprinkler lines, steam and gas lines, and site and foundation plans.

Scheduled Building Maintenance

The initial cost of installed mechanical and electrical equipment of a medical facility may exceed 40 percent of the cost of the building.[7] Therefore, it is important to service and maintain the structure and equipment as called for in building and equipment specifications, to avoid disruption of clinical services. Further, a system of record-keeping for maintenance performed and for scheduled maintenance should be developed. Maintenance in a student health service can be completed in a several ways. One option is to have scheduled maintenance completed by the campus physical plant division/campus utilities-maintenance department; another option is to contract with a local or regional vendor; another is to complete the work in-house; the last is a combination of any of the preceding.*

Painting

Labor may constitute 80 to 90 percent of the cost of painting.[8] It is essential that high-quality paint be utilized for the health service. To minimize the paint supplies in-

---

* At the university of one of the authors' (RW), a program that saves money has been developed within the housekeeping department for planned maintenance and for minor replacement and repairs. In addition to performing assigned custodial duties, staff members also can perform maintenance and repair tasks normally expected of a skilled tradesman. Additionally, a carpentry and repair shop has been added in the basement area, where many items can be constructed or repaired. In addition to budgetary savings, staff morale is enhanced because of the efficiency and expertise exhibited by the housekeeping department. Of utmost importance, service to patients and customers is rarely disrupted.

ventory, a limited number of paint colors should be utilized. By using high-quality paint that is washable, the length of time between painting and repainting is extended.

Carpentry

Every student health service should maintain a supply of hand tools, so staff can perform small repairs. Most health services may require the services of the campus physical plant division's skilled workmen for larger carpentry tasks. Others may contract the work to a local repairman or vendor. However, if a health service has a maintenance repair person on its staff, a small carpentry shop may well be in order. The ability to provide in-house carpentry work and projects can conserve funds for utilization elsewhere.

The size and layout of a shop depends on the size of the student health service and available space. Ideally, a shop should include a workbench, storage cabinets, and hand tools such as an electrical drill, saber saw, and sander. Dust-collecting equipment is essential for sanding, grinding, and sawing. A maintenance repair person can usually perform a variety of related tasks, such as repairing and laying flooring materials and baseboards; replacing and installing acoustical ceiling tiles; and repairing all portable wheeled equipment, in addition to small cabinet-making and carpentry-associated jobs.[9]

Electrical

Most clinics will use an off-campus electrical contractor or the campus physical plant division for electrical repairs or renovation. If possible, it can be cost-effective for the student health service to have a maintenance support worker on staff who can install and relocate electrical receptacles, move and install electrical lighting appliances, repair appliances and replace broken cords, and similar activities. Employee morale escalates when someone in-house can quickly restore a broken appliance or restore electricity.

It is also important to maintain a service record on each piece of electrical equipment utilized for patient care. All electrical equipment in the student health service should be inspected at least annually, including electric coffee makers, electric heaters, and electric fans. Records should be kept of such inspections. The health service workshop should contain a few items of electrical test equipment (e.g., a volt-ohm meter, electrical safety tester, signal generator, and receptacle circuit tester).[10]

For electrical work, many codes or standards must be followed. These include the Standard Building Code, National Electrical Code (NFPA 70), National Electrical Safety Code (NESC), Life Safety Code (NFPA 101), accessibility and usability standards (ANSI A117.1), Americans with Disabilities Act of 1990, and applicable state codes or standards.[11] Therefore, it is mandatory that anyone doing electrical work be legally permitted to perform the work and have full knowledge of all legal/code requirements.

Plumbing

Plumbing repair work, installation work, or plumbing renovations are typically contracted out to an independent licensed vendor, or to the campus physical plant division. As with electrical work, directors and administrators must be somewhat familiar with various local, state, and national codes and standards as they relate to plumbing issues. It is also advisable to have a set of building blueprints showing all water lines, plumbing fixtures, sewage lines, drain lines, steam lines, fire sprinkler systems, and autoclave systems.

It is helpful to have a maintenance repair person or a handyman housekeeper who can complete small plumbing tasks, such as opening a clogged sink, drain line, or clogged toilet drain line, installing new washers in sink faucets, and similar small problems. Useful tools include a plunger, a sewer-cleaning "snake" machine, and an assortment of various pipe wrenches. It is always a good idea to have a standby hot-water tank in case of an emergency, so some hot water is available for continued patient care activities.

Roofing

Obviously, health service buildings are of varied sizes, designs, and architecture. Thus, materials for roofing are of numerous compositions. With exposure to the sun, wind, rain, sleet, snow, and hail, the roof takes the harshest treatment of any exterior surface of a building. Therefore, it is important to examine the roof annually for cracks, breaks, and needed repairs. Also, all roofs are subject to expansion and contraction because of variations in temperature, which can lead to leaks and the need for subsequent repairs.[12] A roofing specialist and a representative of the student health service should conduct annual inspections. Upon completing the inspection, an annual report should be prepared which reflects the condition of the roof, including guttering, flashing, and roof drains. It is important also to place screening over vent ducts and ventilation openings to keep out birds and small animals. The campus physical plant division or a reputable contractor is probably best to complete roof repairs and services.

Landscaping

The appearance of the health services building and grounds directly affects students' perception of the quality of the health care they receive. A well-groomed lawn with trees, flowers, and shrubs does much to relieve a person's apprehension about coming for care. The campus grounds and landscape services usually maintain the mowing and maintenance for all campus outdoor areas as well as any underground lawn sprinkler systems. The health service should make certain that all sidewalks are routinely cleaned and clear and that the lawns are free of paper, bottles, and other debris. Waste receptacles should be emptied frequently. Driveways and parking spaces must be kept clean, either by the health service staff or by campus custodial personnel.

Heating and Air Conditioning

Heating and air conditioning systems are commonly tied in with a complete system called an HVAC (heating, ventilation, and air conditioning) system. Heating and air conditioning problems are best managed by the campus physical plant division or by a licensed and bonded specialist. The key to a successfully balanced system is preventive and scheduled maintenance.

In most health services, air conditioning and heating fixtures are integrated through various complex components. The four basic types of air conditioning systems are direct expansion system, all-water system, all-air system, and air-water system.[13.] To become thoroughly familiar with air conditioning equipment, an individual must have knowledge of various fans, filters, dehumidifiers, pumps, ductwork, special coils, dampers, and a computerized system which can balance the air temperature between different zones within a building. An annual inspection and calibration of all equipment should be completed by service personnel to insure filters are changed as prescribed and that fan bearings are lubricated.

Telephones

In the past several years, all kinds and types of telephone options have been made available by changes in technology. For health services, it is possible to rent telephone service from the local community telephone service, lease or buy the operating equipment from another company, participate as part of a campus network system, or own outright the telephone system. The university communications department or the local telephone company can assist in explaining the options best suited to a specific program.

Emergency Generator

Large student health service facilities should have an emergency power generator; small health facilities are less likely to have this type of equipment. Generators selected for providing emergency power can be gasoline-powered, diesel-powered, or steam turbine-driven. Emergency generators, where required by Life Safety Code, should be tested and maintained in accordance with the National Fire Protection Association (NFPA 110, Standard for Emergency and Standby Power Systems).[14] It is very important for an emergency generator to activate within 10 seconds of power failure and be able to run for a considerable length of time, at least 90 minutes under normal load.[15] JCAHO mandates that an emergency generator be tested monthly and also requires that prudent documentation be maintained on servicing and testing.[16] Preventive maintenance calls for the fuel levels, oil level, and battery power to be checked. Service records should indicate dates of service performed and the responsible individual.

Emergency generators should be enclosed so that they are out of the weather. The generator should be surrounded with enough enclosure so that the engine cover/jacket does not drop below 50 degrees Fahrenheit. It is important also that the generator battery have a starting capacity for at least 60 seconds of continuous cranking. Generators should not be situated in the same general location as components of normal power, and the generator sets should be equipped with alarm signaling devices, which sound when fuel or oil pressure is low.[17]

Administrators and clinical directors need to determine the location for emergency power outlets (and insure that staff know where these outlets are located; coding by red faceplates may be useful), patient support equipment, and other emergency systems to be powered by the emergency generator. This is true whether the health service has its own generator or is part of a larger campus power grid.

Equipment Maintenance

Inventory of Equipment

To conserve resources and maintain accountability, a student health service should maintain an inventory of equipment and property the cost of which exceeds a stipulated or designated dollar amount. Your institution may have regulations governing these levels. The purpose of an inventory listing is twofold: it provides a method of periodic accounting for all institutional property valued over a specified dollar amount, and it provides a total value for all accountable property and equipment. The dollar amount of value for inventory property and equipment should be at its acquisition rate.

One useful method of inventory accountability is to place a barcode decal on all equipment and property, which can then be listed on a computer spreadsheet along with the applicable barcode. At a predetermined interval (commonly annually), property and equipment can be accounted for on a formal basis. Inventory accountability can also be done manually by tagging or numbering each item and then recording the items in a logbook. If pieces of individual equipment are issued to a staff member on a "hand receipt," that person is responsible for its accountability. Items that cannot be located, after reasonable time and search, should be removed from the inventory list following the institution's prescribed methods. Items that are surplus or damaged beyond repair should be removed from the inventory listing as well.

Scheduled Maintenance and Calibration of Equipment

Scheduled maintenance is preventive maintenance. To establish a scheduled maintenance program is a large undertaking requiring time and tenaciousness. This is an essential program for a health facility and must receive a high priority to enable patient care to be provided at consumer expectation levels. A specific inventory of equipment requiring maintenance should be developed along with notation of the manufacturer's guide for maintenance.

Vehicles

Many large student health service programs have their own vehicle(s) or access to a university vehicle. Issues of concern are insurance, preventive maintenance, user responsibility, dispatching, and security. In some cases, the vehicle is used as a patient transport vehicle, so that patients needing transportation may be moved from the student health service to a designated location. Depending on the situation, a clinician may be required to accompany the patient to the referral location, e.g., an emergency room. Therefore, it is necessary to have adequate insurance coverage on passengers, operators, and the vehicle itself. Further, special equipment and accessories may be necessary. Responsibility for the vehicle rests with a designated department, which should be accountable for who uses the vehicle, for what types of trips and purposes it is utilized, and for the overall security of the vehicle. Important items for consideration are:

- Who is responsible for tag acquisition?
- Who is authorized to use the vehicle?
- Who is responsible for routine maintenance?
- Where should the vehicle be taken for repairs?
- Who is responsible for the gas/oil credit card?

Office Equipment Maintenance

Office equipment must be repaired or replaced in a timely and expeditious manner if administrative and business activities are to function smoothly. Most universities will have a campus source for repair, or the health service will have a maintenance contract with a local office-equipment repair vendor. It is important to maintain a repair record on each piece of equipment, so that when new equipment is to be procured, the repair records and costs of the specific brand and model can be reviewed.

Elevator/Escalator Maintenance

The facility or campus usually has a contract arrangement with a vendor for elevator or escalator service and repair. Ongoing preventive maintenance normally calls for oil, grease, inspection, and minor parts. Repair service includes preventive maintenance plus major operating part repairs. Repairs and maintenance should be conducted during hours in which the student health service is nonoperational.

Environmental Factors

Infection Control

Infection control is critical to a health care facility. The primary goal is to provide a safe working environment for patients and staff, based upon scientific knowledge and good hygiene. In a health service, this is accomplished by insuring good environmental hygiene and pollution control by a facility-wide program which is designed to monitor and evaluate those activities. An infection control committee composed of staff representation from various departments of the facility is essential. It should meet regularly and assure, at the minimum, compliance with JCAHO and AAAHC accreditation standards.

The committee should develop, review, and update policies annually and as needed, including those required by state and federal law. Further, it should develop procedures for reporting communicable diseases as required by applicable state and federal laws. Additionally, the committee should develop protocols for evaluation and follow-up of all exposures to blood or body fluids. A plan that insures a defined system for collecting data and maintaining records should be instituted, as well as an ongoing education program for staff members. A staff in-service education program should be conducted annually with a mandatory attendance to insure indoctrination as required by OSHA. An exposure control plan should be updated annually in order to comply with 1992 Occupational Safety and Health Administration (OSHA) Regulation of Bloodborne Pathogens.[18]

The following list provides suggestions for areas of inspection and regular monitoring for improvement in infection control practices:

- Work site clean and sanitary.
- Sharps container—clearly labeled, puncture-resistant, and not overfilled.
- Handwashing sink available with approved soap.
- Trash container conveniently located.
- No food/drink/cosmetics in patient areas.

- Biohazardous waste containers accessible and lined with red plastic bags which are clearly labeled.[18]
- Goggles, masks, gloves, lab coats and gowns, and other protective equipment worn for tasks involving exposure to blood and body fluids.[18]
- Hepatitis B vaccine provided for staff members at risk for exposure to blood or body fluids (or declination signed and filed).[18]
- Documentation of staff education about BBP Exposure Control Plan.[18]
- Patient care refrigerators clean and equipped with thermometer and log sheet, and free of food.
- Clean supplies and dirty supplies are kept separate.
- Clean and sterile products are properly stored.
- Dated supplies are not beyond expiration date.
- Air handlers and airflow equipment are maintained and serviced to reduce air pollution. Maintenance log sheets maintained and properly documented.
- Surveillance of facility water system periodically tested by chemical analysis for organisms.
- Sterilizers continually tested for microorganisms; log is maintained which indicates testing, maintenance, and repairs.

Water and Liquid Wastes

The quality of water supplied to a student health service affects every phase of clinic operations. Chemically acceptable water must be available for optimum operation of equipment and performance of many laboratory tests.[19] Water inlets to a plumbing fixture should end above the highest water level in the plumbing fixture to prevent contamination from back-flowing into clean water. Where this in not possible, a backflow device/preventor must be installed. Overhead drain lines need to be installed in those locations which do not pass over expensive or valuable equipment or supplies, in the event of leaks. New replacement pipes and fittings should be decontaminated before placing them into service. This can be accomplished by flushing/washing with a chlorine solution. A student health service does not normally produce the types and amounts of chemical wastes warranting special examination by a sanitation engineer, but an engineer should review blueprints and physically observe and inspect all drain lines for sanitary water waste and sewage water waste, to ascertain that they are separate. The campus physical plant division should be capable of providing advice and assistance in this area.

Insect and Rodent Control

From time to time, every health service will experience a problem with insects and rodents. Depending upon the weather and state of cleanliness, insects and rodents will attempt to infiltrate the building via cracks or crevices in the building. Wet and cold weather tends to drive insects and rodents into a warmer atmosphere, and the state of cleanliness to a large extent determines the amount of pest control required. Health service managers should frequently examine staff break rooms for food particles and exposed food. Coffee makers should be clean and sanitary. Good housekeeping procedures go a long way toward the prevention of an insect and rodent problem. Frequent mopping with a disinfectant also does much to reduce the insect control.

Landscaping practices which keep bushes and shrubs cut so that they do not touch the building or windows help prevent the entrance of insects from shrubs into the building. Metal trash and refuse containers should also be kept at considerable distance from the building in order to help prevent a rodent problem. Trash containers should be emptied frequently. Most universities will have a pest control specialist or a contracted pest control company to address insect and rodent control problems when they occur.

Solid Waste Systems/Hazardous waste

Hazardous waste and solid waste disposal for a medical facility is an increasingly complex and difficult problem. Health service managers and directors need to become familiar with federal, state, and local codes which regulate the disposal of medical waste. Each college or university physical plant division should be able to provide assistance and guidance on how best to dispose of medical waste. The following general types of wastes present specific hazards in health services:[20]

- Infectious wastes containing microorganisms capable of causing illness to a susceptible host.
- Toxic chemicals, which can cause poisoning when inhaled, ingested, or brought into contact with the skin.
- Flammable liquids and explosive gases, which can cause injury to personnel or damage to the facility structure by fire and explosion.
- Caustic materials (acids or bases), which can cause injury.
- Physically injurious wastes that can produce punctures, cuts, or abrasions.
- Radioactivity-contaminated wastes.

If there is a doubt about waste disposal, contact the local/county health department or a local hospital for assistance in developing a program. In recent years, federal legislative initiatives have been promulgated to make certain that medical facilities fulfill their legal and ethical responsibility to insure proper disposal of hazardous waste materials.

Housekeeping Department Responsibilities

The housekeeping or maintenance department provides multiple services in support of the health care delivery system. Their goal should be to uphold the highest possible quality of patient care through maintaining standards of cleanliness necessary to control infection and to present a clean and neat appearance. In addition to routine cleaning functions, the staff may assist with maintenance, provide courier and patient transport services, and transfer equipment and supplies within the building.

Products and Cleaning Equipment

The selection of cleaning products and cleaning equipment must be conducted with a number of factors in mind, including the cost, ease of use, safety, and storage equipment of these products. An excellent reference book for housekeeping supervisors is *Essentials of Housekeeping in Health Care Facilities.*[21]

SAFETY

Fire Safety

The National Fire Protection Association 101 *Life Safety Code* is a most important reference resource for a health service administrator, concerning fire safety and fire codes.[5] Most accreditation agencies will use or reference this book as their source when mandating certain requirements. Also, state or local fire officials may use the book as their guide for citing code violations and for making recommendations for compliance. The purpose of the Life Safety Code is to set forth minimum guidelines for design, maintenance, and operation of buildings. It is focused on life safety from fire and other emergencies. The Life Safety Code is applicable to both new construction and existing buildings and structures intended for human occupancy. Important relevant chapters for college health facilities include:

- Chapter One—title, purpose, scope, application, occupancy, maintenance and equivalency concepts of the Code.
- Chapter Twelve—life safety requirements for the design of new hospitals, limited care facilities, nursing homes, and ambulatory health care facilities. Of special interest in this chapter are means-of-egress requirements covering doors, locks, stairs, hallways, travel distances, ramps, and vertical openings.
- Chapter Thirteen—requirements for existing buildings or structures occupied as ambulatory health care centers; addresses additions, renovations, conversions, and mixed occupancies.
- Chapter Twenty-six—new business occupancies, including new ambulatory health care centers.

Fire and Disaster Drills

Medical administrators and department supervisors should keep abreast of the latest developments in fire safety. Each health facility should have a safety committee, an emergency disaster committee, or both. The committee should meet at least quarterly and regularly update procedures and written guidelines.

JCAHO has mandated in its 2000–2001 accreditation manual for ambulatory care facilities that the Emergency Preparedness Plan be tested twice a year.[22] This manual provides the focus, instructions, and record-keeping for health centers' fire/disaster drills. The 1998 accreditation handbook for the AAAHC also references the requirements for fire/disaster emergency preparedness (Chapter 8, "Facilities and Environment")[23] and sets forth the requirement for fire drills and periodic training and instruction of all personnel on the proper use of safety, emergency, and fire-extinguishing equipment. It also mandates a plan to address internal and external emergencies when calling for personnel trained in cardiopulmonary resuscitation and use of emergency equipment.

Fire drills should be critiqued and evaluated after each session. Corrections should be immediately instituted after each drill. Reports including evaluations and corrections should be maintained on file for periodic review. All employees should have at least annual instruction on how to operate fire-extinguishing equipment, exit the building properly, handle patient care issues during a fire or fire drills, and properly report a fire.

Concurrently, each treatment facility should schedule and conduct an annual training session on emergency preparedness and disaster drills. This training should include those issues which are relevant to the operation of the specific health service, among which may be how to properly lift litters, transfer patients to a gurney, move patients via elevator, triage patients, tag patients, deal with mental health issues, operate emergency communication equipment, or properly use a backboard; patient accountability and medical records; public relations and press release procedures; transfer of patients; and discharge of patients. The frequent practice of fire drills and disaster drills will insure that staff have been trained and educated to respond quickly and efficiently to a real situation.

Laboratory Safety

Risks in the clinical laboratory include fire, explosions, cuts from glass or sharp objects, chemical burns, inhalation of toxic chemicals and vapors, and accidental falls. The laboratory supervisor is ultimately responsible for the safety procedures established in the laboratory and for periodic monitoring to insure these procedures are carried out and deficiencies reported. Each health service should have its laboratory safety procedures published in a manual and made available to all new employees as part of their orientation process. Annually, all employees should be provided a period of safety training to take advantage of any new equipment or instruments. Records of safety training received by employees should be documented for utilization in future accreditation surveys. Training should also be documented in the individual staff member's credential file.

Protective equipment such as safety eye goggles must be available to laboratory employees. Laboratory coats, protective gowns, or in some cases, rubberized aprons will help keep damaging chemical and solutions off the personal clothing of employees. Protective gloves should also be worn in all situations when warranted. The protective equipment utilized must be appropriate for the task and be free of any flaws which might compromise safety. Equipment should fit properly and snugly. A designated place or area should be available for the disposal of contaminated protective clothing and equipment. The daily pickup of these items must be made to insure proper laundering and disposal of gloves or other items not launderable.

Emergency water supplies should be available in the laboratory so that flushing and irrigation may occur as soon as harmful agents contact the skin or eyes.

Radiation Safety

In the health service setting, radiation safety usually is focused in two areas; environmental surveillance and personnel dosimetry.[24] Fortunately, most tasks performed in the radiology department do not provide great risk of staff exposure to radiation.

Accrediting agencies have safety guidelines for use in areas where diagnostic imagery service occurs. They usually stipulate that the health service have written procedural policies addressing:[25]

- Regulation of the use, removal, handling, and storage of potentially hazardous materials
- Precautions against electrical, mechanical, magnetic, ultrasonic, radiation, and other potential hazards
- Proper shielding where radiation, magnetic field, and other potentially hazardous energy sources are used
- Acceptable monitoring devices for all personnel who might be exposed to radiation, magnetic fields, or otherwise harmful energy (monitoring devices worn by personnel in any area with a potentially hazardous energy field)
- Maintenance of personnel exposure records
- Instructions to personnel in safety precautions and in dealing with emergency hazardous energy field exposure
- Retention of diagnostic images
- Need for proper warning signs, alerting the public and staff to the presence of hazardous energy fields

Environmental surveillance measures are focused on assessing and controlling the level of radiation exposure to visitors and staff. Therefore, radiology facilities must be designed and constructed in a manner which prevents accidental radiation exposure. The central booth and diagnostic radiographic room must be shielded so as not to contaminate adjacent areas with radiation. Ongoing inspections are mandated to insure overall staff and patient safety. The use of a radiology film badge by staff personnel allows an assessment of dose exposure to external radiation. The personnel dosimetry program using film badges worn on the body is mandatory for employees subjected to the risk of external exposure to radiation. Film badges are surrendered at periodic intervals and reviewed by qualified monitoring personnel. A log-book record should be maintained on film badge radiation readings for staff members.[26]

Record Keeping

While the ultimate responsibility for safety issues within a student health service rests with the director, every health service should have a safety committee which meets at least quarterly. All matters of importance relating to safety or to the safety committee should be documented, including fire drills, safety training classes with a roster of attendees, accidents and/or safety injuries, emergency preparedness training, and disaster and fire emergency plans. Accrediting agencies require this documentation during the survey process.

Communications

Communication systems planning in a health service requires the expertise of many individuals. Each director or administrator may have a different set of demands and needs for the various communication instruments that are available. The decision of whether to lease equipment (and services), as opposed to purchasing it, is an individual decision. However, accelerating technology makes current communication equipment obsolete more quickly. When considering communications and data equipment for the health service, the following observations may be useful:

- Television—Waiting-room television set programming can be received from a master antenna or satellite dish as well as closed-loop educational television programming.
- Dictation—Several modes of medical transcription devices are available utilizing various communications systems. Dialing in on the health service telephone system from an external number or utilizing the internal phone system to dictate is possible. Several systems of stand-alone equipment are available.
- Radio—Utilizing the intercom or paging system, background music can be provided using a local radio station, or by featuring a cable network program. An emergency radio which can be utilized for disasters or catastrophic situations should be available to function on police, fire, and emergency channels.
- Pagers—Pagers can be operated on a fixed antenna system, which must be licensed by the Federal Communications Commission, or can be operated on a loop antenna system.
- Cell phones—Commonly, the selection of a vendor is coordinated with the university's communications division. Having one cell phone with a single number, to rotate any on-call personnel, is very useful.
- Data Processing—Using a mainframe computer system or a stand-alone local area network (LAN) is a decision that each health service must make. Choices of hardware, software, and operating programs are critical issues for meeting the diverse needs of various institutions.

Locks and Key Control

Numerous types of locks and security systems exist which can meet the needs of most outpatient health care facilities. Key control for any system of locks is important, and the scheme of control determines how well the system functions. A master with sub-master sets for various departments is usually recommended. A locking cylinder with enough tumblers to incorporate master, sub-master, and individual keying must be provided.[27] It is important that a key log be maintained by the department and that each individual issued a key be required to sign for its receipt. Keys must be returned when a person terminates employment.

Monitoring Systems

A number of types of security monitoring systems are available. Certain areas of the facility may need security surveillance because of their location. These include entrance and exit doors used after-hours, the medical records area, the pharmacy, the personnel and payroll area, the cashier's office, central supply and storage area, or any other space of a sensitive nature.

REFERENCES

1. *You and Your Architect.* The American Institute of Architects, Washington, D.C., 1986.

2. Ibid., p. 11.

3. Isadore Rosenfield, *Hospital Architecture and Beyond* (New York, New York; Van Mostrand Reinhold Company, 1969), p. 73.

4. "Architectural Terms." The American Institute of Architects, via web: http://www.aiaaccess.com/institutional/iterms.asp

5. National Fire Protection Association 101, *Life Safety Code,* 1994 Edition. Quincy, MA: National Fire Protection Association, pp. 101-24–101-25.

6. Ibid., p. 101–17.

7. John R. McGihony, M.D., *Principles of Hospital Administration* (New York: G.P. Putnam's Sons, 1969), p. 317.

8. American Hospital Association, *Hospital Engineering Handbook.* Chicago: American Hospital Association, 1974, p. 73.

9. Ibid., p. 75.

10. Ibid., p. 77.

11. University of Florida Physical Plant Division, *Architecture/Engineering Project Manual.* Gainesville: University of Florida, 1990, p. 16020.1.

12. American Hospital Association, op. cit., p. 81.

13. Ibid., p. 167.

14. National Fire Protection Association 101, op. cit., pp. 101–226.

15. Accreditation Association for Ambulatory Health Care, Inc., *Accreditation Handbook for Ambulatory Health Care,* 1998 Edition. Skokie, IL: Accreditation Association for Health Care, p. 65 (Appendix F).

16. Joint Commission on Accreditation of Healthcare Organizations. *1996 Accreditation Manual for Ambulatory Care,* Oakbrook Terrace, IL: Joint Commission on Accreditation of Healthcare Organizations, p. 226.

17. Accreditation Association for Ambulatory Health Care, Inc., op. cit.

18. Code of Federal Regulations, Title 29, Part 1910.1030. Bloodborne Pathogens. Federal Register, Vol. 56, No. 235, pp. 69175–69182.

19. American Hospital Association, op. cit., p. 104.

20. Ibid., p. 118.

21. J.M. Kurth, Essentials of Housekeeping in Health Care Facilities. Rockville, MD: Aspen Publishers, 1984.

22. Joint Commission on Accreditation of Healthcare Organizations, *2000–2001 Comprehensive Accreditation Manual for Ambulatory Care.* Oakbrook Terrace, IL: Joint Commission on Accreditation of Healthcare Organizations, pp. EC-34 to EC-36.

23. Accreditation Association for Ambulatory Health Care, Inc., op. cit., p. 26 (Chapter 8).

24. William Charney and Joseph Schirmer, *Essentials of Modern Hospital Safety.* Chelsea, MI: Lewis Publishers, 1990, p. 166.

25. Accreditation Association for Ambulatory Health Care, Inc., op. cit., p. 41–42.

26. Charney and Schirmer, op. cit., pp. 166–167.

27. American Hospital Association, op. cit., p. 299.

Index